SOCIAL INJUSTICE AND PUBLIC HEALTH

TO HOWARD MARKEL –

WITH GREAT ADMIRATION FOR YOUR

WORK.

Barry Levy

Vic Sidel

September 28, 2005

SOCIAL INJUSTICE AND PUBLIC HEALTH

Edited by
Barry S. Levy
Victor W. Sidel

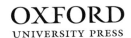

UNIVERSITY PRESS

*Published in Cooperation with
the American Public Health Association*

2006

OXFORD

UNIVERSITY PRESS

Oxford University Press, Inc., publishes works that further
Oxford University's objective of excellence
in research, scholarship, and education.

Oxford   New York
Auckland   Cape Town   Dar es Salaam   Hong Kong   Karachi
Kuala Lumpur   Madrid   Melbourne   Mexico City   Nairobi
New Delhi   Shanghai   Taipei   Toronto

With offices in
Argentina   Austria   Brazil   Chile   Czech Republic   France   Greece
Guatemala   Hungary   Italy   Japan   Poland   Portugal   Singapore
South Korea   Switzerland   Thailand   Turkey   Ukraine   Vietnam

Copyright © 2006 by Oxford University Press, Inc.

Published by Oxford University Press, Inc.
198 Madison Avenue, New York, New York 10016

www.oup-usa.com

Oxford is a registered trademark of Oxford University Press

Library of Congress Cataloging-in-Publication Data
Social injustice and public health / edited by Barry S. Levy and Victor W. Sidel.
p.   cm.
Includes bibliographical references and index.
ISBN-13 978-0-19-517185-3
ISBN 0-19-517185-3
1. Social medicine.   2. Social justice.   3. Public health—Social aspects.
I. Levy, Barry S.   II. Sidel, Victor W.
RA418.S6423 2005
362.1'042—dc22   2004065433

9 8 7 6 5 4 3 2 1

Printed in the United States of America
on acid-free paper

Dedicated to health workers
throughout the world
committed to ending
social injustice.

FOREWORD

Despite the tremendous improvements in overall health and life expectancy during the past century, at the start of the twenty-first century there are unconscionable gaps in health for many vulnerable groups, including racial and ethnic minorities and the poor. These gaps in health thrive in a climate of economic and social inequities. These inequities create the conditions that adversely affect the health of individuals and communities by denying individuals and groups the equal opportunity to meet their basic human needs.

Minority children and children from low-income families continue to lag behind their counterparts in almost every health indicator. Poor children are at least twice as likely as are nonpoor children to suffer stunted growth or lead poisoning. Black children and children from poor families are more likely to have disabling asthma. Infants born to black mothers are more than twice as likely as infants born to white mothers to die before their first birthdays. Black and Mexican-American children living in older (pre-1946) housing are more than twice as likely to have elevated blood lead levels as are white children living in comparable housing.

Quality health care alone, however, cannot prevent children from being poisoned by lead paint in deteriorating homes or developing asthma from fumes emitted by inadequately vented stoves. These disparities in children's health reflect the inequities in social and economic well-being of children and their families. For example, nearly 13 million American children—more than one in six—lived in families with an annual income below the government poverty level in 2003. In that year, 34 percent of black, 30 percent of Latino, 13 percent of Asian, and 10 percent of white children were poor. The racial gaps in the poverty rate testify to generations of social injustice that have created a system of unequal access to many sectors of American life, including education, housing, employment, finance, and criminal justice.

Social Injustice and Public Health calls us to action to improve health through the pursuit of social justice. This book makes a powerful and compelling argument that a primary goal of public health is to address the root causes of social injustice: widening gaps between rich and poor, the unequal distribution of resources within our society, discrimination, and the disenfranchisement of individuals and groups from the political process.

This system of social injustice has contributed to disparities not only in health but also in childhood development, education, employment, income, housing, and family and community safety. The racial and social progress of the last half-century is in peril of being lost. This would be a moral, social, and economic catastrophe for America. If we can remove children from the dangerous intersection of race, poverty, and poor education where so many young lives are wrecked, we would not only improve children's health but we would also help all Americans realize the core values of freedom and justice that make America *America*.

—*Marian Wright Edelman*

PREFACE

Social injustice underlies many public health problems throughout the world. It is manifested in many ways, ranging from various forms of overt discrimination to wide gaps between the "haves" and "have-nots" within a country and between rich and poor countries. It leads to higher rates of disease, injury, disability, and premature death. Public health professionals as well as students of the health professions need a clear understanding of social injustice in order to address these problems, but relatively few books address the wide range of issues involved.

The aim of this book is to offer a comprehensive approach to understanding social injustice and its impact on public health. Part I explores the nature of social injustice and its adverse effects on public health. Part II describes in detail how the health of 10 specific population groups is affected by social injustice. Part III explores how social injustice adversely affects health in 10 different areas, ranging from infectious diseases to mental health, from prevention of assaultive violence and war to occupational health and safety. Part IV provides an action agenda for what needs to done to prevent social injustice and to minimize its impact on health.

This book arose from our experience and observations of the ways in which social injustice underlies public health problems. Previously we edited *War and Public Health* and *Terrorism and Public Health*, in which we identified social injustice as a principal causative factor and as a consequence of war and terrorism. The current book examines social injustice as a principal causative factor and as a consequence of many public health problems.

We conceived this book with the goals of stimulating a better understanding of the relation between social injustice and public health, promoting education and research on these issues, and facilitating effective measures to minimize the impact of social injustice on health and well-being.

B.S.L. and V.W.S
Sherborn, Massachusetts
The Bronx, New York
May 2005

ACKNOWLEDGMENTS

Developing *Social Injustice and Public Health* has involved the combined skills and resources of many people, to whom we are profoundly grateful.

We are indebted to all of the contributors, who worked, often with short deadlines, to write chapters and boxes that reflect their observations, insights, and expertise. Their commitment to social justice and to public health is evident in their work and in their contributions to this book.

We thank many people for their insights that helped extend our knowledge and sharpen our thinking about social injustice and public health. These include Philip Brachman, Paula Braveman, Jack Geiger, and Nancy Krieger.

We express our deep appreciation to Heather Merrell for her excellent work in preparing multiple drafts of the manuscript and coordinating communications with contributors. We also thank Angela Adjei and Deyanira Suarez for secretarial support.

We greatly appreciate the guidance, assistance, and support of Jeffrey House, who was instrumental in the development of this book, as well as Carrie Pedersen, Keith Faivre, and others associated with Oxford University Press, and Jean Blackburn of Bytheway Publishing Services.

Finally, our gratitude and love to Nancy Levy and Ruth Sidel for their continuing inspiration, encouragement, and support.

CONTENTS

Part IV. What Needs to Be Done

CONTRIBUTORS

Carol Easley Allen, PhD, RN
Professor and Chair
Department of Nursing
Oakwood College
7000 Adventist Boulevard
Huntsville, AL 35896
256-726-7297
256-726-8338 (fax)
callen@oakwood.edu

Myron Allukian, Jr., DDS, MPH
Oral Health Consultant
Massachusetts League of Community Health
  Centers and Lutheran Medical Center
46 Louders Lane
Boston, MA 02130
617-654-8920
617-542-0777 (fax)
MyAlluk@aol.com

Lisa Arangua, MPP
Senior Research Analyst
Department of Family Medicine

David Geffen School of Medicine at
  UCLA
Los Angeles, CA 90095-1683
310-794-6094
310-794-6097 (fax)
lisaa@ucla.edu

Robert E. Aronson, DrPH, MPH
Assistant Professor
Department of Public Health Education
University of North Carolina at
  Greensboro
437J HHP Building
PO Box 26170
Greensboro, NC 27402-6170
336-256-0119
336-334-3238 (fax)
rearonso@uncg.edu

Ruth Bell, PhD
Senior Research Fellow
Department of Epidemiology and Public
  Health

University College London
1-19 Torrington Place
London WC1E 6BT
United Kingdom
+44 020 7679 1684
+44 020 7813 0242 (fax)
r.bell@ucl.ac.uk

Talia Bettcher, PhD
Assistant Professor
Department of Philosophy
California State University, Los Angeles
5151 State University Drive
E & T A405
Los Angeles, CA 90032-8114
323-343-4179
323-343-4193 (fax)
tbettch@calstatela.edu

Kathryn L. Bolles, MPH
Child Survival Specialist
Save the Children/US
54 Wilton Road
Westport, CT 06880
203-221-3778
203-221-4056 (fax)
kbolles@savechildren.org

Paula Braveman, MD, MPH
Director, Center on Social Disparities
   in Health
Professor of Family and Community
   Medicine
University of California, San Francisco
500 Parnassus Avenue, Room
   MU-306E
San Francisco, CA 94143-0900
415-476-6839
415-476-6051 (fax)
braveman@fcm.ucsf.edu

Joseph E. Brenner, MA
Director, Center for Policy Analysis
   on Trade and Health (CPATH)
98 Seal Rock Drive
San Francisco, CA 94121-1437
415-933-6204
415-831-4091 (fax)
jebrenner@cpath.org

J. Larry Brown, PhD
Distinguished Scientist, Brandeis
   University
Executive Director, Center on Hunger
   and Poverty
The Heller School for Social Policy
   and Management
Mailstop 077
60 Turner Street, First Floor
Waltham, MA 02454-9110
781-736-8885
781-736-3925 (fax)
jlbrown@brandeis.edu

Colin D. Butler, BMed, MSc, PhD
Research Fellow
National Centre for Epidemiology and
   Population Health
Medical Director, Benevolent
   Organization for Development Health
   and Insight (BODHI)
Australian National University
Canberra, ACT, 0200 Australia
61 2 6125 5624
61 2 6125 0740 (fax)
Colin.Butler@anu.edu.au

Wendy Chavkin, MD, MPH
Professor of Population and Family Health
   and of Obstetrics/Gynecology
Department of Population and
   Family Health
Mailman School of Public Health
60 Haven Avenue, B2
New York, NY 10032
212-304-5220
212-305-7024(fax)
wc9@columbia.edu

Ernest M. Drucker, PhD
Professor, Departments of Epidemiology
   and Population Health, Psychiatry
   and Behavioral Sciences, and Family
   Social Medicine
Division Head, Division of Public Health
   & Policy Research
Albert Einstein College of Medicine
Montefiore Medical Center
111 East 210th Street

Bronx, NY 10467
718-920-4766
emdrucker@earthlink.net

Cheryl E. Easley, PhD, RN
Dean and Professor
College of Health and Social Welfare
University of Alaska Anchorage
3211 Providence Drive
Anchorage, AK 99508
907-786-4407
907-786-4440 (fax)
ceasley@uaa.alaska.edu

Carroll L. Estes, PhD
Professor and Founding Director
Institute for Health & Aging, UCSF
3333 California Street, Suite 340
San Francisco, CA 94118
415-476-3236
415-502-5404 (fax)
cestes@itsa.ucsf.edu

Paul E. Farmer, MD, PhD
Presley Professor of Medical Anthropology
Department of Social Medicine, Harvard
    Medical School
Chief, Division of Social Medicine and
    Health Inequalities, Brigham and
    Women's Hospital
Founding Director, Partners In Health
641 Huntington Avenue
Boston, MA 02115
617-432-3718
617-432-6045 (fax)
paul_farmer@hms.harvard.edu

Henry A. Freedman, LLB
Executive Director
Welfare Law Center
275 Seventh Avenue, Suite 1205
New York, NY 10001-6708
212-633-6967
212-633-6371 (fax)
freedman@welfarelaw.org

H. Jack Geiger, MD, MSciHyg
CUNY Medical School
City College of New York, H-401

138th Street at Convent Avenue
New York, NY 10031
212-650-6860
718-802-9141 (fax)
jgeiger@igc.org

Jeanne Geiger-Brown, PhD, RN
Assistant Professor
Family and Community Health
School of Nursing
University of Maryland at Baltimore
655 West Lombard Street
Baltimore, MD 21202
410-706-5368
jgeiger@son.umaryland.edu

Lillian Gelberg, MD, MSPH
George F. Kneller Professor
Chief, Health Research
Department of Family Medicine
David Geffen School of Medicine at
    UCLA
50-071 CHS Box 951683
Los Angeles, CA 90095-1683
310-794-6092
310-794-6097 (fax)
lgelberg@medet.ucla.edu

Nora Ellen Groce, PhD
Associate Professor
Global Health Division
Yale School of Public Health
College Street, Room 320
New Haven, CT 06520
203-785-2866
203-785-6193 (fax)
nora.groce@yale.edu

Sofia Gruskin, JD, MIA
Associate Professor of Health and Human
    Rights
Program on International Health and
    Human Rights
Francois-Xavier Bagnoud Center for
    Health and Human Rights
Department of Population and
    International Health
Harvard School of Public Health
FXB Building, 7th Floor

653 Huntington Avenue
Boston, MA 02115
617-432-4315
sgruskin@hsph.harvard.edu

John W. Hatch, PhD
Keenan Professor Emeritus
Department of Health Behavior and
    Health Education
University of North Carolina at
    Chapel Hill
Rosenau Hall CB #7440
Chapel Hill, NC 27599-7440
919-966-3761
john5505@aol.com

Alice M. Horowitz, PhD
Senior Scientist
National Institute of Dental and
    Craniofacial Research
National Institutes of Health
45 Center Drive, Room 4AS-37A
Bethesda, MD 20892-6401
301-594-5391
301-480-8254 (fax)
Alice.Horowitz@nih.gov

Sir Richard Jolly, MA, PhD
Professor
Institute of Development Studies
University of Sussex
Brighton BN1 9RE
United Kingdom
44(0)1273 606261
44(0)1273 621202 (fax)
R.Jolly@ids.ac.uk

Nancy Krieger, PhD, MS
Associate Professor
Department of Society, Human
    Development, and Health
Harvard School of Public Health
Kresge 717
677 Huntington Avenue
Boston, MA 02115
617-432-1571
617-432-3123 (fax)
nkrieger@hsph.harvard.edu

Robert S. Lawrence, MD
Edyth H. Schoenrich Professor of
    Preventive Medicine
Associate Dean for Professional Practice
    and Programs
Director, Center for a Livable Future
Johns Hopkins Bloomberg School of
    Public Health
615 N. Wolfe Street, W1033
Baltimore, MD 21205
410-614-4590
410-502-7579 (fax)
rlawrenc@jhsph.edu

Barry S. Levy, MD, MPH
Adjunct Professor
Department of Public Health and
    Family Medicine
Tufts University School of Medicine
PO Box 1230
20 North Main Street, Suite 200
Sherborn, MA 01770
508-650-1039
508-655-4811 (fax)
blevy@igc.org

Emilia Lombardi, PhD
Assistant Professor
Graduate School of Public Health
Department of Infectious Diseases/
    Microbiology
University of Pittsburgh
3520 Fifth Avenue, Suite 400
Pittsburgh, PA 15213-3313
412-383-2233
412-383-1513 (fax)
Emilial@stophiv.pitt.edu

Kay Lovelace, PhD, MPH
Associate Professor
Department of Public Health Education
University of North Carolina–Greensboro
437M HHP Building
PO Box 26170
Greensboro, NC 27402-6170
336-334-3246
336-334-3238 (fax)
klovelace@uncg.edu

Sir Michael Marmot, MBBS, MPH, PhD
Professor
Director, International Centre for Health
and Society
Head of Department
Department of Epidemiology and Public
Health
University College London
1-19 Torrington Place
London WC1E 6BT
United Kingdom
+44 020 7679 1717
+44 020 7813 0242 (fax)
m.marmot@public-health.ucl.ac.uk

Anthony J. McMichael, MBBS, PhD
Professor
Director, National Centre for
Epidemiology and Population Health
Australian National University
Canberra, ACT, 0200 Australia
61 2 6125 4578
61 2 6125 5608 (fax)
Tony.McMichael@anu.edu.au

James A. Mercy, PhD
Associate Director for Science
Division of Violence Prevention
National Center for Injury Prevention
and Control
Centers for Disease Control and Prevention
4770 Buford Highway, NE
Mailstop K-68
Atlanta, GA 30341
770-488-4362
770-488-4221 (fax)
jam2@cdc.gov

Joia S. Mukherjee, MD, MPH
Medical Director, Partners In Health
Assistant Professor, Division of Social
Medicine and Health Inequalities,
Brigham and Women's Hospital
Department of Social Medicine,
Harvard Medical School
641 Huntington Avenue
Boston, MA 02115

617-432-3735
617-432-6045 (fax)
jmukherjee@pih.org

Carles Muntaner, MD, PhD
Professor and Chair
Psychiatry and Addictions
Nursing Research
Culture, Community and Health Studies
Social, Policy and Prevention Research
Department
Center for Addictions and Mental Health
University of Toronto
250 College Street
Toronto, Ontario M5T 1R8
Canada
416-979-6905
416-979-0564 (fax)
carles_muntaner@camh.net

Linda Rae Murray, MD, MPH
Chief Medical Officer–Primary Care
Ambulatory & Community Health Network
Cook County Bureau of Health Services
621 South Wood Street, Suite 331
Chicago, IL 60612
312-864-0748
312-864-9879 (fax)
lindarae@interaccess.com

Alonzo Plough, PhD, MPH
Director, Department of Public Health,
Seattle and King Counties
Professor, School of Public Health and
Community Medicine, University of
Washington
999 Third Avenue, Suite 1200
Seattle, WA 98104-4039
206-296-1480
206-296-0166 (fax)
alonzo.plough@metrokc.gov

Stacey J. Rees, CNM, RN, MA
Former Program Director
Soros Reproductive Health and Rights
Fellowship
Mailman School of Public Health,
Columbia University

Midwife, Clementine Midwifery and
    Natural Birth
247 Mulberry Street, Suite 14
New York, NY 10012
646-519-7209
646-519-7209 (fax)
nycmidwife@verizon.net

Sara Rosenbaum, JD
Hirsh Professor and Chair
Department of Health Policy
The George Washington University
    Medical Center
School of Public Health and Health
    Services
2021 K Street NW, Suite 800
Washington, DC 20006
202-530-2343
203-530-2361 (fax)
sarar@gwu.edu

Ellen R. Shaffer, PhD, MPH
Director, Center for Policy Analysis on
    Trade and Health (CPATH)
98 Seal Rock Drive
San Francisco, CA 94121-1437
415-933-6204
415-831-4091 (fax)
ershaffer@cpath.org

Victor W. Sidel, MD
Distinguished University Professor of
    Social Medicine
Albert Einstein College of Medicine
Montefiore Medical Center
111 East 210th Street
Bronx, NY 10467
718-920-6586
718-654-7305 (fax)
vsidel@igc.org

Andrea Kidd Taylor, DrPH, MSPH
Assistant Professor
Morgan State University
Public Health Program
1700 East Cold Spring Lane
343 Jenkins Hall
Baltimore, MD 21251
443-885-2044
443-885-8309 (fax)
ataylor4@jewel.morgan.edu

Michael Toole, BMedSc
Centre for International Health
The Macfarlane Burnet Institute for
    Medical Research and Public Health
GPO Box 2294
Melbourne 3001, Australia
61 3 9282 2216
61 3 9482 3123 (fax)
toole@burnet.edu.au

Steven P. Wallace, PhD
Professor of Community Health
    Sciences
UCLA School of Public Health
Associate Director, UCLA Center for
    Health Policy Research
10911 Weyburn Avenue, 300
Los Angeles, CA 90024
310-794-0910
310-794-2686 (fax)
swallace@ucla.edu

Peter Weiss, JD
Vice President
Center for Constitutional Rights
5022 Waldo Avenue
Bronx, NY 10471
petweiss@igc.org

Tony L. Whitehead, PhD, MSHyg
Professor of Anthropology
0123 Woods Hall
University of Maryland
College Park, MD 20742-7415
703-620-0515
tonylwhitehead@comcast.net

Derek Yach, MB, ChB, MPH
Professor of Global Public Health
Yale University School of Medicine
Department of Epidemiology and Public
    Health
60 College Street, Suite 319
New Haven, CT 06520
203-785-3927
203-785-6193 (fax)
derek.yach@yale.edu

Chung-Hi H. Yoder, JD, MS
cyoder@law.gwu.edu
yoderch@aol.com

SOCIAL INJUSTICE AND PUBLIC HEALTH

Part I

Introduction

1

THE NATURE OF SOCIAL INJUSTICE AND ITS IMPACT ON PUBLIC HEALTH

Barry S. Levy and Victor W. Sidel

Introduction

Social injustice means a wide variety of different things to different people who are affected by it:

- To children in urban slums and depressed rural areas, it may mean few teachers, crowded classrooms, inadequate curricula, functional illiteracy, and no development of marketable skills.
- To unemployed youth, it may mean decreased likelihood of getting a permanent job.
- To minority workers, it may mean reduced opportunities for advancement, reduced income, and increased exposure to on-the-job health and safety hazards.
- To women, it may mean increased risk of being violently attacked or sexually abused.
- To people forced to migrate within or between countries, it may mean decreased social cohesion and increased stress.
- To many people worldwide, it may mean unsafe food and water, poor sanitation, crowded and substandard housing, exposure to environmental

hazards, decreased protection of human rights and civil liberties, and inadequate access to medical care and public health services.

Social injustice creates conditions that adversely affect the health of individuals and communities. It denies individuals and groups equal opportunity to meet their basic human needs. It violates fundamental human rights.

We define *social injustice* in two ways. First, we define it as the denial or violation of economic, sociocultural, political, civil, or human rights of specific populations or groups in the society based on the perception of their inferiority by those with more power or influence. Populations or groups that suffer social injustice may be defined by racial or ethnic status, socioeconomic position, age, gender, sexual orientation, or other perceived population or group characteristics. These groups are often negatively stereotyped and stigmatized and may be the targets of hate and violence. Part II (chapters 2 to 11) is organized around this definition of social injustice, with each chapter focusing on a population or group whose health is affected by social injustice.

Our second definition of *social injustice* is based on the Institute of Medicine definition of *public health:* what we, as a society, collectively do to assure the conditions in which people can be healthy.[1] This second definition of social injustice refers to policies or actions that adversely affect the societal conditions in which people can be healthy. Although this type of social injustice is often communitywide, nationwide, or even global, the populations and groups described in our first definition of social injustice—especially the poor, the homeless, the ill or injured, the very young, and the very old—usually suffer more than others in the population as a result of these policies and actions. Examples of this form of social injustice include policies or practices that promote

- War and other forms of violence
- Global warming or other widespread environmental damage
- Failure to provide essential public health and medical care services
- Corruption of government or culture
- Erosion of civil liberties and freedoms
- Restriction of education, scientific research, and public discourse.

Part III (chapters 12 to 21) is organized around this definition of social injustice, with each chapter focusing on a different area of public health. Public health is ultimately and essentially an ethical enterprise committed to the notion that all people are entitled to protection against the hazards of this world and to the minimization of death and disability in society.[2]

Under either definition, social injustice represents a lack of fairness or equity, often resulting from the way that society is structured or from discrimination by groups or individuals within the society. Among the roots of social injustice are poverty and the increasing gap between the rich and the poor; maldistribution of resources within the society; racism and other forms of discrimination; weak laws or weak enforcement of laws protecting human rights and other rights; and disenfranchisement of individuals and groups from the political process. Relevant to our two definitions of social *injustice,* concepts and definitions of social *justice* are based on justice, fairness, and equity (box 1-1).

Social injustice leads to a wide range of adverse health consequences, as reflected by disparities in health status and access to health services within or between populations. Within the United States, there have been—and still are—many disparities with regard to health status, such as the following:

- In the 1998–2000 period, the infant mortality rate for blacks was 14 per 1,000 live births, and for whites and Hispanics, 6.
- In the 1999–2000 period, among women aged 20 to 74, blacks had a 50 percent rate of obesity, compared with 40 percent among Mexicans and 30 percent among whites.
- In 2001, 90 percent of white pregnant women received prenatal care early in their pregnancies, compared with 75 percent of blacks and Hispanics.
- In 2001, 35 percent of Hispanics had no health insurance coverage, compared with 20 percent of blacks and 15 percent of whites.[3]

The Department of Health and Human Services through its *Healthy People 2010* initiative has committed the United States to eliminating these and other health disparities.[4]

Social injustice and its manifestations have varied with time and place. In the United States, groups of people with dark skin were denied many opportunities in the past by law. Since the repeal of laws requiring discrimination and the adoption of laws banning discrimination, many opportunities have been often denied these same groups by social patterns and custom, such as by segregation.

Marked disparities also exist internationally (see chapter 21). For example, a female infant born today in Japan will live, on average, 85 years. She will be fully vaccinated and will receive adequate nutrition and extensive education. If she becomes pregnant, she will receive adequate maternity care. If she develops chronic disease, she will likely receive excellent treatment and rehabilitation. If she becomes sick, she will likely receive approximately US$550 in medications. In contrast, a female infant born today in Sierra Leone will live, on average, 36 years. She will have a low probability of being immunized and a high probability of being underweight and malnourished. She will likely marry as a teenager and have six or more children, none of whom will be delivered by a trained birth attendant. One or more of her children will likely die during infancy. She will be at high risk of death during childbirth. If she becomes sick, she will likely receive about US$3 in medications. If she

BOX 1-1 Concepts of Social Justice

While the focus of this book is social *injustice* and methods for preventing and correcting social injustices, it is important to review definitions and concepts of social justice. Many definitions focus on preventing human rights abuses, especially those affecting minority groups, women, and children, and ensuring adherence to international law, especially international law concerning war crimes and crimes against humanity. Social justice refers, in part, to the equitable societal distribution of valued goods and necessary burdens.[1] In a similar vein, social justice can be thought of as an application of the concept of distributive justice to the wealth, assets, privileges, and advantages that accumulate within a society or state.[2] Some describe it as justice that conforms to a moral principle, such as that all people are equal.[3] Some characterize it as full and equal participation of all groups in a society that is mutually shaped to meet their needs, including a vision of society that is equitable and in which all members are physically and psychologically safe and secure.[4] In contrast, some contend that social justice may be distinguished from justice in law and justice embedded in systems of morality, which may differ between cultures.[5]

Many definitions of social justice are based on the premise that all people, in the words of the U.S. Declaration of Independence, have "inalienable rights." In the United States, political and civil rights are usually seen as central. In other countries, economic, social, and cultural rights are emphasized; these include the right to services to meet basic human needs regardless of differences in economic status, class, gender, race, ethnicity, citizenship, religion, age, sexual orientation, disability, and health. The Universal Declaration of Human Rights, adopted by the United Nations General Assembly on December 10, 1948, provides a widely accepted summary of basic human rights (see box 1-2). It served as the foundation for the original two legally binding United Nations human rights documents: the International Covenant on Civil and Political Rights and the International Covenant on Economic, Social, and Cultural Rights.[6,7] Many definitions of social injustice therefore hold that achieving social justice involves eradicating poverty and illiteracy, establishing sound environmental policy, and attaining equality of opportunity for healthy personal and social development.[8]

Social, or civil, justice is largely based on various social contract theories. Most of these theories are a variation of the concept that as governments are instituted among populations for the benefit of their members, they must see to the welfare of their citizens. This concept usually includes, but is not limited to, upholding human rights. In addition, many variants of this concept contain elements demanding more equitable distribution of wealth and resources.

A widely accepted formulation of the basis for these rights rests not on the deism that led the authors of the U.S. Declaration of Independence to state

(continued)

that people are "endowed by their Creator" with these rights, but rather on the concept elaborated by John Rawls in *A Theory of Justice*.[9] Rawls draws on the social contract theories of Thomas Hobbes, Jean-Jacques Rousseau, and John Locke and argues that the "veil of ignorance" that prevents people from knowing *a priori* what position in society they would occupy requires them to insist on basic liberties and to insist that inequalities in wealth and position be arranged so as to benefit the worst-off group in society.

We agree with Paula Braveman and Sofia Gruskin[10] that social justice means equity or fairness and that it is an ethical concept grounded in principles of distributive justice. Equity in health can be defined as the absence of socially unjust or unfair health disparities. For purposes of operationalization and measurement, equity in health can be defined as the absence of systematic disparities in health (or in the major social determinants of health) between social groups that have different levels of underlying social advantage or disadvantage—that is, different positions in a social hierarchy. Health represents both physical and mental well-being, not just the absence of disease. Key social determinants of health include household living conditions, conditions in communities and workplaces, and health care, along with policies and programs affecting these factors. Underlying social advantage or disadvantage refers to wealth, power, and/or prestige—that is, the attributes that define how people are grouped in social hierarchies.[10]

The extent to which social justice and equity exist in a society correlates with the distribution of resources within the population. Equality in distribution of wealth within a society improves population health status and reduces health disparities within that society.[11]

Social justice is inextricably linked to public health. It is the philosophy behind public health.[12] Under social justice, all groups and individuals are entitled equally to important rights such as health protection and minimal standards of income. The goal of public health to minimize preventable death and disability is a dream of social justice.

References

1. V. H. Schmidt. Available at: http://www.nclyn.org/content/blogsection/6/. Accessed on March 6, 2005.
2. Dictionary of Political Thought. Available at: http://www.nclyn.org/index2.php?option=content&do_pdf=1&id=11. Accessed March 7, 2005.
3. Black's Law Dictionary. Available at: http://www.nclyn.org/index2.php?option=content&do_pdf=1&id=11. Accessed March 7, 2005.
4. Al Goldfarb. Available at: http://www.nclyn.org/index2.php?option=content&do_pdf=1&id=11. Accessed March 7, 2005.
5. The Free Dictionary. Available at: http://www.social_justice.exsugo.com. Accessed March 7, 2005.

(*continued*)

BOX 1-1 (*continued*)

6. United Nations Universal Declaration of Human Rights. Available at: http://www.
   un.org/Overview/rights.html. Accessed December 30, 2004.
7. A call to action on the 50th anniversary of the Universal Declaration of Human
   Rights. Health Hum Rights 1998;3:7–18.
8. Green Party. Available at: http://www.europeangreens.org/info/globalgreencharter.
   html. Accessed March 7, 2005.
9. Rawls J. A theory of justice (revised edition). Cambridge, Mass.: Belknap Press, 1999.
10. Braveman P, Gruskin S. Defining equity in health. J Epidemiol Commun Health
    2003;57:254–8.
11. Anderson LM, Scrimshaw SC, Fullilove MT, Fielding JE, and the Task Force on
    Community Preventive Services. The Community Guide's model for linking the
    social environment to health. Am J Prev Med 2003;24:12–20.
12. Foege WH. Public health: moving from debt to legacy (1986 presidential ad-
    dress). Am J Pub health 1987;77:1276–8.

develops a chronic disease, she likely will not have adequate treatment or rehabilitation. She will likely die prematurely of a preventable disease or injury.[5]

Social injustice leads to increased rates of disease, injury, disability, and premature death because of increased risk factors and decreased medical care and preventive services. People and communities affected by social injustice may have, for example,

- Poorer nutrition
- Greater exposure to unsafe water
- Increased contact with infectious disease agents
- Increased exposure to occupational and environmental hazards
- Increased complications of chronic diseases
- Increased alcohol, tobacco, and drug abuse
- Decreased social support
- Increased physiological and immunological vulnerability to disease
- Less access to comprehensive diagnostic, therapeutic, and rehabilitative services
- Lower quality of health care
- Less access to clinical preventive services, such as screening and counseling
- Less access to community-based preventive measures.

It is increasingly recognized that factors related to social injustice, including poverty, inadequate education, and inadequate health insurance, significantly contribute to increased rates of disease, disability, and death. For example, in 1991, the director of the National Cancer Institute declared that poverty is a carcinogen.[6]

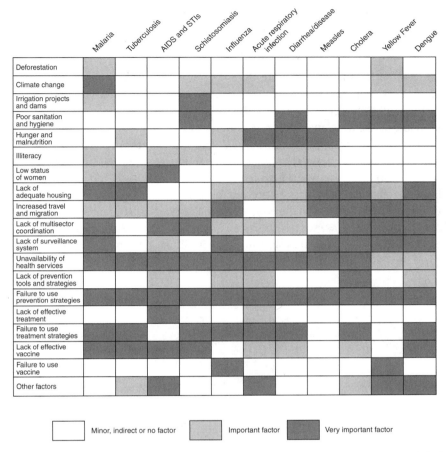

Figure 1-1 Determinants of infectious diseases. (From Kickbusch H, Buse K. Global influences and global responses: international health at the turn of the twenty-first century. In: Merson MH, Black RE, Mills AJ, eds. International public health: diseases, programs, systems, and policies. Gaithersburg, Md.: Aspen Publishers, 2001:708. Copyright 2001 Jones and Bartlett Publishers, Sudbury, Mass. www.jbpub.com. Reprinted with permission.)

The causes of many diseases are a complex interplay of multiple factors, many of which are due to social injustice. This is illustrated in figure 1-1, which describes the impact of multiple causative factors on the occurrence of several different infectious diseases (also see chapters 13 and 21).

Social injustice often occurs when those who control access to opportunities and resources block the poor, the powerless, and those otherwise deprived from gaining fair and equitable access to these opportunities and resources. Social injustice enables those in the upper class to receive a disproportionate share of wealth and other resources—"the good things in life"—while others may struggle to obtain the basic necessities of life.

Special circumstances may increase the level of social injustice. For example, a drought or a flood that diminishes the availability of food supplies often affects some groups more than others, unless social or legal action is taken to prevent this disparity. War or civil conflict may increase social injustice for some groups, especially for those on the losing side. War, or preparation for war, may divert resources and attention from social injustice issues. However, major community emergencies may mobilize and bring together people in ways that ameliorate social injustice.

The disparities between the rich and poor within the United States and between rich and poor nations are greater than they have ever been. And the rich are getting richer, and the poor, poorer. The poor are at greater risk of many diseases and injuries, with resultant disability and premature death. The gap in wealth between the rich and the poor is illustrated in figure 1-2, which

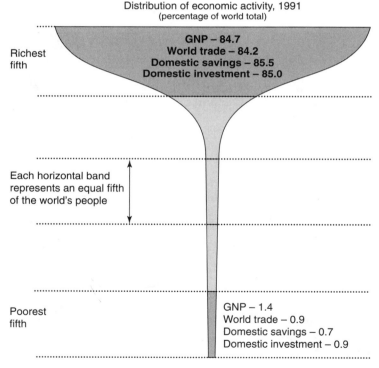

Distribution of economic activity, 1991
(percentage of world total)

Richest fifth

GNP – 84.7
World trade – 84.2
Domestic savings – 85.5
Domestic investment – 85.0

Each horizontal band represents an equal fifth of the world's people

Poorest fifth

GNP – 1.4
World trade – 0.9
Domestic savings – 0.7
Domestic investment – 0.9

Figure 1-2 Global economic disparities. (From United Nations Development Program. Human development report 1994. New York, N.Y.: Oxford University Press, 1994:63.)

demonstrates that the richest quintile (20 percent) of people in the world owns approximately 85 percent of the wealth, whereas the poorest quintile owns approximately 1 percent.

Market justice, which has created many of these disparities and gaps, may be the primary roadblock to dramatically reducing preventable injury and death.[2] It has been asserted that market justice is a pervasive ideology that protects the most powerful or the most numerous from the burdens of collective action.[2] An important role for public health is to challenge market justice as fatally deficient in protecting the public's health and to advocate an ethic for protecting the public's health—giving highest priority to reducing death and disability and protecting all humankind against hazards.[2]

What Needs to Be Done

Humanity, for the first time, has the technical capacity and the human and economic resources to address poverty, ill health, human rights violations, and the social injustice that helps spawn and promote these problems. Some forms of social injustice may be prevented or corrected by individual action, but most forms of social injustice require social or legal action for their prevention or correction.

As reflected in part IV (chapters 22–28), we believe that basic public health approaches need to be further developed and implemented to address the role of social injustice in public health. These approaches include the following:

- *Addressing social injustice in a human rights context:* The Universal Declaration of Human Rights (box 1-2) and the International Declaration of Health Rights (box 1-3) provide a foundation for reducing, and ultimately eliminating, social injustice (also see chapter 22).
- *Promoting social justice by public health policies, programs, and services:* Public health departments and other government bodies at the local, state, national, and international levels can reduce social injustice and promote social justice (see chapter 23).
- *Strengthening communities and the roles of individuals in community life:* Communities—as well as civil-society organizations and individuals within communities—can play vital roles in addressing social injustice and its impact on public health (see chapter 24).
- *Promoting social justice through education in public health:* Schools of public health and educational programs in public health can promote social justice in many ways, including featuring social-justice subjects and issues in their curricula (see chapter 25).

(*text continues on p. 19*)

BOX 1-2 Universal Declaration of Human Rights

On December 10, 1948, the General Assembly of the United Nations adopted and proclaimed the Universal Declaration of Human Rights, the full text of which appears below. It then called upon all member countries to publicize the text of the Declaration and "to cause it to be disseminated, displayed, read and expounded principally in schools and other educational institutions, without distinction based on the political status of countries or territories."

Preamble

Whereas recognition of the inherent dignity and of the equal and inalienable rights of all members of the human family is the foundation of freedom, justice and peace in the world,

Whereas disregard and contempt for human rights have resulted in barbarous acts which have outraged the conscience of mankind, and the advent of a world in which human beings shall enjoy freedom of speech and belief and freedom from fear and want has been proclaimed as the highest aspiration of the commonpeople,

Whereas it is essential, if man is not to be compelled to have recourse, as a last resort, to rebellion against tyranny and oppression, that human rights should be protected by the rule of law,

Whereas it is essential to promote the development of friendly relations between nations,

Whereas the peoples of the United Nations have in the Charter reaffirmed their faith in fundamental human rights, in the dignity and worth of the human person and in the equal rights of men and women and have determined to promote social progress and better standards of life in larger freedom,

Whereas Member States have pledged themselves to achieve, in cooperation with the United Nations, the promotion of universal respect for and observance of human rights and fundamental freedoms,

Whereas a common understanding of these rights and freedoms is of the greatest importance for the full realization of this pledge,

Now, therefore, the General Assembly proclaims this Universal Declaration of Human Rights as a common standard of achievement for all peoples and all nations, to the end that every individual and every organ of society, keeping this Declaration constantly in mind, shall strive by teaching and education to promote respect for these rights and freedoms and by progressive measures, national and international, to secure their universal and effective recognition and observance, both among the peoples of Member States themselves and among the peoples of territories under their jurisdiction.

(*continued*)

Article 1

All human beings are born free and equal in dignity and rights. They are endowed with reason and conscience and should act towards one another in a spirit of brotherhood.

Article 2

Everyone is entitled to all the rights and freedoms set forth in this Declaration, without distinction of any kind, such as race, color, sex, language, religion, political or other opinion, national or social origin, property, birth or other status. Furthermore, no distinction shall be made on the basis of the political, jurisdictional or international status of the country or territory to which a person belongs, whether it be independent, trust, non-self-governing or under any other limitation of sovereignty.

Article 3

Everyone has the right to life, liberty and security of person.

Article 4

No one shall be held in slavery or servitude; slavery and the slave trade shall be prohibited in all their forms.

Article 5

No one shall be subjected to torture or to cruel, inhuman or degrading treatment or punishment.

Article 6

Everyone has the right to recognition everywhere as a person before the law.

Article 7

All are equal before the law and are entitled without any discrimination to equal protection of the law. All are entitled to equal protection against any discrimination in violation of this Declaration and against any incitement to such discrimination.

Article 8

Everyone has the right to an effective remedy by the competent national tribunals for acts violating the fundamental rights granted him by the constitution or by law.

Article 9

No one shall be subjected to arbitrary arrest, detention or exile.

(*continued*)

BOX 1-2 (*continued*)

Article 10

Everyone is entitled in full equality to a fair and public hearing by an independent and impartial tribunal, in the determination of his rights and obligations and of any criminal charge against him.

Article 11

(1) Everyone charged with a penal offence has the right to be presumed innocent until proved guilty according to law in a public trial at which he has had all the guarantees necessary for his defense. (2) No one shall be held guilty of any penal offence on account of any act or omission which did not constitute a penal offence, under national or international law, at the time when it was committed nor shall a heavier penalty be imposed than the one that was applicable at the time the penal offence was committed.

Article 12

No one shall be subjected to arbitrary interference with his privacy, family, home or correspondence, nor to attacks upon his honor and reputation. Everyone has the right to the protection of the law against such interference or attacks.

Article 13

(1) Everyone has the right to freedom of movement and residence within the borders of each state. (2) Everyone has the right to leave any country, including his own, and to return to his country.

Article 14

(1) Everyone has the right to seek and to enjoy in other countries asylum from persecution. (2) This right may not be invoked in the case of prosecutions genuinely arising from non-political crimes or from acts contrary to the purposes and principles of the United Nations.

Article 15

(1) Everyone has the right to a nationality. (2) No one shall be arbitrarily deprived of his nationality nor denied the right to change his nationality.

Article 16

(1) Men and women of full age, without any limitation due to race, nationality or religion, have the right to marry and to found a family. They are entitled to equal rights as to marriage, during marriage and at its dissolution. (2) Marriage shall be entered into only with the free and full consent of the

(continued)

intending spouses. (3) The family is the natural and fundamental group unit of society and is entitled to protection by society and the State.

Article 17

(1) Everyone has the right to own property alone as well as in association with others. (2) No one shall be arbitrarily deprived of his property.

Article 18

Everyone has the right to freedom of thought, conscience and religion; this right includes freedom to change his religion or belief, and freedom, either alone or in community with others and in public or private, to manifest his religion or belief in teaching, practice, worship and observance.

Article 19

Everyone has the right to freedom of opinion and expression; this right includes freedom to hold opinions without interference and to seek, receive and impart information and ideas through any media and regardless of frontiers.

Article 20

(1) Everyone has the right to freedom of peaceful assembly and association. (2) No one may be compelled to belong to an association.

Article 21

(1) Everyone has the right to take part in the government of his country, directly or through freely chosen representatives. (2) Everyone has the right to equal access to public service in his country. (3) The will of the people shall be the basis of the authority of government; this shall be expressed in periodic and genuine elections which shall be by universal and equal suffrage and shall be held by secret vote or by equivalent free voting procedures.

Article 22

Everyone, as a member of society, has the right to social security and is entitled to realization, through national effort and international co-operation and in accordance with the organization and resources of each State, of the economic, social and cultural rights indispensable for his dignity and the free development of his personality.

Article 23

(1) Everyone has the right to work, to free choice of employment, to just and favorable conditions of work and to protection against unemployment. (2) Everyone, without any discrimination, has the right to equal pay for equal work. (3) Everyone who works has the right to just and favorable

(continued)

BOX 1-2 (*continued*)

remuneration ensuring for himself and his family an existence worthy of human dignity, and supplemented, if necessary, by other means of social protection. (4) Everyone has the right to form and to join trade unions for the protection of his interests.

Article 24

Everyone has the right to rest and leisure, including reasonable limitation of working hours and periodic holidays with pay.

Article 25

(1) Everyone has the right to a standard of living adequate for the health and well-being of himself and of his family, including food, clothing, housing and medical care and necessary social services, and the right to security in the event of unemployment, sickness, disability, widowhood, old age or other lack of livelihood in circumstances beyond his control. (2) Motherhood and childhood are entitled to special care and assistance. All children, whether born in or out of wedlock, shall enjoy the same social protection.

Article 26

(1) Everyone has the right to education. Education shall be free, at least in the elementary and fundamental stages. Elementary education shall be compulsory. Technical and professional education shall be made generally available and higher education shall be equally accessible to all on the basis of merit. (2) Education shall be directed to the full development of the human personality and to the strengthening of respect for human rights and fundamental freedoms. It shall promote understanding, tolerance and friendship among all nations, racial or religious groups, and shall further the activities of the United Nations for the maintenance of peace. (3) Parents have a prior right to choose the kind of education that shall be given to their children.

Article 27

(1) Everyone has the right freely to participate in the cultural life of the community, to enjoy the arts and to share in scientific advancement and its benefits. (2) Everyone has the right to the protection of the moral and material interests resulting from any scientific, literary or artistic production of which he is the author.

Article 28

Everyone is entitled to a social and international order in which the rights and freedoms set forth in this Declaration can be fully realized.

(*continued*)

Article 29

(1) Everyone has duties to the community in which alone the free and full development of his personality is possible. (2) In the exercise of his rights and freedoms, everyone shall be subject only to such limitations as are determined by law solely for the purpose of securing due recognition and respect for the rights and freedoms of others and of meeting the just requirements of morality, public order and the general welfare in a democratic society. (3) These rights and freedoms may in no case be exercised contrary to the purposes and principles of the United Nations.

Article 30

Nothing in this Declaration may be interpreted as implying for any State, group or person any right to engage in any activity or to perform any act aimed at the destruction of any of the rights and freedoms set forth herein.

- *Researching critical questions on social justice and public health:* Systematic research approaches can better document social injustice, identify its underlying causes, and help point the way to reducing social injustice and its impact on public health (see chapter 26).
- *Protecting human rights through national and international laws:* National and international laws can be strengthened and better implemented to protect human rights and promote social justice (see chapter 27).
- *Promoting equitable and sustainable human development:* Achievement of social justice requires equitable and sustainable human development (see chapter 28).

The *Healthy People 2010* initiative in the United States and the Millennium Development Goals initiative worldwide provide a framework for making progress in reducing social injustice as it affects public health. (See table 21-7 on p. 394.) The Millennium Development Goals include eradicating extreme poverty and hunger; reducing infant and childhood mortality; improving maternal health; combating HIV/AIDS, malaria, and other infectious diseases; ensuring environmental sustainability; and establishing a global partnership for development.

We believe that the ultimate remedy for social injustice and its adverse effects on health lies in the development, adoption, and implementation of policies and programs that promote social justice and protect individuals and communities from social injustice. Therefore, we believe that advocacy for these policies and programs is the most critical component of an agenda for social justice and public health. Solving problems of social injustice requires

BOX 1-3 International Declaration of Health Rights

We, as people concerned about health improvement in the world, do hereby commit ourselves to advocacy and action to promote the health rights of all human beings.

- The enjoyment of the highest attainable standard of health is one of the fundamental rights of every human being. It is not a privilege reserved for those with power, money or social standing.
- Health is more than the absence of disease, but includes prevention of illness, development of individual potential, a positive sense of physical, mental and social well-being.
- Health care should be based on dialogue and collaboration between citizens, professionals, communities and policy makers. Health services should be affordable, accessible, effective, efficient and convenient.
- Health begins with healthy development of the child and a positive family environment. Health must be sustained by the active role of men and women in health and development. The role of women, and their welfare, must be recognized and addressed.
- Health care for the elderly should preserve dignity, respect and concern for quality of life and not merely extend life.
- Health requires a sustainable environment with balanced human population growth and preservation of cultural diversity.
- Health depends on the availability to all people of basic essentials: food, safe water, housing, education, productive employment, protection from pollution, and prevention of social alienation.
- Health depends on protection from exploitation without distinction of race, religion, political belief, economic or social condition.
- Health requires peaceful and equitable development and collaboration of all peoples.

The International Declaration of Health Rights was created by the faculty, students, and alumni of the Johns Hopkins School of Public Health on the occasion of the School's 75th anniversary. It was first signed at a ceremony on April 23, 1992, by Hiroshi Nakajima, Director-General of the World Health Organization; James Grant, Executive Director of UNICEF; and Alfred Sommer, Dean of the School.

Since then, signing ceremonies have taken place around the world to bring recognition to the need for all peoples to work together to prevent disease, disability, and premature death.

painful costs that the dominant interests in society may be unwilling to pay. Ultimately, what is needed to effectively address social injustice is the popular and political will to address its root causes. A primary goal of public health is to help develop this popular and political will, and to use it to help end social injustice.

References

1. Institute of Medicine. The future of public health. Washington, D.C.: IOM, 1988.
2. Beauchamp DE. Public health as social justice (invited paper). J Inquiry 1976;XII:3–13.
3. U.S. Department of Health and Human Services. Healthy People 2010: Progress review focus area 1. Access to quality health services. Available at: http://www.cdc.gov/nchs/about/otheract/hpdata2010/focusareas/fa01-atqhs.htm. Accessed on March 6, 2005.
4. U.S. Department of Health and Human Services. Tracking Healthy People 2010. Washington, D.C.: U.S. Government Printing Office, 2000.
5. World Health Organization. World health report 2003. Geneva, Switzerland: WHO, 2003.
6. Broder S. Progress and challenges in the National Cancer Program. In: Brugge J, Curran T, Harlow E, McCormick F, eds. Origins of human cancer: a comprehensive review. Plainview, N.Y.: Cold Spring Harbor Laboratory Press, 1991:27–33.

Further Reading

Hofrichter R (Ed.). Health and social justice: politics, ideology, and inequity in the distribution of disease. San Francisco, Calif.: Jossey-Bass, 2003.

Rhodes R, Battin MP, Silvers A (Eds.). Medicine and social justice: essays on the distribution of health care. New York: Oxford University Press, 2002.

Part II

How the Health of Specific Population Groups Is Affected by Social Injustice

2

THE SOCIOECONOMICALLY DISADVANTAGED

Michael Marmot and Ruth Bell

Introduction

In many of the rich countries of the world, social inequalities in health have been increasing. This has happened at the same time as overall health has improved. National data from England and Wales show that although mortality has improved for each social class between the 1970s and the late 1990s, it has improved most for those initially in the highest social class[1] (fig. 2-1). As a result, the life expectancy gap between the bottom and top social classes has increased. Similar results have been seen for many European countries[2] and for the United States[3] (fig. 2-2).

Why is this relevant to a book on social injustice? If differences in health among social groups were an inevitable consequence of the social stratification that comes from living in social groups, we might comment on it but would perhaps not regard it as unjust. But inequalities in health can change over a relatively short time as overall health improves. Such inequalities are therefore unlikely to be inevitable. If they are not inevitable and if we could do something about them, they are unjust.[4]

The starting point for this chapter is that inequality in the conditions under which people live and work translates into inequalities in health. We argue that it is the inequality in these circumstances that is unjust. To take action

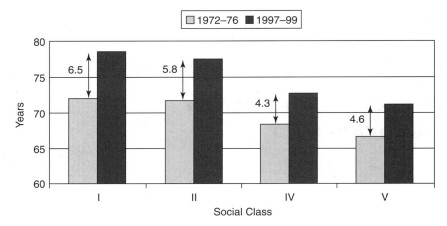

Figure 2-1 Life expectancy for men by social class in England and Wales. (From Donkin A, Goldblatt P, Lynch K. Inequalities in life expectancy by social class, 1972–1999. Health Stat 2002;15:5–15.)

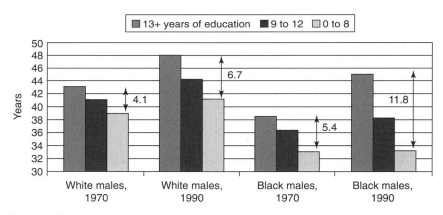

Figure 2-2 Life expectancy at age 30 by education for men in the United States. (Adapted from Crimmins EM, Saito Y. Trends in healthy life expectancy in the United States, 1970–1990: gender, racial, and educational differences. Soc Sci Med 2001;52:1629–1641, table 2. Copyright 2001, with permission from Elsevier.)

against the circumstances that determine ill health, we need a better understanding of what they are and how they come about.

Socioeconomic Disadvantage Is More Than Low Income

One could equate "socioeconomic disadvantage" with poverty, and poverty with lack of money. Socioeconomic disadvantage does indeed imply lack of money, but it also implies more. One cannot understand the relation between socioeconomic disadvantage and health by focusing solely on money or material disadvantage. Other disadvantages are associated with socioeconomic position and these are crucial for health. Amartya Sen, a pioneer in the use of the concept of capabilities, observed that it is not so much what one has that is important but rather what one can do with what one has.[5] Social inequalities in health may be a consequence of inequalities in capabilities.

A second, related, theme pervades this chapter: In considering socioeconomic disadvantage or poverty, there is no sharp dividing line between "the poor" and "the non-poor." Many countries set a threshold level of income for "poverty." Below it, people are considered to be poor, and above it, not poor. A threshold is useful insofar as one can then calculate the prevalence of poverty and make comparisons over time and among countries.[6] Its limitation is that there are degrees of socioeconomic disadvantage. Similarly, social inequalities in health are graded—the lower the social position, the higher is the risk of ill health.

To understand the important, but not comprehensive, role played by money in generating inequalities in health, we provide two crucial distinctions: (a) The importance of income for health depends on how much or how little money an individual or a population has (see below). (b) Income or wealth of individuals has to be separated from income or wealth of populations.

Income Matters If You Have Little of It

If individuals or populations have little money, a small increase may make a big difference. At low incomes, internationally, there is a strong relation between gross national product (GNP) per capita and life expectancy. Much of this is driven by infant and child mortality. In Sierra Leone, the mortality of children under age 5 is about 300 per 1,000 live births. This contrasts with Sweden and Japan, where infant and child mortality is about 4 per 1,000 live births.[6] Extreme poverty is related to extreme bad health. Investment in public health and poverty relief has a major impact on ill health in poor countries.[7] The disparities in health between rich and poor countries represent a gross abuse of human rights[8] (see chapter 21). The remainder of this chapter deals with socioeconomic differences in health within the richer countries of the world.

After Material Deprivation, Absolute Income Matters Less

Among richer countries, differences in absolute income appear to be less important than among poorer countries. Among developed countries, there is no relationship as measured by gross domestic product (GDP) between national income and life expectancy[6] (table 2-1). For example, the United States, for which the GDP in purchasing power is second only to Luxembourg, ranks 26th in life expectancy. Israel, Greece, Malta, and New Zealand—all countries with a GDP of less than $20,000—have a higher life expectancy than the United States. Greece, with a GDP of slightly more than $17,000, has a longer life expectancy than the United States, which has twice the national income. Once a country has solved its basic material conditions for good health, there is evidence that more money does not buy better health.[9]

TABLE 2-1   Life Expectancy at Birth and Gross Domestic Product (GDP) in U.S. Dollars in 2001, Adjusted for Purchasing Power

	Life Expectancy at Birth	GDP
Japan	81.3	25,130
Sweden	79.9	24,180
Canada	79.2	27,130
Spain	79.1	20,150
Switzerland	79.0	28,100
Australia	79.0	25,370
Israel	78.9	19,790
Norway	78.7	29,620
France	78.7	23,990
Italy	78.6	24,670
The Netherlands	78.2	27,190
New Zealand	78.1	19,160
Malta	78.1	13,160
Greece	78.1	17,440
Cyprus	78.1	21,190
Germany	78.0	25,350
Costa Rica	77.9	9,460
United Kingdom	77.9	24,160
Singapore	77.8	22,680
United States	76.9	34,320
Ireland	76.7	32,410
Cuba	76.5	5,259
Portugal	75.9	18,150

From Human development report 2003 by United Nations Development Programme. Copyright 2003 by the United Nations Development Programme. Used by permission of Oxford University Press, Inc.

We have included two poorer countries in the table: Cuba (GDP* adjusted for purchasing power, $5,259) and Costa Rica ($9,460). Life expectancy in Costa Rica, at 77.9 years, is higher than in the United States, 76.9 years, and that of Cuba is only 0.4 year less, despite having less than one sixth the purchasing power.

All of the countries listed in table 2-1 have low infant and child mortality rates—an indication that none of them suffer from the severe material deprivation seen in Sierra Leone. In the United States, for example, infant mortality is about 7 per 1,000 live births.[10] Within countries, there are major differences in health among socioeconomic groups, especially in the middle and older age groups. For example, infants born to mothers with less than 12 years of education (in the 1998–2000 period) had a mortality rate of 8.0 per 1,000, compared with 5.1 per 1,000 for infants born to mothers with 13 or more years of education. Even infants born to African-American mothers with low education, the group with the worst rate of mortality in this analysis, had a mortality rate of 14.8 per 1,000—remarkably better than that of infants in Sierra Leone (182 per 1,000).

This is not to say that socioeconomic disadvantage ceases to be a problem for health in the United States or other rich countries. Despite small differences in infant mortality rate, there are still substantial differences among socioeconomic groups in life expectancy. There is, for example, a 7.4-year gap in life expectancy between the lowest and highest social classes in England and Wales (see fig. 2-1). Not only does length of life show a socioeconomic gradient; so do measures of ill health. For example, in the United Kingdom, at each age there is a remarkable stepwise relation between wealth and poor health[11] (fig. 2-3). Not only do people at the bottom have poor health, but also there is a gradient: The lower one's wealth, the worse is one's level of health. For all groups, ill health increases with age; however, the level of ill health for those in the top quintile of wealth in the 70–74 age group is less than the level of ill health for those in the bottom quintile in the 50–54 age group. We could repeat figure 2-3, substituting income for wealth, and obtain similar findings.

We have then an apparent paradox: Among the rich countries, income of a country is not related to health or life expectancy. However, within a rich country, there is a strong relationship between measures of socioeconomic status and health. Therefore, in rich countries, where the problems of absolute material deprivation have been solved, it is not absolute level of income or wealth that matters for health. What matters is a person's position

---

*Gross domestic product is adjusted for purchasing power in order to make the "meaning" of a dollar comparable across countries.

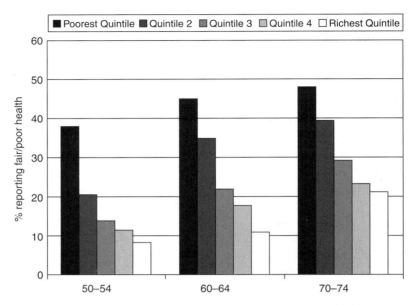

Figure 2-3 Self-reported health by total wealth quintile. (Data from the English Longitudinal Study of Ageing [University College London and the Institute for Fiscal Studies].)

within the social hierarchy. Let us examine which features of socioeconomic position are important for health.

At Higher Levels of Income, Relative Position Remains Important

A focus on the "haves" and "have-nots" leads, understandably, to concern with those toward the bottom of any hierarchy, or with those who are totally socially excluded. The social gradient in health, however, runs all the way from top to bottom of society. In our Whitehall studies of British civil servants, we found a social gradient in health and disease in which those second from the top had worse health than those at the top.[12,13] It would be hard to describe those second from the top as socioeconomically disadvantaged, yet the social gradient in health includes them.

This phenomenon is not confined to British civil servants. In Sweden, for example, men with a doctoral degree had a lower mortality rate than those with a masters degree or professional qualification, even after income was taken into account.[14]

The Impact of Social Injustice on the Socioeconomically Disadvantaged

"Modern" Impoverishment

The ways of doing without have changed. For example, in the early twentieth century, poverty in Britain meant damp, cold, crowded houses, with poor sanitation, unclean water, and lack of nutrition. It meant working in dusty, hazardous, and physically arduous occupations. These living and working conditions provided ample explanation for the high mortality rate of children and high susceptibility of adults to chronic respiratory disease and tuberculosis.

This is no longer the typical picture of the socioeconomically disadvantaged. Here are two quotes from a lower-status civil servant in our Whitehall II study.[9] The first is about work:

> I went to the typing pool, and sat there typing documents. Which was absolutely soul destroying. The fact that we could eat sweets and smoke was absolute heaven, but we were not allowed to talk.

The second is about her life after retirement. Although on a "reasonable" occupational pension, she does not have the resources to engage in a meaningful retirement. She said:

> I've got used to my own company.... I do find the week-ends a bugger.... I've got no incentive.... I sit and read the paper.... and breakfast at 10.30. If you sit watching TV in the afternoon.... I'm at rock bottom.

These quotes were chosen to demonstrate what "impoverishment" means for people not at the bottom of the social hierarchy. For those closer to the bottom, there may be no work and no social isolation so much as living in disordered circumstances. The following comes from a young man living in a deprived neighborhood in the north of England:

> I trust my work mates more than my close mates. I've experienced what they've done with each other, I've watched as they've slagged each other off to me and I think, you know, I'll not say anything to this guy 'cos he'll go and tell him, so I just keep it hush hush, I don't tell 'em much.
>
> I'd never trust anyone else, not in this area. A lot are drug dealers who would rob you, it's as simple as that, they would do anything to get in your house. They would backstab you. They will just turn around and rob you.

The challenge is to understand how the circumstances of impoverished lives lead to poor health, when people have enough to eat, do not drink contaminated water, have adequate shelter, and are not dying, to any major extent, of infectious disease.

Early Life

The work of David Barker has alerted us to the importance of early life for the subsequent risk of adult diseases. He described the effects of exposure in a critical period with long-term subsequent effects. In a series of studies, he showed that the physical dimensions of children at birth and age 1 year— height and thinness—predict diabetes, hypertension, and heart disease in adulthood.[15] The presumed cause is maternal and child nutrition, which, in turn, are likely to be linked to social position of mothers. Although Barker has shown that the relation between low birth weight and subsequent risk of heart disease is independent of the link with *maternal* socioeconomic position, it is, in part, dependent on the *individual's* adult socioeconomic position. In a study in Helsinki, Finland, Barker and colleagues showed that thinness at birth *and* low social position in adulthood were linked to an increased risk of heart disease; adult socioeconomic position was more strongly related to disease if people had also had a low birth weight, and vice versa.[16]

There are at least two other ways in which social and environmental circumstances can affect adult risk of disease: (1) a pathway effect, and (2) accumulation of advantage and disadvantage; for example, the effects of poor nutrition, infections, and psychosocial exposures at different points in life may cumulate to influence adult disease risk.[17] The pathway effect demonstrates that it is not the circumstances of early life, per se, that increase risk of adult disease but rather that circumstances in childhood lead to circumstances in adulthood that affect adult risk. The strong relation between education and adult disease may reflect both accumulation and pathway effects.[18] Indeed, in order to understand the impact of socioeconomic disadvantage on adult disease, circumstances through the entire life span need to be considered.[19–21]

One way we see the evidence of early life effects is by studying adult height. There is a clear relation between social position and height. In the Whitehall studies, the taller the man, the higher was the employment grade.[22] On average, men in the top employment grades were 5 cm taller than men in the bottom. We see a similar phenomenon in the United States.[23] Height of *individuals* is clearly related to genetic inheritance. Heights of *groups*, however, are far more likely to be related to nutritional status at birth and during childhood and adolescence, which is linked to socioeconomic circumstances.

In the Whitehall studies, short height was a potent predictor of adult coronary heart disease.[24,25] The additive effects on prediction of coronary heart disease of short height and adult social position suggest that social circumstances of both adulthood and childhood make important contributions to risk of adult disease.

Medical Care

Equity in health care can be construed as equal access for equal need. In theory, lack of utilization of health care could be related to lack of access or, conversely, personal disinclination to use health care that cannot be attributed to lack of access.[26] Inequity is a reasonable label for lack of access that results from circumstances beyond an individual's control. In practice, as disinclination to use health care can also be attributed to social, cultural, or educational barriers, utilization of health care is used as a proxy for lack of access.

When considering social inequities in health care as a contributor to social inequalities in health, there is a striking contrast between Britain and the United States. In Britain, the whole population has access to the National Health Service, which provides care independent of ability to pay. In the U.S. system, over 40 million people do not have health insurance and, therefore, do not have the same access as those who do. With access to Medicare, differential access may be less important in people over 65. Overall generalizations like these do not reveal the patterns of inequity in relation to need that may occur. Equity of access in theory is not the same as equity of access in practice.

A review in Britain of access in relation to need revealed a mixed picture.[26] In part, the mixed results relate to problems in defining "need." If need for health care is thought of as capacity to benefit from that health care, then a person with advanced malignancy may have no "need" for curative treatment in that he or she has no capacity to benefit from it. This contrasts with the person with less advanced malignancy who has capacity to benefit and, therefore, greater "need" for health care. In practice, health status is taken as a measure of need.

This may account for some of the variation in results. In Britain, most studies show that people from lower socioeconomic groups have higher rates of health service utilization than those from higher socioeconomic groups. But they have greater need. When adjusted for need, the results seem to depend on the type of need. For emergency hospital admissions, lower socioeconomic groups seem to have rates proportional to need. For elective procedures and those involving preventive care, lower socioeconomic groups are underserved.[26]

This issue has been reviewed comprehensively in the United States by the Agency for Health Care Research and Quality.[27] It found that the lower the income, the less satisfactory is entry to the health care system, as reflected by: (a) no or inadequate health insurance, (b) no specific source of ongoing care, and/or (c) difficulties in obtaining care. It also found that low income is associated with (a) reports of poor communication with health care personnel and (b) lower likelihood of having had blood pressure or plasma cholesterol checked as part of preventive health care.

At first, the disparities in health care appear to be greater in the United States than in Britain. In both countries, however, there are large socioeconomic differences in health. Socioeconomic differences in health cannot easily be attributed to lack of access to high quality medical care since they are seen for onset of new disease and for treatment of existing disease. Nevertheless, inequities in medical care are a further cause of morbidity and suffering that will contribute to the disadvantage of having low socioeconomic status.

Lifestyle and Its Effects

The term "lifestyle" commonly conveys a misleading impression. It is common to refer to the diseases that affect the rich countries of the world as diseases of affluence and, in turn, attribute them to lifestyle factors, such as smoking, diet, and sedentary habits. This is doubly misleading. First, the major causes of morbidity and mortality in rich countries affect the socioeconomically disadvantaged to a greater extent than those more affluent. Second, to think of lifestyle as something freely chosen—a style—provides little insight as to why relevant health behaviors now follow a social gradient.

There are two questions in relation to lifestyle: (a) How much of the social gradient in health and disease does it explain? (b) Why should there be a social gradient in lifestyle? Let us consider cigarette smoking. Strikingly, smoking is more prevalent as one descends the social hierarchy.[28] In the Whitehall and Whitehall II studies of British civil servants, smoking accounted for just under one-quarter of the social gradient in coronary heart disease.[29,30] While this leaves much unexplained, smoking is still an important contributor to the social gradient in health. Explanations for why there should be a social gradient in smoking have been somewhat unsatisfactory. It has been suggested that people of lower socioeconomic position are more oriented to the present than the future and hence are less likely to take action that will lead to future health benefits. That leaves open the question of why this should be. Hilary Graham has shown that women's smoking can be linked to problems in their lives that come from their precarious social and economic circumstances.[31,32]

The same may apply to other health behaviors. Cost may be of more direct relevance. Although to smoke cigarettes makes no economic sense, because it costs the smoker money and leads to worse health, the consumption of energy-dense foods may indeed be a cheaper way to find calories. In the United States, there is an inverse association between energy density of foods (in calories per kilogram) and energy cost (per calorie); that is, cheaper foods have more calories per weight. However, high-energy density usually means fats and added sugars.[33] Given that low income means, among other things, lower expenditure on food, this may help explain the link between lower socioeconomic status and obesity. Interestingly, this link is stronger among women than among men,[34] possibly because body weight is under stronger cognitive control in higher-status women, who have the luxury to consider body shape.

The quality of diet is important in other ways. Higher status means greater consumption of fruit and vegetables, which generally reduces risk of disease.

A contributor to socioeconomic differences in obesity is differences in physical activity. As physical activity at work has become less important, leisure-time physical activity has become more important. The higher the social position, the more frequent is participation in leisure-time physical activity.[22,35,36]

In summary, lifestyle does provide a partial explanation for the social gradient in health, but lifestyle is related to socioeconomic situation.

The Circumstances in Which People Live and Work

If inequalities in health cannot be attributed to differences in medical care or lifestyle, what else is there? Work environments are important for health[37] and may play an important role in generating inequalities in health.[30] Two models of the work environment have been shown to be linked to increased risk of cardiovascular disease: (a) jobs characterized by high psychological demand and low control, and (b) jobs that entail high effort and low rewards in terms of esteem, career opportunities, and financial remuneration. These aspects of work may be important links between socioeconomic status and disease.[38] Psychosocial characteristics of work are related not only to cardiovascular disease but also to sickness absence, mental and physical functioning, mental illness, and musculoskeletal disorders.[39–42]

Outside of work, the characteristics of residential areas predict disease beyond the characteristics of the individuals who live in those places.[43] Socioeconomic characteristics of areas are linked to the health status of individuals, even after taking into account individual characteristics.[44–47] Part of the explanation for these effects appears to lie in the degree of social cohesion of neighborhoods.[48,49]

The fact that social and psychosocial characteristics of areas may be important for health does not rule out the contribution of more physical exposures. Lower social status means worse housing quality in ways that may damage health.[50] A recent review, citing evidence from the United States and the United Kingdom, showed that people of lower income are more likely to be exposed to residential crowding, hazardous wastes, ambient and indoor air pollutants, adverse water quality, and ambient noise, in addition to worse working and housing conditions.[51] The review concluded, however, that in the present state of knowledge it is not possible to provide an accurate estimate of how important these exposures might be in generating the social gradient in health.

Roots and Underlying Factors of This Social Injustice

All societies have stratification. Social stratification by its nature means unequal access to resources, privileges, and esteem. Does this mean that social inequalities in health are inevitable? Not to the extent that we now see them. Health inequalities have increased in the United States, Great Britain, and many other countries. If they can increase, they can, presumably, decrease.

Fundamental human needs can be simplified into (a) health and its determinants, (b) autonomy or control over life, and (c) opportunities for full social participation—and these domains are linked.[9] To these could be added respect and self-respect and participation in culture, including the tradition of people,[52] which could easily be linked with autonomy and social participation.[53] If these needs for autonomy and social participation are not met, health suffers. Inequality in the degree to which these needs are met constitutes social injustice. Our contention is that although social hierarchies are universal, the degree of social inequality in meeting these needs varies. Our approach is closely linked to Amartya Sen's concept of capabilities or freedoms.[54]

It is tempting to think that marked economic inequalities are a feature of unbridled markets seen in advanced capitalist countries. Indeed, there is evidence to support the view that income inequalities are not only tolerated but also encouraged in some capitalist countries more than in others. (It is difficult to lay this at the door of markets per se. Much of the accumulation of great wealth can be attributed more or less directly to the distortion of markets. There is nothing like a monopoly position with little market competition for wealth accumulation by a section of the community.)

That said, income inequalities are more marked in developing countries than in established market economies[55] (table 2-2). Although comparison among countries is limited by differences in how data are collected, some general conclusions can be drawn. First, there are large variations in the degree of income inequalities among the rich countries. The top 10 percent of households in Japan, Sweden, and Norway enjoy less than 22 percent of total income; in contrast, in the United Kingdom, the top 10 percent have 28 percent, and in the United States, 31 percent. In both the United Kingdom and the United States, income differentials have grown in recent years.[56,57] Second, income inequalities are smaller in rich countries than in poor countries. The

TABLE 2-2   Percentage Share of Income Distribution of
Bottom 10 Percent and Top 10 Percent of Households

	Bottom 10 Percent	Top 10 Percent
Japan	4.8	21.7
Sweden	3.7	20.1
Canada	2.8	23.8
Switzerland	2.6	25.2
Norway	4.1	21.8
France	2.8	25.1
Italy	3.5	21.8
The Netherlands	2.8	25.1
Greece	3.0	25.3
Germany	3.3	23.7
United Kingdom	2.3	27.7
Costa Rica	1.7	34.6
United States	1.8	30.5
Dominican Republic	2.1	37.9
Paraguay	0.5	43.8
Sierra Leone	0.5	43.6

Adapted from The World Bank. World development report 2003.
Washington, D.C.: The World Bank, 2003.

well-developed market economies of the West have narrower differences
between rich and poor than in the grossly unequal conditions of countries such
as Paraguay and Sierra Leone. Even Costa Rica, with a good health record, has
wider income inequalities than the richer countries listed in the table 2-2.

There has been a vigorous debate as to whether income inequalities, per
se, lead to worse health.[58,59] We do not need to review the arguments here to
note that increasing income inequalities are indicators of increasing divisions
in society. These are likely to be fundamental drivers of inequality in access
to resources. In other words, inequality in income is likely to be correlated
with inequality in meeting needs. Such inequalities are not inevitable but are,
in part, a consequence of decisions taken as to how a society's economic and
social affairs are to be organized.

A second trend that goes along with increased income inequality has been
seen, particularly in the United States, to be the increasing geographic segregation of affluence and poverty.[60] Increasingly, people below the poverty
line live in neighborhoods with a high proportion of poor households; those
at the upper end, increasingly, live in neighborhoods that are more exclusively affluent. Such residential divisions are likely to mean poorer services,
more crime, and more civil disruption in poorer neighborhoods than in
wealthier areas.

In the United Kingdom, similarly, affluence and poverty tend to be spatially segregated. There has, however, been no strong trend for this spatial segregation to increase in recent years.[61]

A third fundamental driver of inequalities in society is education. Inequalities affecting today's adults are passed on via today's children to tomorrow's adults[9] (fig. 2-4). An international literacy survey conducted by the Organization for Economic Cooperation and Development (OECD) demonstrated that the literacy levels of young people are highly correlated with their parents' level of education.[62] This relationship is graded: the higher the parents' education, the better their children perform. The slope of the relation, however, varies: it is much shallower in Sweden than it is in the United States. These findings suggest that family background matters but so does the general environment of the country. In detailed studies, J. Douglas Willms[63] has shown that family background, social capital of the area in which the person lives, and the quality of the school all influence the development of literacy.

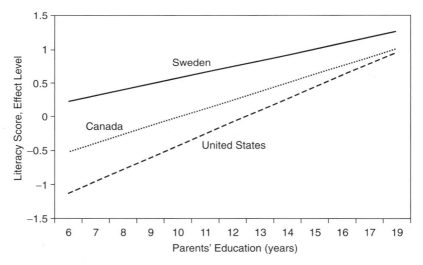

Figure 2-4 Literacy scores of people aged 16–25 according to level of education of their parents in the United States, Canada, and Sweden. (Adapted from Statistics Canada; Inequalities in Literacy Skills Among Youth in Canada and the United States by J. Douglas Willms, Catalogue number: 89-552-MIE, International Adult Literacy Survey No. 6, reference period: September 1999, adapted from Figure A. Statistics Canada information is used with the permission of the Minister of Industry, as Minister responsible for Statistics Canada. Information on the availability of the wide range of data from Statistics Canada can be obtained from Statistics Canada's Regional Offices, its World Wide Web site at http://www.statcan.ca, and its toll-free access number, 1-800-263-1136.)

(Robert Putnam defines social capital as "the connections among individuals—social networks and the norms of reciprocity and trustworthiness that arise from them."[64]) The relevance for our present concern is that various measures of education are strongly related to health. Figure 2-4 presents a mechanism by which socioeconomic disadvantage is passed down from one generation to another; the degree of the intergenerational transmission, however, is less in Sweden than it is in the United States.

What Needs to Be Done

A society without social hierarchy is one that has yet to be observed. Even hunter-gatherer societies that are said to be relatively egalitarian have hierarchies.[65] They are kept in check.[66] More complex forms of social organization have clearer hierarchies. There cannot, therefore, be a realistic program of action that aims to abolish hierarchies. Nor does the history of the twentieth century engender much enthusiasm for the type of communist government seen in central and eastern Europe. If the health records of these countries is a judge, then in the 1970s and 1980s these countries failed to meet human needs on a grand scale.[67,68]

Neither of these cautions—the universality of hierarchies and the disappointing experience of state socialism—should be taken as grounds for thinking that nothing can be done. Health levels and inequalities in health vary over time within countries and vary among countries. There is, therefore, good reason to believe that appropriate social and economic changes can reduce the health disadvantage associated with progressively lower position in the social hierarchy. In the United States, for example, with life expectancy ranked at twenty-sixth among countries despite spending approximately one sixth of GDP on health care, there are scant grounds for complacency.

Britain's record also gives little reason for complacency but recent history is encouraging. In 1997, after a change in government, the new Labor government set up an independent group to inquire into inequalities in health under the chairmanship of Sir Donald Acheson, a former chief medical officer to the government. (One of the authors, M.M., was a member of the scientific advisory group of that inquiry.[57]) The group made 39 recommendations to government, of which only two had to do with health care. Three key recommendations that we made were as follows:

1. We RECOMMEND that as part of health impact assessment, all policies likely to have a direct or indirect effect on health should be evaluated in terms of their impact on health inequalities, and should be formulated in such a way that by favouring the less well off they will, wherever possible, reduce such inequalities.

1.1. We recommend establishing mechanisms to monitor inequalities in health and to evaluate the effectiveness of measures taken to reduce them.

1.2. We recommend a review of data needs to improve the capacity to monitor inequalities in health and their determinants at a national and local level.

2. We RECOMMEND a high priority is given to policies aimed at improving health and reducing health inequalities in women of childbearing age, expectant mothers, and young children.

3. We RECOMMEND policies which will further reduce income inequalities, and improve the living standards of households in receipt of social security benefits. Specifically:

3.1. We recommend further reductions in poverty in women of child-bearing age, expectant mothers, young children and older people should be made by increasing benefits in cash or in kind to them.

3.2. We recommend uprating of benefits and pensions according to principles which protect and, where possible, improve the standard of living of those who depend on them and which narrow the gap between their standard of living and average living standards.

3.3. We recommend measures to increase the uptake of benefits in entitled groups.

We recommend further steps to increase employment opportunities.

In other words, the group took the view that health inequalities are a result of wider social and economic inequalities in society. The group, therefore, recommended that there be a fundamental change in attitude to inequality in society that runs across the whole of government. The recommendations of the group spanned the life course from pregnant women and early childhood to education, skills training for those dropping out of school, workplaces, communities, and support for people beyond retirement age. Lifestyle was put in context and changes were called for in the provision and availability of healthy food, exercise facilities, and nicotine replacement therapy available on prescription to aid those individuals in economic need.

Does the report represent wishful thinking on a grand scale?[69] Perhaps, but there is evidence that government has moved to implement many of these recommendations.[70] To take the most contentious, income redistribution—a subject not popular with the well-to-do—there is evidence that the tax system has been changed to mitigate the effects of growing pretax income inequalities.[71] Figure 2-5 shows the effects of the finance minister's (chancellor of the exchequer's) changes to the tax and benefit regimen since taking office in 1997. The lower the income to begin with, the more favorable have been the changes in the tax and benefit regimen—that is, the greater has been the gain in household income.

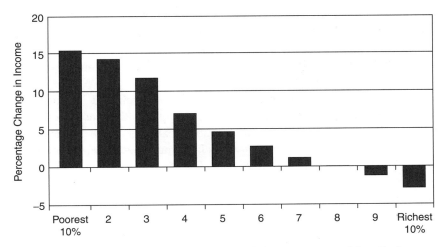

Figure 2-5 The effects on disposable incomes of changes to tax and benefits between 1997 and 2002, by income decile group. (From Bond S, Wakefield M. Distributional effects of fiscal reforms since 1997. In: Chote R, Emmerson C, Simpson H, eds. The IFS Green Budget: January 2003, London, England: Institute for Fiscal Studies, 2003.)

A crucial question relates to improving the chances of the next generation. Child poverty is a particular problem in Britain, and the chancellor has set reduction in child poverty as an aim. There is a new program, Sure Start, aimed at early child development, that is modeled on the U.S. Head Start program.

There is a view that, for society to be affluent, the wealth-producers have to be motivated to generate wealth—rather than hampered with indignities, such as progressive taxation. If this means growing inequalities, it is an acceptable side effect, even if such economic inequalities lead to health inequalities. This view has been characterized as a myth convenient to the interests of those who benefit from inequalities.[72] In fact, the view that growing income inequalities aid economic growth has been seriously questioned.[60]

There is indeed a case to be made that growing income and social inequalities will damage social cohesion.[64] This will, in turn, work to the detriment not only of the socioeconomically disadvantaged but also of everyone in society. A society that is more socially inclusive is likely to be a healthier society.

Conclusion

A usual reaction to the evidence on the social gradient in health is that the causes must have to do with inadequacies of medical care or an unhealthy lifestyle. In fact, inequalities in health relate fundamentally to inequalities in society. Health of a population and inequalities in health are markers of how a society is meeting the needs of its members. There is no reason to believe that the health of today's disadvantaged groups could not improve were that socioeconomic disadvantage to be relieved.

The fact that socioeconomic disadvantage is not relieved is a matter of social injustice. This is not to call for egalitarianism in the sense of everyone being the same—a hopeless and undesirable goal. It is, however, to suggest that society may benefit if our set of social arrangements were to move toward a situation where control over one's life and full social participation are more equitably distributed. Governments can help this occur by the way they channel resources to improve the conditions under which people live and work and in which our children develop and older citizens thrive.

References

1. Donkin A, Goldblatt P, Lynch K. Inequalities in life expectancy by social class, 1972–1999. Health Stat Q 2002;15:5–15.
2. Mackenbach JP, Bos V, Andersen O, et al. Widening socioeconomic inequalities in mortality in six Western European countries. Int J Epidemiol 2003;32:830–7.
3. Crimmins EM, Saito Y. Trends in healthy life expectancy in the United States, 1970–1990: gender, racial, and educational differences. Soc Sci Med 2001;52:1629–41.
4. Marmot M. Do inequalities matter? In: Daniels N, Kennedy B, Kawachi I, eds. Is inequality bad for our health? Boston, Mass.: Beacon Press, 2000.
5. Sen A. Inequality reexamined. Oxford, England: Oxford University Press, 1992.
6. United Nations Development Programme. Human development report 2003. New York, N.Y.: Oxford University Press, 2003.
7. Anand S, Ravallion M. Human development in poor countries: on the role of private incomes and public services. J Econ Perspect 1993;7:133–50.
8. Farmer P. Pathologies of power: health, human rights, and the new war on the poor. Berkeley, Calif.: University of California Press, 2003.
9. Marmot M. Status syndrome. London, England: Bloomsbury, 2004.
10. U.S. Department of Health and Human Services. Chartbook on trends in the health of Americans: Health, United States, 2003. Hyattsville, Md.: National Center for Health Statistics, 2003.
11. Marmot M, Banks J, Blundell R, et al. Health, wealth and lifestyles of the older population in England. The 2002 English Longitudinal Study of Ageing. London, England: Institute for Fiscal Studies, 2003.
12. Marmot MG, Shipley MJ. Do socioeconomic differences in mortality persist after retirement? 25 year follow up of civil servants from the first Whitehall study. BMJ 1996;313:1177–80.
13. Marmot MG, Ryff C, Bumpass L, et al. Social inequalities in health: next questions and converging evidence. Soc Sci Med 1997;44:901–10.
14. Erikson R. Why do graduates live longer? In: Jonsson JO, Mills C, eds. Cradle to grave: life-course change in modern Sweden. Durham, U.K.: Sociology Press, 2001.

15. Barker DJP. Mothers, babies and health in later life. Edinburgh, U.K.: Churchill Livingstone, 1998.
16. Barker D, Forsen T, Uutela A, et al. Size at birth and resilience to effects of poor living conditions in adult life: longitudinal study. BMJ 2001;323:1273–6.
17. Power C, Hertzman C. Social and biological pathways linking early life and adult disease. Br Med Bull 1997;53:210–21.
18. Smith JP. Unraveling the SES-health connection. Population Dev Rev, in press.
19. Kuh D, Ben-Shlomo Y. A life course approach to chronic disease epidemiology. Oxford, England: Oxford University Press, 1997.
20. Kuh D, Hardy R. A lifecourse approach to women's health. Oxford, England: Oxford University Press, 2002.
21. Davey Smith G, ed. Health inequalities: lifecourse approaches. Bristol, England: The Policy Press, 2003.
22. Marmot MG, Davey Smith G, Stansfeld SA, et al. Health inequalities among British Civil Servants: the Whitehall II study. Lancet 1991;337:1387–93.
23. Komlos J, Baur M. From the tallest to (one of) the fattest: the enigmatic fate of the American population in the 20th century. Econ Hum Biol 2004;2:57–74.
24. Marmot MG, Shipley MJ, Rose G. Inequalities in death—specific explanations of a general pattern. Lancet 1984;323:1003–6.
25. Marmot M, Shipley M, Brunner E, et al. Relative contribution of early life and adult socioeconomic factors to adult morbidity in the Whitehall II study. J Epidemiol Commun Health 2001;55:301–7.
26. Dixon A, LeGrand J, Henderson J, et al. Is the NHS equitable? A review of the evidence. LSE Health and Social Care Discussion Paper Number 11. London, England: The London School of Economics and Political Science, 2003.
27. U.S. Department of Health and Human Services. National healthcare disparities report. Rockville, Md.: Agency for Healthcare Research and Quality, 2003.
28. Jarvis MJ, Wardle J. Social patterning of individual health behaviours: the case of cigarette smoking. In: Marmot MG, Wilkinson RG, eds. The social determinants of health. New York, N.Y.: Oxford University Press, 1999.
29. van Rossum CTM, Shipley MJ, van de Mheen H, et al. Employment grade differences in cause specific mortality. A 25 year follow up of civil servants from the first Whitehall study. J Epidemiol Commun Health 2000;54:178–84.
30. Marmot M, Bosma H, Hemingway H, et al. Contribution of job control and other risk factors to social variations in coronary heart disease incidence. Whitehall II Study. Lancet 1997;350:235–9.
31. Graham H, Hunt K. Socio-economic influences on women's smoking status in adulthood: insights from the West of Scotland Twenty-07 study. Health Bull 1998; 56:51–8.
32. Graham H. Hardship and health in women's lives. London, England: Harvester Wheatsheaf, 1993.
33. Drewnowski A, Specter SE. Poverty and obesity: the role of energy density and energy costs. Am J Clin Nutr 2004;79:6–16.
34. Erens B, Primatesta P. The Health Survey for England 1998. Cardiovascular disease. London, England: The Stationery Office, 1998.
35. James WPT, Nelson M, Ralph A, et al. Socioeconomic determinants of health: the contribution of nutrition to inequalities in health. BMJ 1997;314:1545–9.
36. Joint Health Surveys Unit. Health Survey for England 1994. London, England: The Stationery Office, 1996.

37. Marmot M, Siegrist J, Theorell T, et al. Health and the psychosocial environment at work. In: Marmot M, Wilkinson RG, eds. Social determinants of health. New York, N.Y.: Oxford University Press, 1999.
38. Siegrist J, Marmot M. Health inequalities and the psychosocial environment—two scientific challenges. Soc Sci Med 2004;58:1463–73.
39. North F, Syme SL, Feeney A, et al. Explaining socioeconomic differences in sickness absence: the Whitehall II Study. BMJ 1993;306:361–6.
40. Stansfeld S, Bosma H, Hemingway H, et al. Psychosocial work characteristics and social support as predictors of SF-36 functioning: the Whitehall II Study. Psychosom Med 1998;60:247–55.
41. Stansfeld SA, Fuhrer R, Head J, et al. Work and psychiatric disorder in the Whitehall II study. J Psychosom Res 1997;43:73–81.
42. Hemingway H, Shipley M, Stansfeld S, et al. Are risk factors for atherothrombotic disease associated with back pain sickness absence? The Whitehall II Study. J Epidemiol Commun Health 1999;53:197–203.
43. Marmot M. Inequalities in health. N Engl J Med 2001;345:134–6.
44. Diez-Roux A. Bringing context back into epidemiology: variables and fallacies in multi-level analysis. Am J Public Health 1998;88:216–22.
45. Diez-Roux AV, Nieto FJ, Muntaner C, et al. Neighborhood environments and coronary heart disease: a multilevel analysis. Am J Epidemiol 1997;146:48–63.
46. MacIntyre S, Ellaway A, Cummins S. Place effects on health: how can we conceptualise, operationalise and measure them? Soc Sci Med 2002;55:125–39.
47. Stafford M, Bartley M, Mitchell R, et al. Characteristics of individuals and characteristics of areas: investigating their influence on health in the Whitehall II study. Health Place 2001;7:117–29.
48. Stafford M, Bartley M, Boreham R, et al. Neighbourhood social cohesion and health: investigating associations and possible mechanisms. In: Morgan A, Swann C, eds. Social capital and health. Issues of definition, measurement and links to health. London, England: Health Development Agency, 2004.
49. Sampson RJ, Raudenbush SW, Earls F. Neighborhoods and violent crime: a multilevel study of collective efficacy. Science 1997;277:916–24.
50. Blane D, Mitchell R, Bartley M. The "inverse housing law" and respiratory health. J Epidemiol Commun Health 2000;54:745–9.
51. Evans GW, Kantrowitz E. Socioeconomic status and health: the potential role of environmental risk exposure. Annu Rev Public Health 2002;23:303–31.
52. Honderich T. After the terror. Edinburgh, U.K.: Edinburgh University Press, 2003.
53. Sennett R. Respect in a world of inequality. New York, N.Y.: W.W. Norton and Co., 2003.
54. Sen A. Development as freedom. New York, N.Y.: Alfred A. Knopf, 1999.
55. World Bank. World development report 2003. New York, N.Y.: The World Bank and Oxford University Press, 2003.
56. Bernstein J, Mishel L, Brocht C. Anyway you cut it: income inequality on the rise regardless of how it's measured. Briefing paper. Washington, D.C.: Economic Policy Institute, 2000. Available at: http://www.epinet.org/content.cfm/briefingpapers_inequality_inequality. Accessed January 10, 2005.
57. Acheson D. Inequalities in health: report of an independent inquiry. London, England: HMSO, 1998.
58. Wilkinson RG. Unhealthy societies: the afflictions of inequality. London, England: Routledge, 1996.

59. Deaton A. Health, inequality, and economic development. J Econ Literature 2003; 41:113–58.
60. Kawachi I, Kennedy BP. The health of nations: why inequality is harmful to your health. New York, N.Y.: The New Press, 2002.
61. Dorling D, Rees P. A nation still dividing: the British census and social polarisation 1971–2001. Environ Planning A 2003;35:1287–313.
62. Willms JD. Quality and inequality in children's literacy: the effects of families, schools and communities. In: Keating D, Hertzman C, eds. Developmental health and the wealth of nations: social, biological, and educational dynamics. New York, N.Y.: Guilford Press, 1999.
63. Willms JD. Inequalities in literacy skills among youth in Canada and the United States (International Adult Literacy Survey No 6). Ottawa, Canada: Human Resources Development Canada and National Literacy Secretariat, 1999.
64. Putnam R. Bowling alone: the collapse and revival of American community. New York, N.Y.: Simon and Schuster, 2000, p. 19.
65. Erdal D, Whiten A. Egalitarianism and Machiavellian intelligence in human evolution. In Mellars P, Gibson K, eds. Modelling the early human mind. Cambridge, England: McDonald Cambridge, 1996.
66. Wright R. Non zero—The logic of human destiny. New York, N.Y.: Vintage, 2001.
67. Bobak M, Marmot MG. East-West mortality divide and its potential explanations: proposed research agenda. BMJ 1996;312:421–5.
68. Bobak M, Pikhart H, Rose R, et al. Socioeconomic factors, material inequalities, and perceived control in self-rated health: cross-sectional data from seven post-communist countries. Soc Sci Med 2000;51:1343–50.
69. Marmot M. From Black to Acheson: two decades of concern with inequalities in health. Int J Epidemiol 2001;30:1165–71.
70. Exworthy M, Stuart M, Blane D, et al. Tackling health inequalities since the Acheson Inquiry. Bristol, England: The Policy Press, 2003.
71. Bond S, Wakefield M. Distributional effects of fiscal reforms since 1997. In Chote R, Emmerson C, Simpson H, eds. The IFS green budget: January 2003. London, England: Institute for Fiscal Studies, 2003.
72. Galbraith JK. The culture of contentment. London, England: Sinclair-Stevenson, 1992.

3

RACIAL AND ETHNIC MINORITIES

Carol Easley Allen and Cheryl E. Easley

Introduction

Many Americans confront complex, historical, multifaceted disparities as they navigate the U.S. health care system, as documented by an extensive review by the Institute of Medicine of health care inequities experienced by racial and ethnic minorities.[1] Even when access-related factors such as insurance and income are controlled, racial and ethnic minorities receive a lower quality of care than do nonminorities across the broad range of health concerns such as cardiovascular problems, pain management, and preventive health care.[1,2] Perhaps these disparities should lead us to place renewed emphasis on prevention for racial and ethnic minorities to keep them out of the hands of health care providers.[3]

The term "racial and ethnic minorities" as used in this chapter includes any of the nonwhite racial or ethnic groups in the United States as well as people of Hispanic origin: blacks regardless of country of origin (African-Americans); American Indians and Alaska Natives; Asians and Pacific Islanders; Native Hawaiians and Other Pacific Islanders; and Hispanics (Latinos). The terms "Hispanic" and "Latino" are used interchangeably, as are the terms "black" and "African-American," with the recognition that not all blacks in the United States are African-American, such as Haitian-Americans, Jamaican-Americans, and people from African countries. Although the focus of this chapter is on racial and ethnic minorities in the United States, the concerns and solutions presented apply to analogous situations in many other countries.

The federal Office of Management and Budget established guidelines in 1997 to collect and present data on race and Hispanic origin. These guidelines were used in Census 2000. The following terms were used:

Race

The concept of race reflects self-identification by people according to the race or races with which they closely identify. The categories are sociopolitical constructs and are not scientific in nature. Race and Hispanic origin are treated as separate and distinct concepts.

White

A person having origins in any of the original peoples of Europe, the Middle East, or North Africa, including people who indicate their race as white or report on entries such as Irish, German, Italian, or Arab.

Black or African-American

A person having origins in any of the original black racial groups of Africa, including, for example, people who indicate their race as black, African-American, or Negro.

American Indian and Alaska Native

A person having origins in any of the original people of North and South America (including Central America) who maintains tribal affiliation or community attachment.

Asian

A person having origins in any of the original people of the Far East, Southeast Asia, or the Indian subcontinent, including, for example, China, India, and the Philippine Islands.

Native Hawaiian and Other Pacific Islander

Includes people who have origins in any of the original peoples of Hawaii, Guam, Samoa, or other Pacific Islands, or who provided a write-in response of a Pacific Islander group.

Hispanic or Latino

A person who identifies in categories such as Mexican, Puerto Rican, or Cuban or as being of other Spanish origin. Origin can be viewed as heritage, nationality group, lineage, or country of birth of the person or person's parents, or ancestors before a person's arrival in the United States. A person who identifies his or her origin as Spanish can be of any race.

For the first time, in Census 2000, respondents were given the option to identify themselves as belonging to more than one racial group. Given this change, Census 2000 data on race are not directly comparable to previous U.S. census data.[4,5]

African-Americans and Non-American Blacks in the United States

Blacks and African-Americans include a rich diversity of cultural groups. Most have descended from the more than 4 million enslaved persons stolen from Africa, but some are children of blacks who were free in this country before the arrival of the *Mayflower* in 1620.[6] The end of slavery in 1865 was followed by laws that disfranchised blacks and imposed racial segregation. Despite advances in civil rights in the past half-century, blacks continue to experience racism throughout the United States. Current black migrants come to this country from many places in Africa, the Caribbean, Europe, and elsewhere.

In 2002, blacks comprised 12.8 percent of the U.S. population (36 million people).[7] While most live in the South, black Americans live in every region of the country. Over half of blacks live in urban areas beset by the conditions of poverty—overcrowding, inadequate housing, poor public education, and crime.[8,9]

Latinos

Latinos have recently overtaken blacks as the largest minority group in the United States, with a diverse population of 37 million, comprising 13.5 percent of the population in 2002.[7] Significant within-group distinctions exist based on place of origin, length of time in the United States, income levels, family size, educational attainment, and the degree to which members speak Spanish, English, or both.[10] Latinos are geographically concentrated, with the highest concentrations in the western and southern United States. Latinos are a young population, of whom 39 percent are foreign born. They are more likely to live in poverty, to reside in large-family households, to be unemployed, and, if working, to earn less than non-Latino whites.[6]

Asian-Americans

Asian-Americans, one of the fastest growing segments of the population, are a diverse group, claiming descent from 28 different countries in the Far East and Southeast Asia. Although some groups have long histories in this country, others, especially some Southeast Asians, are relatively recent arrivals.[11] Asian-Americans are at the extremes of income and educational scales.[12] Most are foreign born, with some groups, namely the Hmong, Khmer, Laotians, Chinese-Vietnamese, and Vietnamese, being at risk of extreme poverty and health disparities.

Native Hawaiians and Other Pacific Islanders

Native Hawaiians and Other Pacific Islanders (NHOPI) have descended from the original peoples of Hawaii, Guam, Samoa, and other Pacific Islands. Although Hawaii comprises the best known of the Pacific islands, there are many other islands with political or historical ties to the United States in both the North and South Pacific.[13]

Pacific Islanders comprise a very small ethnic group in the United States. Until 2000, they were grouped with Asians under the category Asian-Americans/ Pacific Islanders (AAPI), in which demographic trends and health needs of Pacific Islanders were often hidden.[14] Like Latinos, Pacific Islanders are a young population. Most live in the western states, with the highest concentrations in Hawaii and California. Many Pacific Islanders, especially Samoans, experience high rates of poverty.[13]

Native Americans and Alaska Natives

There are 569 federally recognized American Indian and Alaska Native (AI/AN) tribes and an unknown number that are not recognized—each with its own culture and beliefs. The unique relationships between the tribes and the federal government derive from wars and subsequent treaties that recognize the tribes as sovereign entities.[15] While the histories of these groups vary according to the timing and nature of their encounters with the Europeans, common features include the introduction of infectious disease, ecological alterations, forced relocation, genocidal violence, social and cultural devastation, and poverty.[16]

AI/AN experience some of the most severe health disparities as well as low incomes and limited access to quality education and, in some cases, to health care. Although the Indian Health Service is charged with the provision of their health care, many who live outside reservations cannot access care provided by the Indian Health Service. Increasingly, AI/AN groups are providing their own health services with federal financial support.[15]

The Impact of Social Injustice on the Health
of Racial and Ethnic Minorities

African-Americans and Non-American Blacks
in the United States

Despite overall decreases, the infant mortality rate among blacks has remained at double the rate among whites for many years. Between 1980 and 2000, the percentage decline for whites (10.9 to 5.7 per 1,000 live births) was greater than that for blacks (22.2 to 14.0 per 1,000 live births). Death rates from heart disease, cancer, and many other diseases are significantly higher among blacks. For example, the prostate cancer mortality rate among black men is more than double that of white men. Black women are more likely to die of breast cancer, despite a lower incidence rate and a higher mammography screening rate than for white women. The HIV/AIDS death rate of blacks is more than seven times that of whites. The homicide rate of blacks is six times higher than that of whites.[17,18]

Latinos

The likelihood of dying of diabetes, in 2001, was nearly 63 percent higher for Latinos than for non-Hispanic whites.[19] In 2003, Latinos accounted for over 27 percent of tuberculosis cases, almost 75 percent of which were in foreign-born Latinos.[20] While the overall infant mortality rate for Latinos is lower than that for whites, this situation masks within-group differences. For example, the infant mortality rate among Puerto Ricans is 50 percent higher than that among whites.[18]

Latinos are highly likely to report communication problems with physicians that affect the care they receive, even when they use English as their primary language. They are most likely to fail to follow a physician's advice because of treatment costs, with many Latinos using alternative therapies that they do not report to physicians. Latinos are least likely to have a regular physician and most likely of all major racial and ethnic groups to report feeling that they (a) have been treated with disrespect by physicians and (b) have little or no choice in sources of health care. Latinos are also most likely to report low rates of screening and preventive health services.[21]

Asian-Americans

Prevalent among Asian-Americans are such problems as parasitic infections, tuberculosis, sudden infant death syndrome (SIDS), sudden unexpected nocturnal death syndrome (SUNDS), hepatitis B virus infection, cardiovascular disease, and HIV infection. Many foreign-born Asian-Americans have reduced access to health care due to lack of insurance, as well as cultural, psychosocial, and language barriers. Many find it difficult and confusing to make the transition from their traditional ways of understanding and treating illness to those of Western health care. Often health care providers other than Asian-Americans have a poor understanding of Asian-American cultures and their health care needs, falling back on stereotypes that inhibit adequate responses.[11,14]

Native Hawaiians and Other Pacific Islanders

NHOPI experience poorer health overall than the total U.S. population, with a high risk of cancer, heart disease, diabetes, and other diseases.[22] Significant health disparities among Pacific Islanders include diabetes and cardiovascular disease, both of which are linked to obesity. Contributing factors include a sedentary lifestyle and high-fat diets throughout the Pacific islands. Health care access problems also confront Pacific Islanders, including high poverty rates, linguistic and spatial isolation, and perceived poor quality of health services. Inadequate national sample sizes for the study of NHOPI render understanding of disparities in health care and health status difficult, especially when examining within-group differences.[13,14]

Native Americans and Alaska Natives

In comparison to other ethnic groups, native people in the United States are more likely to die from unintentional injuries, diabetes, chronic liver disease (including cirrhosis), and suicide. In 2000, AI/AN infants died at nearly twice the rate of white infants. These minorities also have disproportionately high rates of SIDS, substance abuse and related problems (including fetal alcohol syndrome), unintentional injuries, and domestic violence.

Among both Native Americans and Alaska Natives, there is a trend toward deaths that occur earlier in the life cycle.[23–25] For example, the 1999 death rate among Alaska Native children aged 1 to 4 years was more than double that for both all Alaskan children and all U.S. children. The 1999 mortality rate per 100,000 population for Alaska Native youth aged 15 to 19 years was 280.6, compared to 110.7 for all Alaskan and 69.8 for all U.S. teenagers in this age group.[26]

The years of potential life lost (YPLL) is a useful measure of the impact of premature death that serves to illuminate disparities in health outcomes for a population. Between 1999 and 2000, the YPLL before age 75 for non-Hispanic whites was 92 percent of the national average, whereas the rate for Native Americans was nearly 107 percent. In Alaska in 2002, the Native population experienced over twice the YPLL before age 75 as the non-Hispanic white population.[23,27] Inadequate national sample sizes for the study of AI/AN render understanding of disparities in health care and health status difficult, especially when examining within-group differences.

Special Health Issues for Minority Women, Children, Elders, and Men

Women

In the United States, women of color comprise the largest number of people with new HIV infections. Among women in the United States during the 1998–2002 period, African-Americans represented approximately 60 percent of new cases, and Latinas, about 20 percent. This difference was most notable among poor women, whose situation is often complicated by family responsibilities. In 2002, the AIDS incidence rate for African-American women was more than 20 times, and for Latinas, more than 5 times, that of white women.[28]

Children

Food-insecure families have reduced diet quality, increased use of emergency food sources, and anxiety about their food supply. In 2001, 0.6 percent of children in the United States lived in households with child hunger and over 4 percent of children lived in food-insecure households, and children from the most populous racial/ethnic minority groups were at higher risk of food insecurity than white children.[29]

Minority children have shorter average survival times than whites for several malignancies, including leukemia. In the 1990s, only 75 percent of black and Latino children with leukemia survived 5 years compared with 84 percent of white children and 81 percent of Asian children, a statistically significant difference,[30] in part because minority children receive less consistent medical care. Apparently, black children are more likely to have a more virulent form of the disease than white children, so genetic differences may affect a child's response to the disease as well as to various drug regimens.[31] A retrospective study of 412 children and adolescents with newly diagnosed acute lymphoblastic leukemia (ALL) revealed that black children were significantly more likely than white children to have factors associated with a poor prognosis, which included a chromosomal translocation. However, the authors of the study concluded that with equal access to effective therapy, black and white children could expect the same high rate of cure.[32]

Older People

In the United States, 16 percent of members of racial/ethnic minority groups are over age 65. This proportion is expected to increase to 22 percent in the next 20 years. Specific ethnicity-related problems include the following:

- Filipinos, Japanese, and Southeast Asian groups in the United States have a high prevalence of hypertension. Hypertension is one of the 10 leading causes of death for men over age 65 only in Asian/Pacific Islanders (ranked ninth) and African-Americans (ranked tenth).[33]
- Obesity and diabetes are increased in Pacific Islanders, American Indians, Alaska Natives, African-Americans, and Latinos. In the 1999–2001 period, obesity among women aged 20 to 74 was much more common among blacks (50.8 percent) and Mexicans (40.1 percent) than among whites (30.6 percent).[34]
- Vietnamese women have the highest incidence of invasive cervical cancer among American women who are Asians or Pacific Islanders—a rate that is three times higher than that of the second-ranked group (Korean women of the same age) and five times higher than that of white women.[35] Cancer is a major concern for this group of women because they are less likely to have annual Pap smears or mammograms.
- Rates of influenza and pneumococcal immunizations are significantly lower for African-American adults (31 percent) and Latino adults (30 percent) than for white adults (57 percent). These disparities have persisted over time.[36]
- Both language and cultural barriers to health care and poverty pose significant and persistent problems for many minority elderly.[18,37]

Men

Men of color are less healthy than any other group, partly due to reduced access to care. They are less likely to be included in programs to reduce disparities in health outcomes.[38] In the United States in 2001, the life expectancy for black men (68.6 years) was lower than that for black women (75.5) and for white men (75.0) and white women (80.2).[39] Black men are at significantly greater risk than white men for death from cardiac and cerebrovascular disease or from HIV/AIDS. In the 1999–2002 period, African-American men accounted for 49 percent of the new HIV cases reported in the United States. In 2000, Latinos represented 13 percent of the population but accounted for 19 percent of the new cases of AIDS—with men accounting for 81 percent of these cases. The two leading instances of HIV infection in the two groups are men having sex with men and injection drug use; however, there is within-group variation among Latinos by place of birth.[40,41] African-American and Latino gay men with AIDS in the United States now outnumber white gay men with the disease.[42]

Men of color are more likely than white men to be poor, less educated, and unemployed and to experience the detrimental effects of residential segregation and other economic and social problems that are associated with poor health. Black and Latino men are less likely than white men to see a physician, even when they are in poor health. Nonelderly black and Latino men are more likely than white men to lack health insurance. Medicaid insures only 6 to 8 percent of black and Latino men. Men of color, regardless of their insurance status, are less likely to receive timely preventive services and more likely to experience the adverse effects of delayed attention to chronic health problems, as reflected, for example, by limb amputation and radical cancer surgery.[38]

The combination of gender and race affects the health of men of color in various ways. The effects of economic marginality and unemployment are especially potent for men, who see themselves as providers. These effects are more pronounced among men of color. Occupational hazards, low-wage jobs, poor educational opportunities, discrimination, and poor housing are among the frequent stressors for men in the United States society.[38]

Environmental Quality

Relatively little research has been done on environmental quality in communities of color. A number of studies since the 1970s, however, demonstrate that African-Americans and other minorities, low-income groups, and working-class persons are disproportionately subjected to pollution and environmental stressors at home and at work. For example, a study of ambient air quality in California revealed that blacks and Hispanics are more likely to live in areas characterized by substandard air quality.[43] Even with social class held constant, studies have found that race is a determining factor in elevated public health risks due to the distribution of air pollution, consumption of contaminated fish, location of municipal landfills and incinerators, abandonment of toxic waste dumps, inadequate clean-up of Superfund sites, and lead poisoning in children. Race has been found to be the single most important determinant in the location of toxic waste sites—more important than income, percentage of home ownership, or property values. Blacks have been shown to be most at risk, with three of five living in communities with abandoned toxic waste sites.[44]

Due to discrimination in housing and lack of economic and political power, minorities live nearest to sources of pollution, such as power plants and industries, and in central cities, where vehicular emissions are often heaviest. African-Americans have fewer chances than low-income whites to escape these conditions because of racial barriers to education, employment, and housing.[44]

The effects of environmental toxins on children that begin in the womb and persist into or emerge in adulthood—such as those due to lead, dioxin, environmental tobacco smoke, and methyl mercury—are examples of the cumulative, life-limiting effects of social injustice.[45,46] The significant long-lasting impacts of environmental exposures are critical risks for children from low-income households, who are more likely to face increased contact with hazardous pollutants in their communities.

Social injustice is also evident in the differential implementation of environmental regulations and other policies that are designed to protect communities, such as cleaning up toxic waste sites and punishing polluters. Unequal protection, favoring white communities over communities of color, occurs whether the community is wealthy or poor.[44] Environmental injustice contributes to the excess burden of a broad array of health problems, such as respiratory, reproductive, renal, and neurological disorders, that affect ethnic minorities in the United States.[47]

Access to and Quality of Health Care

A qualitative study has shown that racial and ethnic minorities have worse first-contact primary care than whites, even after controlling for disparities in sociodemographic and health-status characteristics.[48] This finding suggests complex relationships in the interactions of persons from different backgrounds with the health care system and indicates the need for culturally competent care to remove barriers to access.

The U.S. Census Bureau estimated, in 2002, that 43.6 million Americans were uninsured—this is thought to be underestimated because it only measured those who were uninsured at the time the census was taken. If the report had counted all who had been uninsured for any part of 2001 and 2002, it would have shown that 74.7 million were without insurance. The numbers of those without insurance increased by 2.4 million between 2001 and 2002, the fastest rate in a decade.[49]

Latinos represent the largest group without health insurance, with nearly half of those under 65 years reporting that they had no health insurance at some point during the previous year. This problem is widespread among people of Central American and Mexican descent[50] because many Latinos work in low-wage jobs that do not provide health insurance, have questionable immigration status, or live in states with stringent eligibility standards for Medicaid.[51] In 2003, approximately 44 percent of Latino children in low-income families were uninsured for all or part of the year, compared with 33 percent of all U.S. children in low-income families.[49]

Disparities in quality of health care have also been documented comprehensively. For example, the odds of blacks and women with chest pain being referred for cardiac catheterization are 60 percent of those for whites and men. Black women with chest pain have only 40 percent the chance of white men of being referred for catheterization.[1]

Roots and Underlying Issues of This Social Injustice

Poverty, Income, and Wealth/Assets

From 2001 to 2002, the number of poor people in the United States increased by 1.7 million, from 11.7 percent to 12.1 percent of the population—34.6 million people were living below the poverty line in 2002. Blacks and Hispanics sustained the greatest increase in poverty during this period. [52]

Although income disparities are significant, and are currently widening, the most compelling difference between majority and minority populations lies in the area of assets or wealth. More than 33 percent of nonwhite households in the United States today do not have any positive wealth, compared with approximately 12 percent of white households.[53]

Social policies for asset development have been used for centuries in the United States to benefit whites and disadvantage minorities, and the discriminating impacts of these policies have cumulated over time. Three salient examples of past discriminatory social policies whose effects persist are the Homestead Act of 1862, the G.I. Bill of 1944, and a series of federal initiatives designed to enable homeownership in the 1940s and 1950s. Racial discrimination and segregation inherent in the implementation of these programs provided opportunities for asset development among whites that were denied to blacks and other ethnic minorities. And the more recent policy of redlining by banks continues to discriminate against blacks and other minorities.[54] ("Redlining" is the practice of designating a particular residential area for preferential or prejudicial treatment based on race or ethnicity.)

Today, institutional policies related to asset development favor those with incomes of $50,000 or more, who receive approximately 90 percent of the benefits from tax deductions or "breaks." These deductions are actually tax expenditures that include tax credits, preferential tax rates, tax deferrals, and exclusions from taxation. Such deductions represent approximately 50 percent of direct federal expenditures on a yearly basis. The largest of these tax expenditures, which help the rich to accumulate financial and real assets, are in the areas of home ownership, retirement accounts, and preferential treatment of gains from investments. The housing tax exemption policy, for example, provides the nonpoor with substantial subsidies that assist them to become homeowners, while the overwhelming majority of the housing subsidies directed to the poor, such as Section 8 of the housing code, rental vouchers, and public housing, enable them only to rent housing, not to own homes.[54–56]

Social Exclusion

Like poverty, social exclusion has a major impact on health and mortality. Social exclusion stems from racism, discrimination, stigmatization, hostility, and unemployment. Persons experiencing these mechanisms are barred from full participation in education and from access to services and community activities, and they experience harm to their overall health.[57]

Geographical Location and Residence Patterns

Segregated residential location has been linked to health and well-being in a number of ways. Living within one's ethnic community has many benefits, such as social support, but the fact that many communities of color are beset by the damaging conditions of poverty affects the health of all community residents.[38] A project to investigate race- and ethnicity-based discrimination in housing reported persistent discrimination against African-Americans, Hispanics, and Asians and Pacific Islanders in both sales and rentals of homes.[58]

Employment Status and Occupational Health Issues

Blacks with an associate degree are unemployed at almost twice the rate as are whites with the same education.[59] Unemployment can lower a person's motivation and can lead to emotional and physical damage.[60] Although data relating minority status with occupational disease are not adequate, there are disproportionately higher rates of disease in occupations and specific occupational activities that employ workers of color[61] (see chapter 19).

Health Literacy Issues

The average American adult reads at the eighth- to ninth-grade level, whereas most health education and information materials are written above the tenth-grade level. Health literacy—the ability to read, understand, and act on health information—is a stronger predictor of health status than age, income, employment status, educational level, or racial or ethnic group. Health literacy problems affect a disproportionate number of ethnic minorities and immigrants, especially those who speak English as a second language.[62] Low health literacy results in higher health care costs, problems with self-management of health care, and increased risk of hospitalization.[62–66]

Specific Implications of Social Injustice for Racial and Ethnic Minorities

Minorities Are at Greater Risk for the Imposition of Social Injustice

The same problems that contribute to discriminatory practices in the larger society also influence the experience of minorities in their encounters with the health care system. These problems include individual and institutional racism in health care and the legal, regulatory, financial, and political environments in which health care decisions are made and implemented, all of which can operate to deny social justice to minorities who seek the benefits of the U.S. health care system.

The health inequities that exist in every nation are largely due to the social injustice that leads to unequal access to societal resources. These inequities are caused by unjust social arrangements that often discriminate against minority groups.[67] The health trends of disadvantaged minorities are extremely sensitive to economic, social, and political trends. Whether a country is rich or poor, better health is associated with higher social position.

In important ways, a nation's health inequities may be seen as a barometer of its citizens' experiences of social justice and human rights. Health equity is best thought of not as a separate social goal but as a measure of social justice.[67]

What Needs to Be Done

Ensuring Cultural Competence Among Health Professionals and Institutions

An expert panel appointed by Physicians for Human Rights made 24 policy recommendations to address the problem of racial and ethnic disparities in the quality of medical care, based on a comprehensive survey of peer-reviewed medical literature:[68]

- The federal government should create an Office of Health Disparities within the Office of Civil Rights of the Department of Health and Human Services to determine if health disparities are the products of discrimination and to take appropriate action.
- The federal government should collect data on race, ethnicity, and primary language in health plans to assure analysis of data on racial and ethnic disparities and to provide resources to agencies addressing racial and ethnic health disparities.

- National professional organizations, educational institutions, accrediting bodies, and health care provider associations should take appropriate action to assure that health professionals are educated on health disparities and cultural competence, and these competencies should be evaluated for licensure and individual and institutional credentialing purposes.
- Research should be performed on patient-provider interactions, provider attitudes and behaviors related to race and ethnicity, health care system disparities in care, and interventions to eliminate disparities.

Language sensitivity that accounts for appropriate words for subpopulations speaking the same language is important. For example, the use of *condones* for "condoms" is acceptable to Puerto Ricans, but for Dominicans, *profilacticos* should be used. Qualified medical interpreters are required for accurate and appropriate care.[42]

Increasing Recruitment and Retention of Minority Youth Into Health Professions

The inadequate number of minorities in health care professions contributes to racial and ethnic minorities receiving unequal treatment, and thus higher rates of morbidity and mortality from chronic diseases. Sensitivity to culture and language is critical to quality health care.[69,70] Recruiting and retaining minority students in the public health and health care professions should be supported through an increased number of scholarship programs and mentoring relationships.

Attention to Clear Health Communication to Address Health Literacy Problems

Public health efforts, such as the Ask Me 3 campaign (www.AskMe3.org) developed by the Partnership for Clear Health Communication, should be directed specifically to minority and immigrant communities that are at significantly greater risk of low health literacy. The American Public Health Association is a founding member of the Partnership, which is now in the first phase of national effort to improve health communication between patients and providers. The Ask Me 3 campaign is a solution-based initiative that promotes three simple, but essential, questions that patients should ask providers during every health care interaction: (a) What is my main problem? (b) What do I need to do? (c) Why is it important for me to do this? [62] In addition, more systemic advocacy is needed to address such issues as the disparities in public education that place poor and minority children at risk of poor literacy skills.

Reducing Poverty and Addressing Factors That Create Poverty

Poverty reduction should begin with monitoring of health outcomes related to poverty and the education of health care providers on the relationship between social injustice and health. Collaborative efforts are necessary with a range of other sectors to address human rights issues, such as adequate food, housing, safe communities, employment, health care, and full social, economic, and political participation. Policies should be changed and resources equitably distributed to ensure an adequate level of public education for all children in the United States, regardless of ethnicity, residential location, or socioeconomic status. The most effective policy change would be a per-capita educational allocation rather than basing educational expenditures on community of residence; the likelihood of this happening in the foreseeable future, however, appears to be remote.

Community-based interventions tailored to specific community contexts can help reduce poverty and improve health outcomes. Such interventions are characterized by the use of multisector and multistrategy approaches and building on community assets, such as enlisting local residents to bridge cultural gaps.[70] It is also important to support capacity-building, the provision of access and opportunity in the areas of health and economic opportunity in minority communities. In terms of the economy, capacity-building includes such things as access capital in the form of small business loans and education in business management for minority group members so they will be able to handle business opportunities. Economic opportunity also includes transportation to the inner city for minority group members who have been relocated to the suburbs due to the renovation and takeover of the inner city by affluent majority groups. Often the suburbanite minorities have no transportation to the inner-city jobs on which they depend. Capacity-building in the area of health involves increasing the numbers of minority group members who are educated in the health professions, especially in the higher-income and higher-status occupations. Capacity-building also includes the provision of health education and information to minority community members so they can assume greater responsibility for their own health status and serve as health resources to others in their communities. Capacity-building can be supported by both government and private initiatives and funding.

Public policy should remove barriers to affordable housing in neighborhoods of choice. Residential segregation, unless forced, is not inherently bad. Indeed, many ethnic minorities prefer to live in neighborhoods of their own race.[38] Problems occur when ethnic neighborhoods are composed solely of the poor, where the accumulated ills of poverty and institutional neglect are compounded by substandard public education, unemployment, and the lack of positive role models, transportation, and opportunities for economic development.

All people should be protected by minimum income and wage guarantees and access to gainful employment. Unemployment benefits should be set at a level that protects individuals and families from drifting into poverty. Education and accessible retraining are important in the prevention of unemployment.[57]

Public and private mechanisms, such as credit unions and credit counseling, may help to reduce indebtedness among the poor. Low-income households should have access to the institutional mechanisms, incentives, and subsidies that exist to assist those who are not poor to save, such as employment-matched pension plans, payroll-deduction savings programs, and mortgage-financed home purchases. The poor generally do not receive the tax benefits for mortgage-interest deductions and, if they are homeowners, they typically receive lower rates of return for their housing investments. The main federal social welfare program to which the poor have access, Temporary Assistance for Needy Families (TANF), actually discourages saving by setting asset limits above which benefits are denied.

Matched savings accounts—known as Individual Development Accounts (IDAs)—enable low-income families to save enough money for a down payment on a home, pay for post–secondary education, or obtain start-up capital for a small business. There are more than 500 community-based asset-building programs, with over 20,000 account-holding beneficiaries in 49 states. These programs have begun to stimulate saving, enable the use of IDAs to purchase assets expected to have high returns, and increase future-oriented thinking.[54,57] One study revealed that 28 percent of matched withdrawals from the IDAs were used to purchase homes; 23 percent to start businesses; 21 percent for post–secondary education; and 18 percent for home repair. Participants reported that the acquisition of assets improved their outlook and helped them to think less about getting through the next day and more about what they might want to do in 5 years.[71]

Addressing Racial Discrimination

Many whites have no awareness of their privileged status even as they protect their interests in every area of social interaction. Although they may admit that disparities exist, they attribute them to lack of ambition or effort by minorities rather than the structural favoritism for whites that has always been an integral part of American society. David Wellman, professor of community studies at the University of California, Santa Cruz, and co-author of a text on racial discrimination, states, "You don't need to be a racist to promote qualities that are race-conscious. Most whites don't see white as a race. Like a fish in water, they don't think about whiteness because it's so beneficial to them."[59]

Camara Jones, a former professor at the Harvard School of Public Health, has presented three levels of racism:

1. *Institutionalized racism* is "differential access to the goods, services, and opportunities of society by race" (p. 1212).[72] It is structured into the norms, customs, and sometimes the laws such that there need be no perpetrator for it operate. Institutional racism is seen in both (a) material conditions, such as lack of equal access to quality education, sound housing, gainful employment, and adequate health care; and (b) access to power, such as differential access to information, resources, and voice (voting rights, representation in government, and control of the media). The historical association between socioeconomic status and race in the United States is perpetuated by contemporary structural arrangements that foster the continuation of those historic injustices.
2. *Personally mediated racism* is prejudice and discrimination—that is, differential assumptions about others based on race and differential actions toward others according to race. It is what many people mean by "racism." Personally mediated racism may be intentional or unintentional and may include acts of commission or omission. It may be evidenced as lack of respect, suspicion, avoidance, devaluation, scapegoating, or dehumanization. Like institutionalized racism, personally mediated racism is condoned by societal norms and maintains structural barriers: Personally mediated racism is manifested in everyday customs of interaction that may range from poor service in a department store to police brutality. Individual practices of avoidance based on race serve to perpetuate structural barriers between racial groups.
3. *Internalized racism* occurs when members of the stigmatized race accept the negative messages of racism about themselves and engage in devaluation of themselves and others of their race. This leads to hopelessness, resignation, and helplessness.

Jones advocates first addressing institutionalized racism. If institutionalized structures no longer support racism, those disadvantaged by such structures would be relieved and it is possible that personally mediated racism would be lessened in succeeding generations.

Performing Research

Comprehensive research is needed on the roots and effects of racial and ethnic discrimination, as well as on the impact of individual and institutional racism on the broad range of health outcomes. Adequate surveillance systems should be developed to obtain data on the determinants and distribution of physical, mental, social, and environmental health outcomes due to racial and ethnic disparities. Data collection should account for the diversity of subgroups within each minority category in the census. Research should be enhanced by the inclusion of data on such issues as residential segregation, occupational health problems, employment discrimination, individual exposure to discrimination and related coping mechanisms, physiological effects of racism and discrimination, and health care provider behaviors that contribute to disparities. Research that explores the relationship between race/ethnicity and occupational health and safety is needed; however, such research will serve a descriptive function only if it is not used to facilitate policy changes that will reduce the increased occupational health risks that confront workers of color.[61]

Researchers must be sensitive to the particular cultural perspective on genetic research of the various ethnic groups in terms of handling of human tissues, confidentiality, and appropriate questions to pursue.[23]

Conclusion

The most important immediate action in response to social injustice against racial and ethnic minorities that leads to disparate health outcomes is the equitable provision of health care (see chapter 12). We must enact legislation that ensures better quality of and access to health care through the provision of basic health care for all people in an atmosphere of acceptance and respect.

Initiatives that address the specific areas of health disparities for ethnic minorities should be promoted, including the collection of data on barriers to equitable care and the monitoring of progress in the elimination of disparate outcomes.

The Institute of Medicine report *Unequal Treatment* contains several recommendations that could be implemented quickly:

- Increasing the awareness of disparities among the general public, key stakeholders, and health care providers
- Integrating cross-cultural education into the training of all current and future health professionals
- Providing patient education on how to access health care and participate in individual health care planning
- Using evidence-based guidelines to promote consistency and equity of health care, with financial incentives to ensure evidence-based practice
- Structuring payment systems that ensure adequate services to minorities and limiting provider incentives that promote disparities
- Providing resources to the Office of Civil Rights of the Department of Health and Human Services to enforce civil rights legislation.[1]

The solution to the problem of disparate health care based on race and ethnicity requires attention not only to its immediate consequences but also to the many contextual issues that have caused and now perpetuate its devastating effects. Health care providers must collaborate with people in other disciplines, the business community, the general public, and minority groups to reach an effective and sustainable resolution to this problem.

References

1. Smedley BD, Stith AY, Nelson AR, eds. Unequal treatment: confronting racial and ethnic disparities. Washington, D.C.: National Academies Press, 2003.
2. Agency for Healthcare Research and Quality. National healthcare disparities report. Rockville, Md.: AHRQ, 2003.
3. Kyle J. Cities without walls: the institutional response to ethnic health care disparities. Healthy People 2004 Conference, Loma Linda University School of Public Health, Loma Linda, Calif., March 11, 2004.
4. U.S. Census Bureau. Overview of race and Hispanic origin, 2000. Washington, D.C.: U.S. Census Bureau, 2001.
5. Grieco EM, Cassidy RC. Overview of race and Hispanic origin. Washington, D.C.: U.S. Census Bureau, 2001.
6. Spector RE. Cultural diversity in health and illness. 6th ed. Upper Saddle River, N.J.: Pearson, 2004.
7. American community survey change profile, 2001–2002. Washington, D.C.: U.S. Census Bureau. Available at: http://www.census.gov/acs/www/Products/Profiles/Chg/2002/0102/. Accessed February 23, 2005.
8. Dalaku J. Poverty in the United States: 2000. U.S. Census Bureau current population reports series P60-214. Washington, D.C.: U.S. Government Printing Office, 2001.
9. U.S. Census Bureau. Census 2000 redistricting data (P.L. 94-171) summary file, Table PL1. Washington, D.C.: Department of Commerce, 2001.
10. Rodriguez-Trias H, Bracho A, Gil RM, et al. Eliminating health disparities: conversations with Latinos. Santa Cruz, Calif.: ETR Associates, 2003.
11. Dhooper SS. Health care needs of foreign-born Asian Americans: an overview. Health Soc Work 2003;28:63–73.
12. Ro M. Moving forward: addressing the health of Asian American and Pacific Islander women. Am J Public Health 2002;92:516–9.
13. Aiu P, Blaisdell K, Pretrick EK, et al. Eliminating health disparities: conversations with Pacific Islanders. Santa Cruz, Calif.: ETR Associates, 2004.
14. Grieco E. The Native Hawaiian and Other Pacific Islander population: 2000. Census 2000 brief. Washington, D.C.: U.S. Department of Commerce, Economics and Statistics Administration, U.S. Census Bureau, 2001.
15. American Indian and Alaska Native (AI/AN) populations. Atlanta, Ga.: Office of Minority Health, Centers for Disease Control and Prevention. Available at: http://www.cdc.gov/omh/Populations/AIAN/AIAN.htm. Accessed May 19, 2005.
16. Olsen B. Culture, colonization, and policy making: issues in Native American health. Presented at the Symposium in the Politics of Race, Culture, and Health, Ithaca College, Ithaca, N.Y., November 13 and 14, 2003.

17. Umar KB. Disparities persist in infant mortality: creative approaches work to close the gap. Closing the Gap, a newsletter of the Office of Minority Health. Washington, D.C.: U.S. Department of Health and Human Services, 2003.

18. U.S. Department of Health and Human Services. Healthy people 2010 (conference edition, in two volumes). Washington, D.C.: U.S. Government Printing Office, 2000.

19. Health, United States, 2003, Table 29, 2003. Atlanta, Ga.: Department of Health and Human Services, Centers for Disease Control and Prevention, National Center for Health Statistics. Available at: http://www.cdc.gov.nchs/data/hus/tables/2003/03hus029.pdf. Accessed May 13, 2004.

20. Surveillance reports, 2003. Atlanta, Ga.: Centers for Disease Control and Prevention, Division of Tuberculosis Elimination, National Center for HIV, STD and TB Prevention. Available at: http://www.cdc.gov/nchstp/tb/surv/surv2003/PDF/Table15.pdf; cdc.gov/nchstp/tb/surv/surv2003/PDF/Table18.pdf. Accessed January 6, 2005.

21. Collins KS, Hughes DI, Doty MM, et al. Diverse communities, common concerns: assessing health care quality for minority Americans. Findings from the Commonwealth Fund 2001 Health Care Quality Survey. New York, N.Y.: The Commonwealth Fund, 2002.

22. Native Hawaiians and Other Pacific Islander (NHOPI) populations. Atlanta, Ga.: Centers for Disease Control and Prevention, Office of Minority Health. Available at: http://www.cdc.gov/omh/Populations/NHOPI/NHOPI.htm. Accessed May 19, 2005.

23. Bird ME, ed. Eliminating health disparities: conversations with American Indians and Alaska Natives. Santa Cruz, Calif.: ETR Associates, 2002.

24. 15 Leading causes of death for American Indians/Alaska Natives, 1999. Atlanta, Ga.: Centers for Disease Control and Prevention. Available at: http://www.omhrc.gov/healthgap2003/amIn.pdf. Accessed March 7, 2004.

25. Fact sheets. Disparities in infant mortality. Atlanta, Ga.: Centers for Disease Control and Prevention. Available at: http://www.cdc.gov/omh/AMH/factssheets/infant.htm. Accessed January 6, 2005.

26. Alaska Department of Health and Social Services. Healthy Alaskans 2010: targets and strategies for improved health. Juneau: State of Alaska, 2002.

27. America's health: state health rankings: 2003 edition. United Health Foundation. Available at: http://www.unitedhealthfoundation.org/shr2003/HealthDisparity.html. Accessed May 19, 2005.

28. HIV/AIDS surveillance supplemental report: cases of HIV infection and AIDS in the United States, by race/ethnicity, 1998–2002, volume 10, number 1. Atlanta, Ga.: Centers for Disease Control and Prevention, National Center for HIV, STD and TB Prevention, Divisions of HIV/AIDS Prevention. Available at: http://www.cdc.gov/hiv/stats/hasr link.htm. Accessed January 6, 2005.

29. America's children: key national indicators of well-being 2003. Federal Interagency Forum on Child and Family Statistics. Available at: http://www.childstats.gov/ac2003/pdf/ac2003.pdf. Accessed January 6, 2005.

30. Kadan-Lottick NS, Ness DD, Bhatia S, et al. Survival variability by race and ethnicity in childhood acute lymphoblastic leukemia. JAMA 2003;290:2008–14.

31. Marcotty J. Studies show equal access to care helps even the odds for minority kids with leukemia. *Star Tribune*. Available at: http://startribune.com /viewers/story.php?template=print_a&st. Accessed May 19, 2005.

32. Pui C, Sandlund JT, Pei D, et al. Results of therapy for acute lymphoblastic leukemia in white and black children. JAMA 2003;290:2001–7.

33. Data warehouse on trends in health and aging. Atlanta, Ga.: Department of Health and Human Services, Centers for Disease Control and Prevention, National Center for Health Statistics. Available at: http://www.cdc.gov/nchs/agingact.htm. Accessed January 6, 2005.

34. NCHS data on racial and ethnic disparities. Atlanta, Ga.: National Health and Nutrition Examination Survey, 1999–2000. Centers for Disease Control and Prevention, National Center for Health Statistics. Available at: http://www.cdc.gov/nchs/data/factsheets/racialandethnic.pdf. Accessed January 6, 2005.

35. Lam TK, McPhee SJ, Mock J, et al. Encouraging Vietnamese-American women to obtain Pap tests through lay health worker outreach and media education. J Gen Intern Med 2003;8:516-24.

36. Centers for Disease Control and Prevention. Racial/ethnic disparities in influenza and pneumoccal vaccination levels among persons aged >65 years—United States, 1989–2001. MMWR Morb Mortal Wkly Rep 2003;52:958–62.

37. Ross H. Growing older: Health issues for minorities. closing the gap. Washington, D.C.: Office of Minority Health, U.S. Department of Health and Human Services, 2000.

38. Facts of life. The forgotten population: health disparities and minority men. Facts of Life: Issue Briefings for Health Reporters, May 2003. Available at: http://www.cfah.org/factsoflife/vol8no5.cfm. Accessed May 19, 2005.

39. National vital statistics reports, Vol 52, No. 14, February 18, 2004. Atlanta, Ga.: Department of Health and Human Services, Centers for Disease Control and Prevention, National Center for Health Statistics. Available at: http://www.cdc.gov/nchs/data/nvsr/nvsr52/nvsr52_14.pdf. Accessed May 19, 2005.

40. HIV/AIDS among African Americans, 2002. Atlanta, Ga.: Department of Health and Human Services, Centers for Disease Control and Prevention, National Center for HIV, STD and TB Prevention, Divisions of HIV/AIDS Prevention. Available at: http://www.cdc.gov/hiv/pubs/Facts/afam.htm. Accessed January 6, 2005.

41. HIV/AIDS among Hispanics, 2002. Atlanta, Ga.: Department of Health and Human Services, Centers for Disease Control and Prevention, National Center for HIV, STD and TB Prevention, Divisions of HIV/AIDS Prevention. Available at: http://www.cdc.gov/hiv/pubs/facts/hispanic.htm. Accessed January 6, 2005.

42. Lee K. The toll of HIV/AIDS on Minority Women. HIV impact. a closing the gap newsletter of the Office of Minority Health. Washington, D.C.: U.S. Department of Health and Human Services, 2000.

43. Wernette DK, Nieves LA. Breathing polluted air: minorities are disproportionately exposed. EPA J 1992;18:16-7.

44. Bullard RD. Dumping in Dixie: race, class, and environmental quality. Boulder, Colo.: Westview Press, 2000.

45. Shettler T. Human health and the environment: lessons from the children. Presented at the Alaska Health Summit, Anchorage, Alaska, December 2, 2003.

46. Sattler B, Lipscomb J, eds. Environmental health and nursing practice. New York, N.Y.: Springer, 2003.

47. Children's Environmental Health Network. Training manual on pediatric environmental health: putting it into practice. Washington, D.C.: Children's Environmental Health Network, 1999.

48. Shi L. Experience of primary care by racial and ethnic groups in the United States. Med Care 1999;37:1068–77.

49. About half of U.S. Hispanics were uninsured in 2001; two-thirds of those in low-wage jobs, study says. Kaiser Daily Health Policy Report. Kaiser Family Foundation. Available at: http://kaisernetwork.org/daily_reports/rep_index.cfm?hint=3&DR_ID=20392. Accessed May 19, 2005.

50. Doty JJ, Ives BL. Quality of health care of Hispanic populations: findings from the Commonwealth Fund 2001 Health Care Quality Survey. New York, N.Y.: The Commonwealth Fund, 2002.

51. Quinn D. Working without benefits: the health insurance crisis confronting Hispanic Americans. New York, N.Y.: The Commonwealth Fund, 2000.

52. U.S. Census Bureau. Poverty in the United States: 2002. Washington, D.C.: U.S. Department of Commerce, 2003.

53. Wolff EN. Top heavy: the increasing inequality of wealth in America. New York, N.Y.: The New Press, 1995.

54. Bailey J. Assets, the poor and democracy. Unpublished paper presented at the American Academy of Religion annual meeting, Atlanta, Ga., November 24, 2003.

55. Sherraden M. Assets and the poor: implications for individual accounts and Social Security. Invited testimony to the President's Commission on Social Security, Washington, D.C., October 18, 2002.

56. Howard C. The hidden welfare state: tax expenditures and social policy in the United States. Princeton, N.J.: Princeton University Press, 1997.

57. Wilkerson R, Marmot M, eds. The solid facts: social determinants of health. 2nd ed. Copenhagen, Denmark: World Health Organization, 2003.

58. Turner MA, Ross SL. Discrimination in metropolitan housing markets: phase 2—Asian and Pacific Islanders, final report. Washington, D.C.: U.S. Department of Housing and Urban Development, 2003.

59. Lehrman S. Colorblind racism. AlterNet. Available at: http://www.alternet.org. Accessed September 17, 2003.

60. Darity WJ Jr. Employment discrimination, segregation, and health. Am J Public Health 2003;93:226–31.

61. Murray LR. Sick and tired of being sick and tired: Scientific evidence, methods, and research implications for racial and ethnic disparities in occupational health. Am J Public Health 2003;93:221–5.

62. Weiss BD. Health literacy: a manual for clinicians. Chicago, Ill.: American Medical Foundation, 2003.

63. Partnership for Clear Health Communication. Health literacy: statistics-at-a-glance. New York, N.Y.: Partnership for Clear Health Communication.

64. Weiss BD, ed. 20 Common problems in primary care. New York, N.Y.: McGraw-Hill, 1999.

65. Williams MV, Baker DW, Honig EG, et al. Inadequate literacy is a barrier to asthma knowledge and self-care. Chest 1998;114:1008–15.

66. Baker DW, Parker RM, Williams MV, et al. Health literacy and the risk of hospital admission. J Gen Intern Med 1998;13:791–8.

67. Evans T, Whitehead M, Wirth M, et al. Challenging inequities in health: from ethics to action, summary. New York, N.Y.: Rockefeller Foundation, 2001.

68. Right to equal treatment. Physicians for Human Rights, Panel on Racial and Ethnic Disparities in Medical Care. Available at: http://www.phrusa.org/research/domestic/race/race_report/other_05.html. Accessed January 6, 2005.

69. Scott BS, Umar KB. Start 'em early, start 'em young: introducing minority youth to health professions. Closing the Gap, a newsletter of the Office of Minority Health, Washington, D.C.: U.S. Department of Health and Human Services, 2003.

70. Policy Link. Reducing health disparities through a focus on communities. Oakland, Calif.: Policy Link, 2002.
71. Schreiner M, Clancy M, Sherraden M. Final report: saving performance in the American Dream Demonstration, a national demonstration of individual development accounts. St. Louis, Mo.: Center for Social Development, Washington University in St. Louis, 2002.
72. Jones CP. Levels of racism: a theoretic framework and a gardener's tale. Am J Public Health 2002;90:1212–5.

4

WOMEN

Stacey J. Rees and Wendy Chavkin

Introduction

Women are often characterized as a special subgroup for purposes of health research and data analysis; witness the presence of this chapter in a section of the book devoted to "Specific Population Groups." Women as a population, however, have been the targets of discrimination and disadvantageous treatment. A too-narrow focus on women's reproductive and mothering roles has been central to this discrimination; however, the assertion of women's inequality in all spheres has been a fundamental organizing principle of social relations and economic and family life. Resulting social injustice has had a profound impact on women's health status. Misogynist cultural and social norms have led to limitations on women's access to abortion and contraceptive services; ignorance of the differences between disease processes in women and men; the exclusion of women from much medical research (as both research subjects and researchers); and the disproportionate effects of both poverty and violence on the health of women. This chapter will attempt to highlight some of the ways that social injustice, rooted in beliefs about women's inequality, has affected women's health.

The health needs of a group as heterogeneous as women vary widely. Nonetheless, all women share reproductive capacity and the potential for engaging in sexual activity. All therefore have significant needs related to the avoidance and treatment of sexually transmitted infections (STIs), including HIV/AIDS; contraception and pregnancy care; and the prevention and treatment of reproductive organ cancers and other reproductive system diseases.

An estimated 26 percent of HIV-infected people in the United States are women. From 1996 through 2001, an average of 10,500 cases of AIDS were annually diagnosed in women and adolescent girls in the United States.[1] As of 2002, an estimated 19.2 million women worldwide were living with HIV/AIDS. In sub-Saharan Africa, North Africa, and the Middle East, the estimated percentage of HIV-positive adults who are women ranges from 55 to 58 percent.[2] Women also shoulder a disproportionate burden of serious health consequences from curable STIs, including infertility and preterm birth.[3]

Pregnancy prevention remains one of women's most pressing health needs. The average age of first childbearing increased in the United States from 21.4 years in 1970 to almost 25 years in 2000.[4] Globally, a demographic transition from high to low fertility is taking place. In less-developed regions, fertility rates have dropped from 6.2 children per woman in 1950 to less than 3 per woman in 1999.[5] Although decreasing fertility rates indicate that progress has been made, up to half of the 175 million pregnancies that annually occur worldwide are either unwanted or ill-timed.[5]

Different issues arise when women struggle to achieve, rather than prevent, pregnancy. Many women, in the United States and elsewhere, put childbearing on hold to accommodate education and career expectations that are not commensurate with early motherhood. The desire for pregnancy later in life has increased demand for assisted reproduction technologies (ART). Lesbian and single women are also seeking access to ART to achieve their childbearing goals. Should we guarantee access to services desired in response to societal pressures on women to delay childbirth? ART is costly; limited health care resources force difficult choices between making such "high-tech" care available to some and making high-quality primary care available to all.

Women who do become pregnant need access to high-quality prenatal and intrapartum care. In the United States, the persistence of higher rates of infant and maternal mortality (compared with most other industrialized countries) and disparities between white and minority women underscore our country's continued failure to equitably meet maternity care needs.

Later in the life cycle, women need access to routine care and screening for reproductive organ cancers, treatment for symptoms of menopause, and osteoporosis care. Eighty percent of people with osteoporosis are women, and the rate of hip fracture is two to three times higher in women than in men. Sustained weight-bearing exercise helps build bone mass and reduce the risk of hip fracture later in life.[6] Because women were traditionally discouraged from participating in athletic activity, older women now face a serious health problem rooted in discriminatory beliefs that kept women from exercising.

Women of all ages face challenges maintaining health insurance that would allow them to seek needed care. Women are more likely to work in low-income, service-industry jobs that rarely provide health insurance benefits. Women who do not work outside the home may be dependent on insurance provided by their husbands' employers. In addition, women who leave the Temporary Aid for Needy Families (TANF) program for jobs may lose health insurance if it is not provided by their employers.

How Social Injustice Affects the Health of Women

Constraints on Choice, Access to Abortion, and Family Planning Services

A careful look at abortion and contraception reveals overt and wide-ranging effects of social injustice on women's health. In 20 states, local laws intrude into the informed consent process by means of state-directed counseling and mandatory waiting periods; more states require counseling but forego the waiting period.[7] For minors, the problem of access to abortion is further exacerbated by parental consent or notification laws.

As of late 2003, 19 states required parental consent and 14 additional states required parental notification before a minor could obtain an abortion. A new parental notification law, which took effect at the end of 2003 in New Hampshire, may be the start of a trend that will likely continue as other states consider restrictive legislation. Only eight states and the District of Columbia do not require parental involvement when a minor child seeks abortion services.[8] For minors unable or unwilling to talk to their parents about their need for an abortion (in some cases out of fear of physical abuse or because the pregnancy was the result of incest), these laws put one more roadblock in the path to an earlier—and therefore safer—abortion. No parental consent is required by any state for childbirth.

Other laws restrict certain kinds of abortion procedures altogether. In 2000, the Supreme Court heard *Stenberg v. Carhart*, a challenge to Nebraska's "partial-birth" abortion ban. The court found the Nebraska ban unconstitutional but did outline a two-pronged test of constitutionality for other such laws: they must include an exception protecting the life or health of the woman and they may not impose an undue burden on a woman's right to choose late-term abortion. Four states currently have laws banning some form of late-term abortion procedure that meet the Stenberg requirements. Twenty-seven states have bans that are unenforceable under the Stenberg test, and in 19 of these states courts have specifically blocked these measures.[9]

Congress enacted and President George W. Bush signed the Partial Birth Abortion Ban of 2003, a bill that contains no exception to protect the health of the mother—one of the two necessary tests of constitutionality under the Stenberg ruling. Reproductive rights advocates have challenged the law in court.

The harassment and physical assaults on both women who seek abortions and those who provide abortion services have had an adverse effect on access to abortion services. The numbers of abortion providers declined by 11 percent between 1996 and 2000.[10] To counter this trend, groups such as Medical Students for Choice and Physicians for Reproductive Choice and Health (PRCH) have galvanized support for abortion training for physicians during medical residencies. Clinicians for Choice advocates for expanding the pool of abortion providers to include midwives, nurse practitioners, and physician assistants.

In the 1990s, a wave of Catholic and secular hospital mergers resulted in religious proscriptions on reproductive health care services. Services such as contraception, sterilization, abortion, and some infertility services were often discontinued in the merger process. In addition, victims of sexual assault who come to Catholic merger-affected hospitals for care have been denied access to emergency contraception to prevent pregnancy from rape. This has led to significant loss of access to such care in many communities.

Access to reproductive health care services is also restricted by managed-care health insurance plans owned by religious groups. These plans serve both the private and Medicaid insurance markets. Fifteen of 48 Catholic managed-care plans identified in a recent report participate in Medicaid managed care.[11] Many argue that refusing to provide reproductive health services on religious grounds is unacceptable if agencies receive state or federal funding. Protections must be built in for women, especially the most vulnerable Medicaid recipients, so that they understand the limitations of such plans before enrolling.

Young women need accurate information about their health and sexuality. Funds are increasingly being made available for abstinence-only education; about 33 percent of teachers in one survey describe their school's main message as abstinence-only until marriage. Such programs do not include any information about contraception or STI prevention strategies.[12] Denying young women (and men) important information about reproductive health impairs their decision-making ability and has potentially negative health consequences. Not teaching young people about the consequences of unprotected sex, including HIV infection, puts them at grave, and unnecessary, risk. Moreover, abstinence-only education has been shown to be ineffective at reducing teen sexual activity and teen births, while comprehensive sex education has a positive impact on these indicators.[13]

Unfortunately, the current chilly climate for women's reproductive health care extends well beyond the borders of the United States. Policies restricting access to services in the United States are echoed by policies limiting U.S. funding for services abroad. In 1984, President Ronald Reagan implemented the Mexico City Policy, better known as the "Global Gag Rule." This policy prevents the United States Agency for International Development (USAID) from giving funds to nongovernment organizations that perform abortions or actively promote abortion as a method of family planning in other nations. This policy remained in effect until 1993, when it was rescinded by President Bill Clinton, but in 2001 one of President Bush's first acts was to reinstate this policy.

The 1985 Kemp-Kasten Amendment prohibits the disbursement of U.S. funds to any group that supports or participates in coercive abortion or involuntary sterilization, as determined by the president. This amendment has been used as a tool to deny funding to the United Nations Population Fund (UNFPA). Funds were withdrawn from UNFPA over its support for China's allegedly coercive population policies, despite a 2002 State Department investigation documenting that the UNFPA does not provide direct support for abortion services in China and has, in fact, worked to stop coercive practices. Congressional passage of the Smith amendment in 2003 prevented payment of $100 million to UNFPA in fiscal years 2004 and 2005, denying crucial reproductive health funding to many women throughout the world.

Disproportionate Impact of Poverty

Although women have gained some ground in earning power over the last decade, women in the United States still earn only $0.76 for every $1.00 that men earn. The gap is wider for single mothers: Over 26 percent of single mothers live below the poverty level, compared with less than 12 percent of the general population. The rate is even higher for African-American and Hispanic single mothers, over 35 percent of whom live below the poverty level.[14]

Access to reproductive and other basic health care is particularly tenuous for women living in poverty. Federal funding for abortion has not been available—except in cases of rape, life endangerment, or incest—since passage of the Hyde Amendment in 1977. Currently, just 16 states have a policy to use their own funds to pay for all or most medically necessary abortions sought by Medicaid recipients. In these 16 states, "health" is broadly defined to include both physical and mental health concerns.[15] An analysis of the number of abortions to Medicaid-eligible women in two states before and after the Hyde Amendment concluded that about 20 percent of the women who would have obtained an abortion, had funding been available, were unable to do so and carried their pregnancies to term.[16]

The 1996 Personal Responsibility and Work Opportunity Reconciliation Act (PRWORA) has effectively eliminated poor women's entitlements to income supports while attaching strings—in the form of strictures on reproductive behavior and employment requirements—to the limited benefits they may still receive. This change in welfare legislation has affected the health of poor women in two ways: through changes in access to care and through changes resulting from reproductive-related provisions of PRWORA.[17]

As advocates had warned, one result of PRWORA has been reduced Medicaid enrollment. Many families who were dropped from, or failed to enroll in, cash assistance programs have not enrolled in Medicaid, despite continued eligibility.[18] Declines in Medicaid enrollment for women have been dramatic with low-income single mothers experiencing the largest decrease.[19] Because nearly half of all publicly funded family planning services in 1994 were paid for by the Medicaid program, declines in Medicaid enrollment mean a subsequent decline in revenues for family planning providers and an increase in uninsured patients whose care must be subsidized. If this trend continues, it may jeopardize the ability of clinicians to continue to provide family planning services. Eighteen states have attempted to prevent the decline in the use of Medicaid family planning services by issuing waivers that extend women's eligibility for such services.[20]

As of late 2003, 13 percent of white women, 23 percent of black women, and 37 percent of Latinas were uninsured.[21] Women without health insurance coverage often fail to make family planning or well-woman visits. They are thus less likely to benefit from routine preventive services, such as Pap smears, mammograms, STI screening, and screening for chronic diseases, such as hypertension.

Mandates expanding Medicaid eligibility during pregnancy have been in effect since 1990, but over 28 percent of pregnant women living in poverty were uninsured in late 2003, as compared with only 3 percent of those earning at least three times the poverty level. Of uninsured pregnant women, 77 percent were eligible for Medicaid in 1997.[22] Why aren't more of these eligible women being reached?

Although not thought of as preconceptional or prenatal care per se, access to the Special Supplemental Nutrition Program for Women, Infants and Children (WIC) and the Food Stamp Program (FSP) before and during pregnancy can have a significant impact on reproductive health. Women with low prepregnancy weights and/or those without sufficient weight gain during pregnancy are at higher risk for low birth weight or preterm birth.[23]

Welfare reform drastically reduced the food safety net for women. The food stamp benefits of poor women, who have been forced into low-wage jobs as a result of welfare reform work requirements, are reduced because these women now have earnings. Such reductions can cause them to decrease spending on food and adversely affect their spending on housing, clothing, and medical care.[24] The net effect of welfare reform on women's nutritional status and reproductive health remains a concern.

Several other elements of welfare reform policy attempt to directly influence women's reproductive choices. For several years, states were offered an illegitimacy bonus under PRWORA for decreases in nonmarital births without a concomitant increase in abortion rates. Twenty-three states have enacted a cap on additional benefits when a new child is born into a family receiving welfare. [25]

Despite little evidence to support their efficacy in reducing teen pregnancy rates, PRWORA also includes an allocation of $50 million over 5 years to fund abstinence-only sex education programs. States are required to match every $4 of federal funds with $3 in state money, bringing the total closer to $90 million.[26]

The reproductive-related components of PRWORA are direct attempts by policy-makers to control the reproductive lives of low-income women and, in the case of abstinence-only education, to forward an agenda for all families that restricts sexual activity to monogamous heterosexual relationships within marriage. Such efforts at social control are an egregious and anachronistic attempt to interfere in women's reproductive decisions, with serious potential to negatively affect the health of low-income women and their families.

The Disproportionate Impact of Violence

Women suffer disproportionately from violence and often face health consequences from sexual abuse and domestic violence that endure years beyond the acute episode of violence. Such violence is global in scope, with at least one in every three women worldwide having been beaten, coerced into sex, or abused in some other way. As many as 5,000 women and girls die each year in so-called "honor killings." Identifying the use of violence against women as a weapon of war, the International Criminal Court added, in 1998, a statute classifying rape, sexual slavery, enforced prostitution, forced pregnancy, enforced sterilization, and other forms of sexual violence as grave breaches of the Geneva Convention.[27]

Most violence suffered by women occurs at the hands of intimate partners. In a U.S. survey, 76 percent of women who reported being raped and/or physically assaulted since the age of 18 were victimized by a current or former husband, cohabiting partner, date, or boyfriend, and 22 percent of all women polled reported an assault perpetrated by an intimate partner in their lifetime.[28] Female victims reported only about half of incidents of violence by an intimate acquaintance to the police.[29] Although over 500,000 women were treated in emergency departments for physical assault in the year preceding one national survey, many more women do not receive any medical care for injuries received as a result of rape or other physical assault.[28]

Violence affects women of all ages, but young women are particularly vulnerable. More than half of female rape victims identified in one survey were younger than 18 years old when they were first sexually assaulted.[28]

The long-term physical and mental health consequences of violence against women are significant. Sexual assault increases the odds of substance abuse by a factor of 2.5, and rape victims are 11 times more likely to be clinically depressed than are others.[30] The importance of integrating sexual abuse therapy into treatment for chemically dependent women is demonstrated by the frequency with which drug-dependent women have been abused sexually and the relationship between such abuse and the severity of addiction.[31]

In addition, rape victims suffer from physical symptoms that can persist years after the attack, including pelvic pain, sleep disturbance, chronic headaches, and sexual dysfunction.[26–32] Sexual abuse has also been identified as a risk factor for HIV infection.[33] Domestic violence in pregnancy may result in pregnancy loss, preterm labor, low birth weight, fetal injury, and fetal death.[34]

Although resistance to recognition of sexual abuse has decreased in recent years, disagreement on the definition of sexual abuse continues to hamper the collection of accurate prevalence data. Insufficient data collection, women's resistance to disclosing abuse histories because of stigma and fear, and the lack of consensus about the definition of sexual abuse have necessarily led to underreporting and increased risk for neglected survivors of abuse.[35]

Campaigns for comprehensive federal policy–based responses to the problem of violence against women began in earnest in 1990. The 1994 Violence Against Women Act (VAWA) created new penalties for gender-related violence and funded grant programs supporting state efforts to address domestic violence and sexual assault. The provisions of VAWA were reauthorized for an additional 5 years in 2000, continuing existing programs, with some improvements, additions, increases in funding, and requirements that several studies be completed, including one addressing insurance discrimination against victims of domestic violence.

Underlying Causes and Roots of Social Injustice Against Women

Gender Discrimination and the Assumption of a Male Norm

Assumptions that male sex is the norm and that female sex is a complication of that norm have had a profoundly negative impact on the health of women. These assumptions have led, until very recently, to the exclusion of women from clinical trials and a dearth of research on specific women's health issues, including differences in prognosis, diagnosis, and progression of diseases that affect both men and women. Such discrimination has also resulted in a missed opportunity for greater understanding of diseases that affect both sexes. A recent Institute of Medicine report asserts that studying sex differences, like other biological variations, can yield greater insight into underlying biological disease mechanisms,[36] leading, in turn, to improved treatments and outcomes.

Few people are aware that cardiovascular disease (CVD) is the leading cause of death in women. Despite the prevalence of CVD among women, early research often failed to provide useful information about key gender differences in risk factors, outcomes, and manifestations among women.[37] Research on gender differences in other disease states that affect both men and women has revealed significant differences in the manifestations and progression of HIV[38] and the increased prevalence among women, compared with men, of diseases such as irritable bowel syndrome,[39] and type 2 diabetes.[40] Major depression or a depressive disorder affects approximately twice as many women as men,[41] and pregnancy as well as gender differences in pharmacokinetics can affect dosage of antidepressant medications for women.

It is clearly essential to include members of both sexes in sufficient numbers to permit analysis and detect gender differences. Otherwise, the medical and scientific community remains uncertain as to whether findings from male-only studies can be generalized to women, and thus uncertain about the course of disease and applicability of treatment to women.[42]

In recognition of this problem, the U.S. Public Health Service Task Force on Women's Health Issues reported, in 1985, that the lack of research specifically addressing women had compromised the quality of health care.[43] Five years later, the National Institutes of Health (NIH) created the Office of Research on Women's Health, and, in 1991, instructions to NIH grantees first included requirements to include women and members of racial/ethnic minorities as research subjects. In 1993, the U.S. Congress passed the NIH Revitalization Act, which included funding for women's health research and policy statements supporting the inclusion of women in federally funded research.[42]

Several decades ago, public concern over the untoward effects of thalidomide and diethylstilbestrol (DES) led to an increased emphasis on the protection of pregnant women in research. In 1975, Department of Health and Human Services regulations were instituted that limited research on pregnant women and that classified them as a vulnerable population. However, when pregnant women are excluded from clinical trials, health care providers end up treating disorders in pregnant women with medications for which the pregnancy-altered pharmacokinetics and the consequences for fetal development are not known.[42] To encourage the participation of women in research, the Food and Drug Administration revised this restriction in 1993.[44]

The impact of gender discrimination affects the very formulation of research questions by muting the voices of women scientists.[45] Although women now constitute almost half of all medical students in the United States,[46,47] a much smaller fraction of faculty members in U.S. medical schools are women—only one-fourth were faculty members in 1995.[48]

Women's underrepresentation in academic medicine, business, public policy endeavors, and government may well contribute to roadblocks encountered when legislation or policy that primarily benefits women's health is considered. The struggle for contraceptive coverage provides a particularly salient example. While most employment-related insurance policies in the United States cover prescription drugs and outpatient medical care, most do not cover contraceptive drugs and devices or the medical care to provide them. Yet, in 1998, more than half of all prescriptions for Viagra, a prescription medication to treat erectile dysfunction, were covered by health insurance.[49] This glaring inequity fueled efforts to mandate contraceptive coverage legislatively at the state and federal level. Nonetheless, the Equity in Prescription Insurance and Contraceptive Coverage Act (EPICC), first introduced in Congress in 1997, has not yet, as of mid 2004, been passed.

There is a delicate balance between protectionism and discrimination in legislation concerning female reproductive capacity. Policies have often valued fetal protection over maternal benefit, as was the case with initial FDA restrictions barring women from clinical drug trials. Antiabortion forces advocate for granting the fetus limited rights of personhood, characterizing pregnant women as so selfish and irresponsible that their indifference to fetal welfare must be constrained by outside intervention.

The antiabortion movement is not alone in using this line of argument; it has also been adopted by those who have advocated for punitive solutions to the problem of women who abuse drugs during pregnancy. Opponents of such sanctions argue that this approach has grave consequences for the social status of women and that it is likely to be ineffective.[50] Policies that assume or foster the construction of maternal-fetal or maternal-child conflict use women's reproductive capacity as the basis for further disadvantage of women.

Overall, U.S. policies on childbearing are inconsistent. Sometimes they have been pro-natalist; for example, Medicaid covers prenatal care but not abortion. At other times, they have been anti-natalist; for example, family cap limitations deny poor women additional income support. The family cap debate has been characterized by a symbolic focus on women coupled with a programmatic lack of interest in them. Welfare policies attempt to dramatically alter the reproductive, parenting, and economic behaviors of poor women, with little compassion for them, while simultaneously asserting concern for the "innocent children," who will now face poverty without public assistance.

What Needs to Be Done

> The advancement of women and the achievement of equality between women and men are a matter of human rights. This is a basic condition for social justice, and should not be seen in isolation as just a women's issue. Indeed, this is the only way to build a sustainable, just and developed society. Empowerment of women and equality between women and men are prerequisites for achieving political, social, economic, cultural and environmental security among all peoples.
> —Platform for Action, 1995 Fourth World Conference on Women, Beijing

To improve women's health and eliminate social injustice, it is necessary to eliminate policies and practices that reduce women's options regarding education, employment, access to resources, and control over their health and choices. At the 1994 International Conference on Population and Development (ICPD) in Cairo and again at the Fourth World Conference on Women (FWCW) in Beijing in 1995, 179 nations agreed to platforms—action plans—to achieve these objectives. The Vienna Declaration, adopted at the 1993 World Conference on Human Rights, had laid the groundwork for the Cairo and Beijing conferences by asserting women's rights as inalienable human rights. Out of the Cairo and Beijing conferences, a worldwide consensus emerged that population and development goals are inextricably linked and that improving the status of women is central to promoting sustainable development.

The enormous significance of the Cairo and Beijing action plans was twofold: (a) gender discrimination and its wide range of manifestations were acknowledged as depriving half of the world's population of basic human rights, and

(b) this deprivation was understood to be a central impediment to economic development and improvements in global health. The Cairo and Beijing conferences brought the issue of gender discrimination to the center of the global stage. For the first time, by signing onto the platforms, nations agreed to actively work toward reducing gender discrimination and its manifestations.

The 16 chapters of the Cairo action plan outline priority actions in areas, including (a) gender equality, equity, and empowerment of women; (b) reproductive rights and health; (c) morbidity and mortality, including women's health and safe motherhood objectives; and (d) population, development, and education. Public health professionals can and must play a vital role in continuing to implement the Cairo vision as it concerns women, social justice, and health. Among the objectives of the Cairo action plan for which the expertise of public health professionals is needed are the following:

- To build the capacity of women and incorporate gender perspectives in all programs related to population and development
- To assist women to establish and realize their rights with regard to sexual and reproductive health
- To develop procedures and indicators for gender-based analyses of development programs and for assessment of the impact of these programs on women's health
- To collect data to raise awareness of all forms of exploitation, abuse, harassment, and violence against women with the objective of ending such practices
- To assist in documentation and condemnation of rape as a weapon of war
- To assist in the development of women-controlled methods to prevent HIV infection, such as microbicides and vaccines
- To ensure that women are involved in the planning, leadership, decision-making, management, implementation, organization, and evaluation of all reproductive and sexual health programs
- To develop and evaluate curricula that adequately cover gender sensitivity and equity, reproductive choices and responsibilities, and sexually transmitted infections, including HIV/AIDS, in order to ensure that education about population issues begins in primary school and continues through all levels of education
- To strengthen training of population specialists at the university level and incorporate content relating to interrelationships of demographic variables with development planning in the social sciences, economics, health, and environmental disciplines.[51]

The Beijing conference was focused on the empowerment, rights, and advancement of women. The Beijing declaration asserted a commitment to ensuring "the full implementation of the human rights of women and of the girl child as an inalienable, integral, and indivisible part of all human rights and fundamental freedoms." (The complete declaration is available.[52]) The chapter of the Beijing Platform for Action that is devoted to women and health identifies five strategic objectives:[53]

1. To increase women's access throughout the life cycle to appropriate, affordable, and quality health care, information, and related services
2. To strengthen preventive programs that promote women's health
3. To undertake gender sensitive initiatives that address sexually transmitted diseases, HIV/AIDS, and sexual and reproductive health issues
4. To promote research and disseminate information on women's health
5. To increase resources and monitor follow-up for women's health.

The input and active participation of public health professionals is essential to fulfill these key aspects of the Beijing conference action plan.

Political consensus about the fundamental importance of combating gender discrimination represented a dramatic step forward. The next series of steps must convert this vision into reality. The Cairo and Beijing action plans called for an unprecedented commitment of funds devoted to implementing the reproductive health–related recommendations of the documents in the developing world. Unfortunately, much of this funding commitment has yet to materialize. The United States lags well behind other developed countries in its level of contributions thus far.

An important element of the holistic approach advocated by the Cairo and Beijing action plans is increasing women's levels of education. Increasing access to education for women is not only key to improving women's prospects but also can positively affect the health of children. Surveys in 25 developing countries demonstrate that minimal education (1 to 3 years of schooling) for a mother can reduce child mortality rates by 15 percent, compared with reductions of just 6 percent when fathers have the same level of education.[54] Such benefits demonstrate the importance of recognizing the many links between efforts to improve women's status and to improve global health. Public health workers can bring these data to the attention of policymakers and the general public, and in so doing can shift the terms of the debate regarding the interrelationships between the status of women and global health.

As we highlight ways to improve women's status and public health globally, it is important to recognize shortfalls that remain in the United States. Seventy-seven percent of uninsured pregnant women were eligible for Medicaid in 1997.[55] Public health professionals can work to ensure that more of those eligible for Medicaid are enrolled in this program.

To reduce the women's health consequences of social injustice, public health workers must continue to serve as advocates for women—both in the United States and elsewhere in the world. They must initiate research that demonstrates the adverse health effects of ill-advised public policies and speak out for change. They must be prepared to respond to and counter disinformation campaigns with sound empirical evidence. Among the many roles that public health professionals can play to reverse the adverse impact that social injustice continues to have on women's health are serving as a resource for advocacy groups and participating in policy formation, including providing congressional testimony.

Teaching and research roles also provide many opportunities for public health professionals to make a difference. Professors and researchers in public health can highlight associations between social injustice and women's health. In so doing, they can influence the debate on women's health issues and continue to encourage progressive social change.

In developing countries, public health professionals, among other key roles, have been at the forefront of efforts to increase access to reproductive health care for women in refugee settings; to develop high-quality sustainable emergency obstetric care and health infrastructure; and to decrease morbidity and mortality associated with illegal abortions. Modest successes have been achieved in these areas, but much work remains. Public health professionals must continue to focus international attention on women's health, especially by advocating for increased international funding for programs that attempt to promote equity for women and mitigate the effects of social injustice, such as those proposed in the Cairo and Beijing action plans.

While efforts to improve the lives of women in developing countries must include ensuring access to basic citizenship rights, resources, and education, social policies must simultaneously address dramatic changes in social roles and the form of families worldwide. Decreasing social injustice and improving the health of women necessitate engaging with a world in transition.

In the second half of the twentieth century, women's participation in the paid workforce rose worldwide, mandating that social policies strive to make parenthood compatible with employment. The concurrent steep decline in childbearing rates globally—although uneven—further underscores the urgency of promoting policies that improve child-care benefits for working parents and support the widespread availability of adequately compensated part-time work that provides health benefits. Other initiatives that support parents' engagement in family life and meaningful employment must also be developed.

Technological developments that separate sex from procreation have resulted from and fueled these trends. Such developments include means of fertility control, such as contraception and abortion, with the recent advances of emergency contraception and medical abortion. These developments also include fertility enhancement, such as ART, which have special relevance to women who defer childbearing to older ages, when infertility risks increase. Although alternatives to later childbearing—including true family-friendly workplace policies that support women as key employees while simultaneously recognizing the importance of their childbearing role—could be a way out of this bind, there is little public pressure to implement such changes. Instead, ART and related technologies have become symbols of profoundly contentious societal transformations, thus often being caught in the center of political storms. The participation of public health professionals is needed to help answer key questions about health equity and access to ART, associated health risks, ethics of ART, and cost burdens.

Because of societal expectations and limited state-sponsored services for care of the elderly, women bear a disproportionate share of caregiving responsibilities for elderly spouses, parents, or disabled children. They often do so while coping with, and sometimes neglecting, their own ill health.[56] Public health professionals can contribute to the creation of other viable options so that this burden does not fall disproportionately on women. They can play an active role in formulating equitable solutions and creating or evaluating pilot programs that can test these solutions. They can also provide data to policy-makers that document the unique health challenges faced by female caregivers.

Uncomfortable as changes may be in matters as intimate as gender roles, family constellations, childbearing, and caregiving, these changes are long term and irreversible. They require societies to formulate policies and provide services that support these altered realities to narrow disparities in health and opportunity.

Conclusion

Many negative health consequences for women are rooted in social injustice. Changes in discriminatory policies, such as those that kept women from participating in clinical trials in the United States, have taken place, but women are still underrepresented in the ranks of research scientists. Welfare reform policies and policies that prevent public funding for abortions in the United States have demonstrated adverse health impacts but nevertheless remain in effect—thus continuing the legacy of social injustice.

Globally, HIV/AIDS continues to spread among women who are monogamous but whose husbands are not. Women still die too often in childbirth and have insufficient access to contraception. Female children's access to education and even adequate nutrition remains restricted in too many parts of the world.

In combating the negative effects of social injustice on women's health, public health professionals have much to do. Many long-term actions were outlined earlier in this chapter. In the short term, what needs to be done seems to constantly shift, often being influenced by changes in the political climate. That women's health is so vulnerable to political gamesmanship is, in itself, an example of social injustice. Recent disturbing examples include the federal partial-birth abortion ban and debates over the appropriateness of making emergency contraceptives available over the counter. To be effective in the short term, public health professionals must pay close attention to the political climate and respond to challenges quickly. For public health professionals and others working to combat the adverse health effects of social injustice on women, making a commitment to effecting positive social change for women is most important.

References

1. Centers for Disease Control and Prevention. HIV/AIDS surveillance in women. Atlanta, Ga.: CDC. Available at: http://www.cdc.gov/hiv/graphics/images/l264/l264-1.htm. Accessed January 11, 2005.
2. UNAIDS. Report on the Global HIV/AIDS epidemic 2002. Geneva, Switzerland: UNAIDS, July 2002.
3. Centers for Disease Control and Prevention. Tracking the hidden epidemics: trends in STDs in the United States 2000. Atlanta, Ga.: CDC. Available at: http://www.cdc.gov/nchstp/dstd/Stats_Trends/Trends2000.pdf. Accessed January 11, 2005.
4. Centers for Disease Control and Prevention. American women are waiting to begin families, National Center for Health Statistics. Atlanta, Ga.: CDC. Available at: http://www.cdc.gov/nchs/releases/02news/ameriwomen.htm. Accessed January 11, 2005.
5. UNFPA. State of the world's population 1999. New York, N.Y.: UNFPA, 1999.
6. Wallace LS, Ballard JE. Lifetime physical activity and calcium intake related to bone density in young women. J Women's Health Gender Based Med 2002;11:389–98.
7. Alan Guttmacher Institute. State policies in brief: mandatory waiting periods for abortion New York, N.Y.: The Alan Guttmacher Institute. Available at: http://www.guttmacher.org/pubs/spib_MWPA.pdf. Accessed January 11, 2005.
8. Alan Guttmacher Institute. State policies in brief: parental involvement in minors' abortions New York, N.Y.: The Alan Guttmacher Institute. Available at: http://www.guttmacher.org/pubs/spib_PIMA.pdf. Accessed January 11, 2005.
9. Alan Guttmacher Institute. State policies in brief: bans on "partial birth" abortion New York, N.Y.: The Alan Guttmacher Institute. Available at: http://www.guttmacher.org/pubs/spib_BPBA.pdf. Accessed January 11, 2005.
10. Finer LB, Henshaw SK. Abortion incidence and services in the United States in 2000. Perspect Sexual Reprod Health 2003;35:6–15.
11. Catholics for a Free Choice. The Access Series: Catholic HMOs and reproductive health care. Washington, D.C.: Catholics for a Free Choice, 2001.
12. Hoff T, Greene L. Sex education in America: a view from inside the nation's classrooms. Menlo Park, Calif.: Kaiser Family Foundation; 2000.

13. Kirby D. Emerging answers: new research findings on programs to reduce teen pregnancy. Washington, D.C.: The National Campaign to Reduce Teen Pregnancy, 2001.
14. Proctor B, Dalaker J. U.S. Census Bureau, current population reports, poverty in the United States: 2001. Washington, D.C.: U.S. Government Printing Office, 2002.
15. Alan Guttmacher Institute. State policies in brief: state funding of abortion under Medicaid New York, N.Y.: The Alan Guttmacher Institute. Available at: http://www.guttmacher.org/pubs/spib_SFAM.pdf. Accessed January 11, 2005.
16. Boonstra H, Sonfield A. Rights without access: revisiting public funding of abortion for poor women. The Guttmacher Report on Public Policy 2000;3:8–11.
17. Handler A, Zimbeck M, Chavkin W, et al. The effects of welfare reform on the reproductive health of women. In: Wallace M, Green G, Jaros K, eds. Health and welfare for families in the 21st century. Sudbury, Mass.: Jones and Bartlett Publishers, 2003.
18. Garret B, Holohan J. Health insurance coverage after welfare. Health Affairs 2000; 19:175–84.
19. Wyn R, Solis B, Ojeda V, et al. Falling through the cracks: health insurance coverage of low-income women. Menlo Park, Calif.: Kaiser Family Foundation, 2001.
20. Alan Guttmacher Institute. State policies in brief: Medicaid family planning waivers New York, N.Y.: The Alan Guttmacher Institute. Available at: http://www.guttmacher.org/pubs/spib_MFPW.pdf. Accessed January 11, 2005.
21. National Women's Law Center. Women and health insurance. Available at: http://www.nwlc.org/pdf/WomenAnd HealthInsuranceApril2003.pdf. Accessed January 11, 2005.
22. Thorpe KE. The distribution of health insurance coverage among pregnant women, 1990–1997. Available at: http://www.modimes.org/PublicAffairs2/distribution.htm. Accessed January 11, 2005.
23. Worthington-Roberts BS, Klerman LV. Maternal nutrition. In: Merkatz I, Thompson JE, eds. New perspectives on prenatal care. Thompson, N.Y.: Elsevier Science Publication Co., 1990.
24. Gunderson C, LeBlanc M, Kuhn B. The changing food assistance landscape. Agricultural economics report no. 773. Washington, D.C.: US Department of Agriculture, 1999.
25. Wise P, Chavkin W, Romero D. Assessing the effects of welfare reform on reproductive and infant health. Am J Public Health 1999;89:1514–21.
26. Association of Maternal and Child Health Programs. Abstinence education in the states. Implementation of the 1996 Abstinence Education Law: results of a survey of state Title V programs. Washington, D.C.: Association of Maternal Child Health Programs, 1999.
27. UNFPA. State of the world's population 2000. New York, N.Y.: UNFPA, 2000.
28. Tiaden P, Thoennes N. Full Report of the prevalence, incidence and consequences of violence against women. Washington, D.C.: U.S. Department of Justice, Office of Justice Programs, National Institute of Justice, 2000.
29. Greenfeld LA, Rand MR, Craven D, et al. Violence by intimates: analysis of data on crimes by current or former spouses, boyfriends, and girlfriends. U.S. Department of Justice Bureau of Justice Statistics. Available at: http://www.ojp.usdoj.gov/bjs/pub/ascii/vi.txt. Accessed January 11, 2005.
30. Kilpatrick DG, Best CL, Saunders BE, et al. Rape in marriage and in dating relationships: how bad is it for mental health? Ann N Y Acad Sci 1988;528:335–44.
31. Paone D, Chavkin W, Willets I, et al. The impact of sexual abuse: implications for drug treatment. J Women's Health 1992;2:149–53.
32. Golding JM. Sexual assault history and women's reproductive and sexual health. Psychol Women Q 1996;20:101–21.

33. Paone D, Chavkin W. From the family domain to the public health forum: Sexual abuse, women and risk for HIV infection. SIECUS Rep 1993;April/May:13–6.

34. Bohn DK. Domestic violence and pregnancy: implications for practice. J Nurse Midwifery 1990;35:86–98.

35. Paone D, Chavkin W. From the family domain to the public health forum: sexual abuse, women and risk for HIV infection. SIECUS Rep 1993;April/May:13–6.

36. Wizemann TM, Pardue M-L, eds. Exploring the biological contributions to human health: does sex matter? Washington, D.C.: National Academy Press; 2001.

37. Lenfant C. Heart disease in women: a look back and a view to the future. In: National Institutes of Health, Office of Research on Women's Health. An agenda for research on women's health for the 21st century: a report of the Task Force on the NIH Women's Health Research Agenda for the 21st century. Vol 2. Bethesda, Md.: National Institutes of Health, 1999. (NIH publication 99-4386.)

38. Sterling TR, Vlahov D, Astemkborski J, et al. Initial plasma HIV-1 RNA levels and progression to AIDS in women and men. N Engl J Med 2001;344:720–5.

39. Horwitz BJ, Fisher RS. The irritable bowel syndrome. N Engl J Med 2001;344: 1846–50.

40. Campaigne BN, Wishner KL. Gender-specific health care in diabetes mellitus. J Gender Specific Med 2000;3:51–58.

41. National Institute of Mental Health. The numbers count: mental disorders in America. Available at: http://www.nimh.nih.gov/publicat/numbers.cfm. Accessed January 11, 2005.

42. Chavkin W. Women and clinical research. JAMWA 1994;49:99–100.

43. US Public Health Service: Report of the Public Health Service Task Force on Women's Health Issues. Public Health Rep 1985;100:73–106.

44. Guideline for the study and evaluation of gender differences in the clinical evaluation of drugs; notice. Fed Register 1993;58:39406–16.

45. Jensvold MF, Hamilton JA, Mackey B. Including women in clinical trials: how about the women scientists? JAMWA 1994;49:110–2.

46. Hughes DM. Changing a masculinist culture: women in science, engineering and technology. In: Morgan R, ed. Sisterhood is forever. New York, N.Y.: Washington Square Press, 2003.

47. Martin JR. Climbing the ivory walls: women in Academia. In: Morgan R, ed. Sisterhood is forever. New York, N.Y.: Washington Square Press, 2003.

48. Minority students in medical education: facts and figures IX. Washington, D.C.: Association of American Medical Colleges, Division of Community and Minority Programs, 1995.

49. Alan Guttmacher Institute. Uneven and unequal: insurance coverage of reproductive health services. New York, N.Y.: The Alan Guttmacher Institute, 1994.

50. Chavkin W, Wise P, Elman D. Policies towards pregnancy and addiction: sticks without carrots. Ann N Y Acad Sci 1998;846:335–40.

51. Programme of Action of the International Conference on Population and Development. Available at: www.unfpa.org/icpd/icpd_poa.htm. Accessed January 11, 2005.

52. Fourth World Conference on Women: Beijing Declaration. Available at: http://www.un.org/womenwatch/daw/beijing/platform/declar.htm. Accessed January 11, 2005.

53. Fourth World Conference on Women: Platform for Action. Strategic Objectives and Actions: Women and Health. Available at: http://www.un.org/womenwatch/daw/beijing/platform/health.htm. Accessed January 11, 2005.

54. Paden M (ed.). Women. Washington, D.C.: World Resources Institute, 1996.

55. Thorpe KE. The distribution of health insurance coverage among pregnant women, 1990–1997. Available at: http://www.modimes.org/PublicAffairs2/distribution.htm. Accessed January 11, 2005.

56. The Commonwealth Fund. Women's health fact sheet: informal caregiving, fact sheet from The Commonwealth Fund 1998 Survey of Women's Health. Available at: http://www.cmwf.org/programs/women/ksc%5Fwhsurvey99%5Ffact2%5F332.asp. Accessed January 11, 2005.

5

CHILDREN

Sara Rosenbaum and Chung-Hi H. Yoder

Introduction

This chapter deals primarily with the impact of social injustice on children in the United States, emphasizing children's rights in a legal context.

The Legal Status of Children in Society

International Standards

The United Nations Convention on the Rights of the Child (CRC) is an international treaty establishing the human rights of children, including the right to an education and health care and protection against execution and life imprisonment for crimes committed by individuals under age 18.[1] Although the United States has signed the CRC, the U.S. Senate has yet to ratify it: among all countries in the United Nations, only the United States and Somalia have failed to ratify the CRC.[2] Analysts speculate that the U.S. Senate's failure to ratify the treaty reflects its concern that the CRC will undermine the authority of parents to control the upbringing of their children.[3]

The availability of the death penalty and life imprisonment under state law for crimes committed by children also may be factors in the Senate's unwillingness to ratify the CRC. It is likely that the availability of the death penalty for child offenders also played a role in the Senate's decision. Although in March 2005, the U.S. Supreme Court held that the death penalty, for juvenile offenders under age 18 was unconstitutional,[4] as of January 2004, more than 70 juvenile offenders were on death row in the United States for crimes committed before age 18.[5] Of all executions of child offenders worldwide since 1995, 65 percent took place in the United States.[6]

Children's Rights Under U.S. Law

The U.S. Constitution protects individuals who are recognized as legal "persons." Thus, for example, U.S. law does not recognize fetuses as "persons," although it accords government considerable powers to protect its interest in potential life once a fetus becomes viable.[7] Children who are born are recognized as legal persons, and the U.S. Supreme Court has recognized that children possess certain constitutional rights independent from those of their parents.[8]

At the same time, however, children who have not reached the age of legal majority under state law are restricted considerably in their legal autonomy on decisions involving family living arrangements, education, and health care. Because children are not autonomous individuals and rely on adults economically and physically, they lack full legal personhood under U.S. law.

Where children are concerned, the United States Supreme Court has stated,

> the constitutional rights of children cannot be equated with those of adults [because of] the peculiar vulnerability of children; their inability to make critical decisions in an informed, mature manner; and the importance of the parental role in child rearing.[9]

The Supreme Court's holdings recognize that states may validly restrict children's freedom to make important decisions for themselves because children lack the maturity and experience "to recognize and avoid choices that could be detrimental to them."[9] In general, children's rights are assigned to the parents or to the state in loco parentis.

The Court's holdings establish parents' liberty interest in directing the education of their children.[10] Similarly, the Court will accord considerable deference to a parent's substantive due process right to determine what is in a child's best interest and has declared such parental rights to be "fundamental."[11]

Furthermore, although children are persons within the meaning of the Constitution and thus must be accorded procedural and substantive due process, the Supreme Court has held that a state has no constitutional duty of rescue—a duty to protect a child from his or her parent, even when the state knows the child's safety is at risk.[12] The Court stated that the 14th Amendment does not require the state to protect individuals from violence between private individuals but is meant as a safeguard from state actions intruding on the liberty interests of private persons.[12] The state has no affirmative duty to protect individuals from private violence; however, when states have limited individual autonomy, they have a duty to provide basic medical services to prisoners and a duty to protect the involuntarily committed.[13]

Children have very limited rights to make their own medical decisions. Informed consent presumes that the individual giving consent is mature enough to understand a choice of treatment and its consequences. Many courts have held that children under the age of 18 do not have the intellectual or emotional capacity to make those decisions, and consequently, their parents are given the discretion to consent or refuse medical treatment for their children. At the same time, the Supreme Court has recognized that parental consent is not absolute and that states are required, in some instances, to provide procedural due process to children. Thus, for example, a parent does not have absolute discretion over a decision to institutionalize a child in a state facility, and commitment can be ordered only following an independent review procedure that meets procedural due process standards.[14]

Children have somewhat greater rights in the areas of abortion and reproductive health. Under rulings of the U.S. Supreme Court, states may constitutionally require that a minor receive parental consent for an abortion, but the state may not grant absolute veto power to a parent or guardian for such a decision and must provide a judicial bypass procedure.[15]

The Impact of Social Injustice on Children's Health

The Health Needs of Children

Although a complex set of factors influences children's health, what children need to promote optimal health is relatively straightforward.[16] Overall, children are healthier than adults. When acute or chronic health threats occur, their symptoms are generally milder and more easily overcome or ameliorated. A very small proportion of children do suffer from highly definable and serious illnesses and conditions, but the prevalence of these conditions in children is lower than that in adults.[16]

Development is the most socially and biologically significant dimension of childhood. Modern social expectations of children are not that they will be self-sufficient and productive in a grown-up sense; rather; society expects that children will develop and evolve toward productivity during adulthood.[16] For this reason, utilitarian norms of functionality for adults have only a limited role in evaluating children's health needs.[16]

Furthermore, conditions that express themselves as overt health problems in adults may manifest themselves as problems of physical, cognitive, or mental development in children. Because poor health in children tends to be expressed in developmental, rather than overt and diagnosable, terms, the health status and needs of children differ from those of adults.[16]

Children in the United States are a generally healthy population.[16] (See box 5-1 concerning children in other developed countries and box 5-2 concerning children in developing countries.) Infant mortality is considered a seminal measure of population health. From 1998 to 2000, the U.S. infant mortality rate reached a historic low of 7.0 deaths per 1,000 live births, higher than in other industrialized countries[17] (fig. 5-1 on p. 97). It remained comparatively elevated for minority infants, especially black and American Indian infants. Indeed, the black–white gap in infant mortality rate actually widened between 1983 and 2000, although minority infants experienced a significant decline in deaths between 1980 and 2000.[17] However, the incidence of low birth weight (less than 5.5 pounds), a key indicator of child health, was higher in 2001 than a decade earlier.[18]

Simple measures of health in childhood also show positive trends in health status. In 2001, an estimated 77 percent of all children aged 19 to 35 months were fully immunized against preventable diseases, a rate that was below the national goal but a significant improvement.[19] The vast majority of children are considered in good to excellent health by their parents and caregivers, and more than 95 percent of all children are reported to have a regular source of health care.[20] In the United States and western Europe, deaths among children are rare. In the earliest years, childhood deaths tend to be associated with congenital anomalies and low birth weight.[16] As children grow, injuries and deaths from defined illnesses and conditions become a factor.[16]

On closer examination, however, the health profile of children becomes much more problematic. A significant proportion of the child population in the United States has a special health need. Studies of child health define the concept of special need in various ways, from the narrowest of definitions (a specific recognized class of diagnosis or a severe disability) to broader conceptualizations (such as having an impairment in functioning[21] or having fair to poor self-assessed health status).[16] Not surprisingly, the health profile of children declines as the definition of *special need* is expanded to encompass more modern concepts of child development and as the measurement tools broaden.[21]

Measurement systems, such a vital statistics, parental interviews, health examinations, and surveys, indicate a broad range of health problems among children.[16] Based on parental assessments, 2.1 percent of U.S. children were estimated, in 1997, to be in fair to poor health—an improvement from the beginning of the decade.[22] However, this figure is higher when the definition is expanded to assessments done by others.

The most widely used current definition of *special needs*, developed by the U.S. Department of Health and Human Services, classifies them broadly to

BOX 5-1 How the United States Compares With
Other Developed Countries

While the social justice agenda can be improved in virtually every nation, there are major differences in how far many nations have come compared with others. This difference is manifest among developed countries. Perhaps the most comprehensive analysis of these variations is depicted by the longitudinal Luxembourg Income Study (LIS), which compared and contrasted poverty within a cohort of 18 nations—both overall and for subpopulation groups, such as children and older people. Countries included in this study were the United States, Great Britain, Germany, France, Israel, Denmark, Sweden, Austria, Belgium, and Italy. A look at LIS outcomes for children among these nations is instructive in terms of how different nations approach the goal of social justice.

In the United States, approximately 25 percent of children live in households whose incomes are below the federal poverty level. Over the past 20 years, the trend in child poverty has been worsening. From 1969 through 1986, for example, child poverty in the United States rose from 13.1 percent to 22.9 percent. Even during the peak economic years of the 1990s, child poverty decreased only slightly, and it has now risen again to more than 25 percent of children. But what, we might ask, happens to child poverty rates when we factor in government benefits, such as income transfer programs and food stamps? The answer is that government programs reduce child poverty (defined as half of the median income after taxes and government benefits) only minimally—to 21.5 percent. Their economic impact, in other words, is quite minimal. They do relatively little to help lift poor children (and their households) out of poverty.

By contrast, France also begins with a child poverty rate equal to that in the United States. But government policy in France slashes that 25 percent rate to 6.5 percent once the impact of national programs are factored in. Most of the other nations in the cohort also fare well. In 11 of the nations surveyed, government programs reduce child poverty by at least 50 percent. And nearly half the nations surveyed—Austria, Belgium, Denmark, Finland, Luxembourg, Norway, Sweden, and Switzerland—have succeeded in keeping child poverty rates below 5 percent. With more than 20 percent of its children in poverty, the United States leads what LIS refers to as "the child poverty league." The world's wealthiest nation has the poorest record in reducing child poverty. Only four other LIS nations have child poverty rates above 10 percent: Australia, Canada, Ireland, and Israel. And each of their records is better than that of the United States.

(continued)

Three related factors are associated with the higher child poverty rates in the United States compared with other developed countries.

The first factor is what economists refer to as differences in the "political economy." In many, if not most, other nations, there is a stronger history of government involvement in rounding off the sharp edges of inequality. While averring attempts to create similar economic outcomes, other nations see inherent dangers in growing gaps between rich and poor. They use their tax systems to control or prevent growing disparities. The United States, on the other hand, has a more laissez-faire approach to income differences, more typically holding that income disparities are reflections of hard work and self-worth.

The second factor is embedded in the first. Taxes in the United States are unpopular, so much so that for nearly two decades no significant political leader has called for an increase in federal taxes. In European and other LIS nations, taxes—at least begrudgingly—are accepted as the price of civilization. They hold society together and are the means to provide a moral bottom line against unacceptable disparities. As a result of these divergent traditions, the tax burden on U.S. households is the lowest in the industrial world. The United States, as a consequence, fails to do what other nations do to reduce poverty.

The third, and final, factor is that the United States relies far more on "welfare programs" to reduce poverty than do other nations. Rather than developing categorical programs designed only for the poor, other nations typically rely far more on their national tax systems to temper the economic extremes. Truly progressive taxes in these countries levy a higher rate on the wealthiest tier, far more than in the United States. At the same time, tax programs also are used to bolster the incomes of otherwise impoverished households. The United States has such programs—the Earned Income Tax Credit (EITC), the most significant, provides tax credits to working families whose annual incomes fall below a certain line. But the United States, unlike most other developed countries, manifests its limited approach to social justice primarily through its regressive tax system. As a result, little is done to reduce poverty. It is almost as if the nation has decided to live with the extremes of social injustice that are now unknown among other developed countries.

include "chronic physical, developmental, behavioral, or emotional conditions [which] require health and related services of a type or amount beyond that required by children generally."[21] Using this modern definition, the magnitude of the problem grows. It includes not only physical conditions but also developmental and mental health needs. As a result, the estimates of children with health problems rise to 14.8 to 18.2 percent of all children under age 18.[21]

More than 10 million children under age 5 die each year from diseases that could be prevented at little or no cost. For example, 2 million children die each year from pneumonia, while life-saving antibiotics are available for US$0.15 per child. The primary causes of children's deaths in developing countries—diarrhea, pneumonia, malaria, measles, and underlying malnutrition—are the same today as they were 20 years ago, despite the wide availability of simple, effective, and low-cost interventions that could save most of these children's lives. Unfortunately, as people worldwide become increasingly—and appropriately—aware of the impact of HIV/AIDS, and as governments dedicate more resources for HIV/AIDS prevention and treatment, efforts to reduce other causes of infant and child mortality are decreasing.

Which Children Are at Risk?

Many factors contribute to placing children at risk of early death, beginning with where they are born. Most child deaths occur in the poorest countries of the world. For example, 10 percent of the world's population lives in sub-Saharan Africa, but 43 percent of child deaths occur there. High levels of absolute poverty—an income of US$1 or less daily—prevent families from having adequate food, appropriate housing, sanitation, safe drinking water, basic health care, and education. In addition, within these countries, the poorest 20 percent of the population are four times more likely to die than the least-poor. Poorer families have less knowledge of healthy behaviors, less access to health services, such as vaccination programs or treatment for malaria, and the available services are often of lower quality.

Poverty also affects a child's mental health and development. In Asia and Africa, families put children to work at young ages to have them contribute to household income—sometimes as young as 6 years of age. In Indonesia, for example, over 8 million children under age 15 are employed. Girls are particularly affected by child labor practices: millions are employed as domestic servants, are forced into prostitution, or sold by their families into indentured servitude. Children who begin working at an early age are often unable to continue their schooling, which results in illiteracy, early age at marriage, and early childbirth. Ten percent of births worldwide occur to teenage mothers; these girls are twice as likely to die in childbirth as are older women. In addition to poverty, lack of education, long geographic distance from health facilities, language barriers among ethnic minorities, low caste, female gender, and the effects of war all lower a child's—and a mother's—chances of survival.

(continued)

What Have We Achieved So Far?

The first month of an infant's life is critical. Forty percent of all children's deaths occur during this period. Mothers in many developing countries postpone naming their children because they are so accustomed to the possibility of an infant dying early. However, health programs that offer simple, life-saving interventions, such as tetanus toxoid immunization during pregnancy, delivery of the infant by a trained birth attendant, access to basic obstetric services, and even drying and keeping a baby warm after delivery all can reduce the newborn death rate. Oral rehydration therapy (ORT), with a simple solution of salt and sugar, has reduced deaths due to diarrhea by half; it can prevent almost 1 million deaths annually. Breastfeeding promotion programs that encourage exclusive breastfeeding for the first 6 months of an infant's life can prevent 13 percent of all children's deaths. And effective immunization campaigns can prevent serious illness or death from diseases like measles, tetanus, and polio.

Finishing the Unfinished Agenda

Although effective and low-cost vaccines are available and can save lives, over 30 million children are not vaccinated each year. Although sleeping under insecticide-treated bednets can reduce one-third of child mortality from malaria, fewer than 2 percent of children sleep under these treated bednets. In the 1980s, global support for the Child Survival Agenda increased the availability of these interventions and saved millions of lives. In the past decade, however, funding and enthusiasm have lagged and the rates of decline in mortality that were once approximately 2.5 percent a year, have slowed to 1 percent. The goal of the World Summit for Children—a one-third reduction in mortality from 1990 to 2000—was not completely achieved; therefore, in 2000, all United Nations member countries set Millennium Development Goals (see table 21-7 on p. 394) that pledged to reduce child deaths by two-thirds and maternal deaths by one-half by 2015. This recommitment to saving the lives of mothers and children has already demonstrated some success. Many governments, even when struggling with continued political instability or insurgency, have committed to increasing the opportunities for girls' education—a proven strategy to reduce both maternal and child death. Since the fall of the Taliban, the government of Afghanistan and its Ministry of Health, in a country with one of the highest rates of maternal and child mortality, have prioritized education and basic health care for girls and the poorest of the poor. The government of Indonesia and counter-trafficking organizations are drafting legislation to prohibit child trafficking and offering programs that provide alternatives to poor families. Newly formed collaborations in developing countries among NGOs, foundations, governments, health care providers, and community groups have brought about positive change, ranging from village health programs to national

(continued)

BOX 5-2 *(continued)*

policy changes. Still, much needs to happen before 2015. It will take collaboration, sufficient funding, and sustained international commitment to reach the Millennium Development Goals and to save lives. (See also chapters 11, 14, 17, 18, 19, 21, and 28.)

Further Reading

Children Having Children: The State of the World's Mothers, Save the Children, 2004. Available at: http://www.savethechildren.org/mothers/report_2004. Accessed January 10, 2005.

Information on the Millennium Development Goals and the association between poverty and health. Available at: http://www.worldbank.org. Accessed January 10, 2005.

Information on the rights of women and children. Available at: http://www.unicef.org and http://www.hrw.org. Accessed January 10, 2005.

State of the World's Children, UNICEF, 2004. Available at: http://www.unicef.org/publications/index_18108.html. Accessed January 10, 2005.

The Child Survival Series. Lancet 361, 2003. Available at: http://www.thelancet.com/journal/vol361/iss9376/child_survival. Accessed January 10, 2005. Note: This special series has five articles within it.

Nearly 20 percent of all children aged 3 to 17 have been estimated to have at least one mental health problem.[23] Furthermore, as children age, the incidence of health problems associated with risk-taking behaviors tends to rise, particularly in the areas of addiction and alcoholism, obesity, unprotected sex and sexually transmitted diseases, teenage pregnancy, suicide, and homicide.[16]

Recent studies of child health recommend that health problems in children be reconceptualized in their relationship to the child population as a whole. These studies suggest that problems of child health and development tend to be co-occurring and concentrated in certain children and that these problems tend to persist over time. Therefore, child health problems need to be understood as long-term, persistent, multilayered, and concentrated in specified cohorts of children.[16]

Threats to Children's Health

To be healthy, children need access to regular, continuous, comprehensive, and stable health care from a health system capable of identifying problems in growth and development at the earliest possible stages and positive and supportive interaction with parents.[24] Parents also need the ability to pay for immediate and appropriate care when the need arises. Even more fundamentally perhaps, children need freedom from the conditions that raise the risk of poor health and diminish developmental potential and attainment.

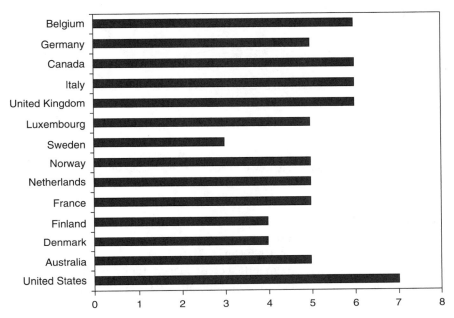

Figure 5-1 Infant mortality rate for industrialized countries for 1999. (From United Nations Children's Fund. The state of the world's children 2001, table 1, basic indicators. New York: UNICEF, 2001.)

Child health is being free not only from specified illnesses and conditions but also from the community and social threats that can profoundly affect long-term development.

Poverty and Health

Among children there is a strong association between low socioeconomic status of children and their poor health—an association that appears to exist in all stages of child and adolescent development and almost all preventable child and adolescent disorders.[16] Therefore, freedom from poverty may be the single most important determinant of child health and development. Child poverty affects a large proportion of children in the United States. In most parts of the country, income at least twice the federal poverty level, which was $18,400 for a family of four in 2003, is essential to ensuring adequate food, clothing, housing, and other basics of life.[25] In 2001, family income below this basic threshold affected nearly 40 percent of all children in the United States, nearly 60 percent of African-American children, and 62 percent of Latino children.[25] In 2000, more than 6 percent of all children, and more than 7 percent of children under age 6, lived in families with incomes below 50 percent of the official federal poverty level.[26] After accounting for food, rent assistance, and

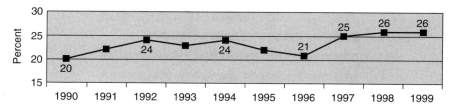

Figure 5-2 Percentage of poor children who live below half the poverty line after accounting for food and rent assistance and taxes, 1990–1999. (From Children's Defense Fund. The state of America's children: 2001 yearbook. Washington, D.C.: Children's Defense Fund, 2001, p. 9. Copyright © 2001 by Children's Defense Fund. All rights reserved.)

taxes, the proportion of children living in deep poverty has grown steadily since 1990, with the largest increases following the enactment of federal welfare reform legislation in 1996 (fig. 5-2).

Poverty carries with it two important consequences for the health of children. First, it creates and maintains poor living conditions for children. Poverty threatens access to adequate food, shelter, health care,[27] child care, family time, and other aspects of daily life that make a child's surroundings safe and stable. Poverty threatens the ability of families to invest in the necessary tangibles of daily life, which, in turn, promotes a sense of well-being and stability. Inadequate income (both cash and in-kind) hampers families' ability to deal with adversity and health threats in a prompt and comprehensive manner.

Second, poverty is associated with stress that robs children and adults of their health and deprives children of their parents as functional and strong caregivers. Perhaps the worst form of childhood poverty in the United States is the concentrated poverty found in the poorest communities in urban America. This intense and concentrated poverty creates geographically identifiable health adversity for the children and their parents who experience it, with elevated rates of illness, disability, and death. Community-ridden poverty leads to "weathering," that is, "the grinding every day stress that flows from such adverse conditions."[28]

Environmental Health Threats

Children's unique developmental status makes them particularly vulnerable to environmental health threats. Young children are more likely to absorb more toxins, such as lead and pesticides in food, water, and air, because they breathe faster and eat and drink more in proportion to their body weight than do adults.[29] Furthermore, children tend to play close to the ground and tend to engage in hand-to-mouth behavior that increases their contact with toxins in soil, dust, and carpets.[30] Also, their hand-to-mouth behavior heightens their likelihood of ingesting toxins in dust or from the ground.

According to the Centers for Disease Control and Prevention (CDC), approximately 890,000 children in the United States aged 1 to 5 have elevated blood lead levels (BLLs), and more than one fifth of African-American children who live in homes built before 1946 have elevated BLLs.[31] Research shows that children sustain impaired intellectual development as a result of lead exposure below what the CDC currently considers safe (10 μg/dL).[32] Children living in poorer communities bear the greatest risk; while poor children represent about 19 percent of all children under age 6,[33] among young children who have elevated BLLs, 60 percent are poor.[32]

Hazardous waste is a danger to children. As of 2000, about 0.8 percent of children in the United States lived within 1 mile of a Superfund hazardous waste site that had not been cleaned up or controlled and another 500,000 children lived within 1 mile of a controlled Superfund site.[34] The Agency for Toxic Substances and Disease Registry estimates that 3 to 4 million children live within 1 mile of at least one hazardous waste site and therefore face a greater chance of exposure and increased risk for health problems.[35]

Poor air quality also is a significant danger to children. In 2001, approximately two fifths of all children were residents of counties that exceeded officially acceptable ozone standards.[36] In 1999, 31 percent of Hispanic children, 25 percent of Asian children, and 16 percent of black children lived in counties in which air quality standards were exceeded.[37]

Air pollution triggers asthma attacks, one of the most common and potentially serious of all childhood conditions. In 2001, 6.3 million children in the United States had asthma. In 2000, there were 214,000 hospitalizations of children below the age of 18 due to asthma. Asthma prevalence and mortality are higher among blacks than among whites.[38] In 2000, asthma prevalence among black children was 10 percent higher than among their white counterparts, while age-adjusted asthma mortality was 200 percent higher.[39]

Other major environmental threats can be found. Elevated mercury levels, chiefly as a result of its unregulated release into the air from coal-burning power plants, are widespread. The CDC estimates that 8 percent of women of childbearing age have levels of mercury higher than what the U.S. Environmental Protection Agency considers safe because they have eaten contaminated fish. As a result, approximately 300,000 infants are at increased risk for brain damage and learning disabilities.[40]

Poor water quality is another problem faced by U.S. children, millions of whom reside in areas without adequate treatment and filtration systems or served by public water systems with health-based violations.[37]

Finally, the presence of pesticides in food is a major health threat. In 2001, 19 percent of fruits, vegetables, and grains had detectable residues of organophosphate pesticides, which can impair the absorption of food nutrients necessary for growth.[41] Furthermore, the underdeveloped digestive system of children may be unable to adequately excrete toxins from the body.[42]

Social injustice linked to maldistribution of family income and of public health risks takes a heavy toll on the health of U.S. children. Table 5-1 summarizes some of the most important known health risks and adverse health conditions associated with childhood poverty, up to quadruple the risk of death from specific diseases. Children who are poor are at elevated risk for a range of preventable and manageable conditions, including complications of appendicitis and diabetes, severely impaired vision, severe anemia, delayed immunization, meningitis, and deaths from accidents.

Children of low-income families are more likely to be born prematurely, at low birth weight, and to women who received inadequate or no prenatal care. One of every six teenagers aged 15 to 18 lacks health insurance, and teenagers are (a) five times as likely as younger children to lack a regular source of health care; (b) four times more likely to have unmet health needs; and (c) twice as likely to have no yearly contact with physicians.[43] Teenagers from families who face the highest social risks have more alcohol

TABLE 5-1   Relative Frequency of Health Problems in Low-Income Children Compared With Other Children

Health Problem	Relative Frequency in Low-Income Children
Low birth weight	Double
Delayed immunization	Triple
Asthma	Higher
Bacterial meningitis	Double
Rheumatic fever	Double to triple
Lead poisoning	Triple
Neonatal death	1.5 Times
Postneonatal death	Double to triple
Child death due to accidents	Double to triple
Child death due to disease	Triple to quadruple
Complications of appendicitis	Double to triple
Diabetic ketoacidosis	Double
Complications of bacterial meningitis	Double to triple
Conditions limiting school activity	Double
Lost school days	40% More
Severely impaired vision	Double to triple
Severe iron deficiency anemia	Double

From Starfield B. Child and adolescent health status measures. U.S. Health Care for Children [serial on line]. 1992;2:225–40, table 5. Available at: http://www.futureofchildren.org/information2827/information_show.htm?doc_id=77358. Accessed January 10, 2005.

and drug abuse, cigarette smoking, unprotected sexual activity, and sexually transmitted diseases, and they more frequently become single parents.[23]

Table 5-2 underscores the magnitude of the nation's failure to invest in children. The United States stands alone among 24 industrialized nations in its failure to guarantee universal health insurance and health care, paid maternal and parental leave at childhood, and a family allowance/child dependency grant.

Underlying Factors and Roots of Social Injustice

Numerous factors contribute to childhood poverty. The first is a maldistribution of income as a result of the failure of U.S. policy to intervene in the market.

TABLE 5-2   How U.S. Child Safety Net Policies Compare With Those of 23 Other Industrialized Countries

Country	Universal Health Insurance/Health Care	Paid Maternal/Parental Leave at Childbirth	Family Allowance/Child Dependency Grant
Australia	Y	Y	Y
Austria	Y	Y	Y
Belgium	Y	Y	Y
Canada	Y	Y	Y
Czech Republic	Y	Y	Y
Denmark	Y	Y	Y
Finland	Y	Y	Y
France	Y	Y	Y
Germany	Y	Y	Y
Hungary	Y	Y	Y
Ireland	Y	Y	Y
Italy	Y	Y	Y
Japan	Y	Y	Y
Luxembourg	Y	Y	Y
The Netherlands	Y	Y	Y
New Zealand	Y	Y	Y
Norway	Y	Y	Y
Poland	Y	Y	Y
Portugal	Y	Y	Y
Spain	Y	Y	Y
Sweden	Y	Y	Y
Switzerland	Y	Y	Y
United Kingdom	Y	Y	Y
United States	N	N	N

From Children's Defense Fund. The state of America's children: 2001 yearbook. Washington, D.C.: Children's Defense Fund, 2001; p. xxix.

The second is a failure of income replacement policies, both cash and in-kind. The third is a low level of commitment at all levels of government to the types of societal investments in families and children, such as paid maternity and parental leave, high-quality child care and education, and supports for vulnerable families. These societal investments help strengthen families and communities, helping them to raise children who are healthy, ready to learn, and capable of the maximum possible growth and achievement. As a result, the problem of childhood poverty, rather than abating over time, has grown more intense in the United States.

Maldistribution of Income

In U.S. history, the gulf between rich and poor families is as wide now as it has ever been. Figure 5-3 illustrates the change over a 40-year time period in the average income of rich and poor families in constant dollars and by economic quintiles. Between 1959 and 1979, the average real income of the lowest 20 percent of all families grew by 75 percent, while families in the top 5 percent of the income bracket experienced real income growth of 54 percent— the real income of poorest families not only grew but also grew in relation to the income growth of the nation's wealthiest families. The nation's industrial base, as well as its governmental policies, fueled real improvements in living conditions among the poorest families. Between 1979 and 1999, the reverse occurred: Real income of the poorest families declined by 4 percent, while that

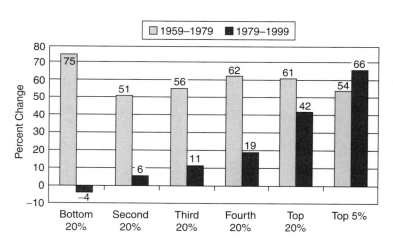

Figure 5-3 Change in the average income of rich and poor families (in constant dollars), 1979–1999. (From Children's Defense Fund. The state of America's children: 2001 yearbook. Washington, D.C.: Children's Defense Fund, 2001, p. 3. Copyright © 2001 by Children's Defense Fund. All rights reserved.)

of the wealthiest families grew by 66 percent—a sharp departure from the previous period (fig. 5-3).

Several factors account for this widening economic gap between wealth and poverty in the United States and this increasing skewing of family income. First, education now represents a "growing fault line in the economy." Workers with limited educational attainment find themselves increasingly relegated to the lowest wage jobs, disproportionately vulnerable to economic slowdowns and job layoffs, and at risk for underemployment. Among non–high school graduates, the median wage for full-time work dropped by 26 percent between 1979 and 2000; for high school graduates, the median wage declined 13 percent. Among black and Hispanic workers, the wage declines were even greater, and unemployment rates, higher.[23]

The failure of the government to intervene in the market is another major contributor to depressed income among such a large proportion of families with children. The minimum wage has failed to keep pace with inflation. In 1970, a minimum wage worker could earn enough from a full-time, year-round job to lift her family above 100 percent of the official federal poverty level—a bare subsistence to be sure, but significant. By 2001, the same full-time, year-round work yielded income equal to only 75 percent of the federal poverty level.[23]

A third cause of declining economic conditions for children has to do with family composition. In the United States, approximately one-fourth of children live with only one parent, a fraction that has risen steadily over the past decade. Between 1990 and 2001, the proportion of all U.S. births that were to unmarried women rose from 28 to 34 percent.[44] Only 8 percent of children who live with both parents are as likely to be poor compared with 42 percent of those who live with single mothers.[23] Numerous factors account for the prevalence of children living with single parents, especially greater social acceptability of both divorce and births to unmarried women of all ages. Whatever the underlying causes, single parenthood—which typically involves a single mother—almost automatically means lower economic prospects for both parent and child.

Failure to Invest in the Neediest Families

Given the market conditions that feed low wage and poverty-level work and promote formation of families at risk for poverty, direct economic interventions aimed at infusing both cash and in-kind income into low-income families thus become critical. Child support collections help. But collection is small in relation to the number of lower-income children living in single-parent families, principally because of inadequate resources to aid in collection of child-support payments and the low income of absent parents.[44] Direct government economic transfers, both cash and in-kind, become key for households headed by a single parent and for low-wage workers generally, regardless of structure of parental presence within the household.

There are several sources of economic cash transfer programs, including welfare assistance and income transfers based on the U.S. tax code. By far, the most important source of cash transfer has become the U.S. tax code, particularly true in the wake of the 1996 welfare reform legislation, which by 2001 had reduced already-low welfare rolls by another nearly 50 percent.[44] Studies suggest that most families work after leaving welfare; two-thirds of low-income children live in households in which someone works.[45] Jobs, however, are unstable, and wages, low.[23]

In this regard the Earned Income Tax Credit (EITC), which is available to low-income families under U.S. tax law, represents a critical source of family support. In 1999, the EITC resulted in a transfer of $31 billion to poor families and lifted 2.6 million of the nation's 16 million poor children entirely out of poverty. But as of 2001, the credit ended at $28,000, and only 15 states supplemented it.[23] In 18 of 42 states that impose a state income tax, poor families continued to owe income taxes in 2002.[46] The economic downturn that began in 2001 and has ravaged state economies poses a fundamental threat to further relief.

Some of the most critical income-transfer programs represent in-kind assistance, such as food stamps, housing assistance for rental housing (which would compensate for the failure of the U.S. tax code to recognize a renter's deduction comparable to the home mortgage deduction), and health insurance. Indeed, housing and health care assistance are two supports that are available to and heavily skewed toward affluent families. In the United States, the value of the home mortgage deduction increases as the value of homes rises and without regard to family income. In the case of health care insurance coverage, employer contributions to private insurance are not treated as taxable income, regardless of the income level of the family receiving assistance.

However, these favorable policies do not reach poor families who do not own homes or have employer-sponsored health insurance. Parents who have low-wage jobs tend to work for employers who offer no health care insurance coverage; as a result, these families receive no employment-based coverage, nor does the tax code provide them with refundable credits to secure affordable group coverage elsewhere. All states extend health insurance to poor and near-poor children under Medicaid and its smaller companion, the State Children's Health Insurance Program (SCHIP). But in 2003, only 39 states extended coverage to all children living at 200 percent of poverty while coverage for parents stood at approximately 71 percent of the federal poverty level.[47] Thus, despite advances in the expansion of public health insurance programs for children, 12 percent of all children, and over 20 percent of poor children, remained without health care insurance in 2002.[48] Minority children and adolescents are at particular risk for lack of coverage (fig. 5-4).

Housing statistics are particularly grim. In 2001, nearly 5 million families in 2001 paid over half their income for rent or lived in substandard housing.[23]

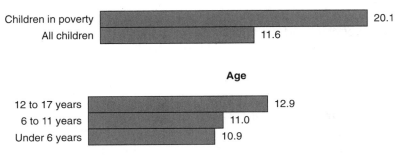

Age

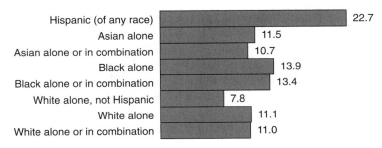

Race and Ethnicity

Figure 5-4 Percentage of children without health care insurance by poverty status, race, ethnicity, and age for 2002. (From U.S. Census Bureau. Health insurance coverage in the United States: 2002, p. 8, figure 4.)

According to a 2003 report, in only seven states could a person working full-time for the minimum wage afford the cost of a two-bedroom rental unit at fair market rental rates. In 40 states, workers needed twice the prevailing minimum wage to afford a two-bedroom rental unit. In the six most expensive states, workers needed to earn three times the minimum wage to afford the rent of a two-bedroom apartment.[49]

In recent years, access to food stamps has fallen sharply. Between 1996 and 2001, the number of food stamp recipients fell by 29 percent, from 24 million to 17 million.[23] More than half of the decrease occurred among the poorest recipients, a phenomenon attributed to the rollover effects of welfare reform on families' access to all forms of benefits, not merely cash welfare. Across-the-board termination of all types of assistance, as well as diversion of families away from seeking assistance for which they remained eligible (such as Medicaid or foods stamps), was pervasive.

Even the most disabled children have not been spared. The welfare reform amendments of 1996 included new restrictions on the Supplemental Security Income (SSI) program, which provides cash assistance to children with severe disabilities.[50] The effect of these changes, which involved new and restrictive criteria for determining disability, has been to remove hundreds of thousands of children from the rolls.

Finally, the effects of welfare reform arguably have been at their most draconian where immigrant children are concerned. As a result of the 1996 legislation, recently arrived, legally resident children no longer can qualify for either Medicaid or SCHIP. Only 19 states have adopted replacement programs for children barred from Medicaid and SCHIP eligibility as a result of the 1996 changes in immigration law.[51]

In addition, an increasingly aggressive stance by the federal government toward immigrant families has elevated their already-high concerns about the potential adverse impact on their legal U.S. status that could result from efforts to secure cash or medical or food assistance—even for eligible children born in this country.

The cumulative result of U.S. economic policies on families is startling. The United States leads industrialized nations in the percentage of children who are poor and lags behind all such nations in the proportion who are lifted out of childhood poverty by government policies (fig. 5-5).

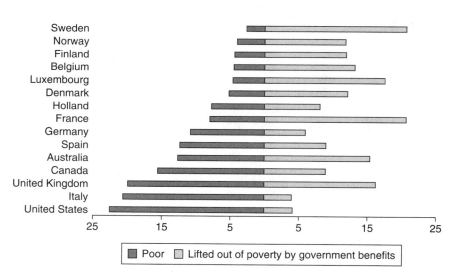

Figure 5-5 International poverty among all children: percent in poverty and percent lifted out of poverty by government benefits. (From Children's Defense Fund. The state of America's children: 2001 yearbook. Washington, D.C.: Children's Defense Fund; 2001, p. 10. Copyright © 2001 by Children's Defense Fund. All rights reserved.)

What Needs to Be Done

Improving the health of children in the United States means moving toward a time when all children live under conditions that foster strong growth and development, rather than act as impediments. It is one thing to say that the nation affords equal opportunity to all residents, but it is quite another to carefully, consciously, and affirmatively pursue the types of policies that make such assertions meaningful. Our national rhetoric is eloquent, but in meaningful follow-through our nation stumbles badly.

The United States has never been particularly good at community investment, but circumstances have grown far worse in recent years. Beginning in 2001, Congress has borrowed more than $4.5 trillion against the country's future, representing additional debt of more than $15,000 for every person in the United States.[52]

Promoting child health means a fundamental rejection of these choices in favor of investments in the families who will most benefit from them. Tax-based economic supports for workers, such as the EITC, could be further broadened to ensure that all families who work can escape low income. Programs for families who do not work because of illness and disability could be established that combine economic supports with education and job training to promote self-sufficiency. The same funds that have been plowed into lavish tax cuts for people who do not need them could instead be invested in maternity and parental leave policies for moderate-income families, the provision of high-quality child care services, universal health care coverage for children and their parents, education improvements (particularly for the poorest communities), and housing assistance. Rather than economically starving our most vulnerable families, the nation needs to invest in them, just as other nations with strong industrial economies have done.

Furthermore, protection of the environment ultimately is a child's issue in the United States. Air, water, and food quality investments may have their biggest payoffs in the lives and health of children, and the diminution and relaxation of standards take their worst toll on children.

Finally, vigilance toward the rights of children is essential. Strong, stable, and loving parents represent perhaps the most important asset to children. At the same time, children need to be safe in all environments, whether controlled by government, industry, or families. Even as the United States places primary emphasis on family-centeredness in the development of children, children deserve to be protected in all settings when necessary. Child welfare programs aimed at strengthening and supporting families through social investments and at providing rapid and preventive services to families under stress are critical to the overall health of children.

The Roles of Health Professionals

Health professionals must be vigilant and committed on behalf of children. Health professionals bring a unique power to the debate over the well-being and future of children because their opinions regarding the factors that underlie threats to children, as well as what can be done to ensure children's healthy growth and development, carry much weight with decision-makers at every level of public policy-making. Whether the issue is building a playground, expanding public health insurance programs, raising the minimum wage, or investing in children and their families in other ways, the power of health professionals must be brought to bear in public debate.

Accomplishing this goal means building a sustained and visible presence with decision-makers through ongoing communication strategies with elected and appointed officials. It also means ensuring that elected and appointed officials see both the conditions under which the poorest children live and success in action through visits to local programs that are making a difference in children's lives. In addition, it means organizing such visible activities as "get out the vote" efforts to support political candidates with strong track records of investment in services and programs that make a difference in the lives of children.

Finally, health professionals can make more personal investments, such as accepting publicly insured children into pediatric practices, volunteering at clinics serving low-income families, participating in community health outreach efforts to identify children at risk, promoting wellness activities in local schools and child care programs, and investing time and energy in other ways that promote concern about and commitment to the future of children.

Conclusion

This chapter has reviewed the impact of social injustice on children's health. It has summarized the rights of children under U.S. law, particularly the legal standards that determine children's personhood status and the corresponding duties that personhood status confers on government. This chapter has also examined important child health indicators, the factors that influence child health, and the pivotal role played in health determinants by measures of growth and development. The well-being of children is critically influenced by far more than medical care. Indeed, the well-being of children depends on many investments, such as adequate family income, safe housing and neighborhoods, and caregivers whose own lives are sufficiently supported to be able to invest time in and nurture their children.

While most children lead healthy lives punctuated by episodes of acute illness, a substantial proportion of children experience significant disabilities and functional limitations that require ongoing investments to foster growth and development.

There is no more serious threat to children and their families in this country than poverty and its consequences, which largely result from societal policies that compare poorly with those of other nations. Health professionals and others can play critical roles in promoting social justice and the health of children by advocating for progressive social policies and personally investing time and energy in activities to promote children's health and well-being.

References

1. G.A. Res. 44/25, U.N. GAOR, 44th Sess., Supp. No. 49, at 167 U.N. Doc. A/44/49 (1989).
2. Office of the United Nations High Commissioner for Human Rights. Status of ratifications of the principal international human rights treaties (Nov. 2003). Available at: http://www.unhchr.ch/pdf/report.pdf [last modified Nov. 2003]. Accessed January 10, 2005.
3. Woodhouse BB. Speaking truth to power: challenging the power of parents to control the education of their own. 11 Cornell J.L. & Pub. Policy 481, 499 (Spring 2002).
4. *Roper v. Simmons*, 125 S. Ct. 1833 (2005) (holding that the death penalty for offenders under the age of 18 violates the 8th Amendment's prohibition of "cruel and unusual punishments").
5. Amnesty International. Death penalty facts. Available at: http://www.amnestyusa. org/abolish/juveniles.html. Accessed January 10, 2005.
6. Amnesty International. United States of America: rights of children must be respected, April 25, 2003. Available at: http://www.web.amnesty.org/library/index/ ENGAMR510582003. Accessed January 10, 2005.
7. See *Roe v. Wade*, 410 U.S. 113 (1973) and *Planned Parenthood v. Casey*, 505 U.S. 833 (1992).
8. See *In re Gault*, 387 U.S. 1 (1967) (juvenile offender has procedural due-process rights); *Tinker v. Des Moines Indep. Cmty. Sch. Dist.*, 393 U.S. 503, 506 (1969) (free speech right to wear armbands in school to protest war); *Brown v. Bd. of Educ.*, 347 U.S. 483 (1957) (14th Amendment applies to school children).
9. *Bellotti v. Baird*, 443 U.S. 622, 634, 635 (1979).
10. *Meyer v. Nebraska*, 262 U.S. 390 (1923) (invalidation of state laws that prohibited teaching a class below the eighth grade in any other language other than English— violation of parents' 14th Amendment liberty interest to control the education of their children); *Pierce v. Soc'y of Sisters*, 268 US 510 (1925) (state law requiring parents to enroll their children in public rather than private elementary schools struck down— violation of parents' substantive due process rights to control education of their children); *Wisconsin v. Yoder*, 406 U.S. 205 (1972) (1st and 14th Amendment allows parents the right to educate their children at home according to their faith. In *Yoder*, the Court held that state compulsory education law violated the constitutional rights of Amish parents to educate their children at home according to their religion).

11. *Troxel v. Granville*, 530 U.S. 57, 65 (2000) (state statute allowing "any person" to petition the court for visitation rights violated parent's substantive due process rights).

12. *DeShaney v. Winnebago County Dep't of Soc. Serv.*, 489 U.S. 189, 196 (1989).

13. *Estelle v. Gamble,* 429 U.S. 97 (1976) (states have a duty to provide basic medical services to prisoners); *Youngberg v. Romero*, 457 U.S. 307 (1982) (states have a duty to protect the involuntarily committed).

14. *Parham v. J.R.*, 442 U.S. 584 (1979).

15. *Bellotti v. Baird*, 443 U.S. 622, 643 (1979). See also, *Planned Parenthood of Central Mo. v. Danforth*, 428 U.S. 52 (1976) and *Ohio v. Akron Ctr. for Reprod. Health*, 497 U.S. 502, 510-19 (1990).

16. Children are individuals under 18 years. See Starfield B. Child and adolescent health status measures, the future of children: U.S. Health Care for Children 2:2 (1992), pp 25–40. Available at: http://www.futureofchildren.org/information2827/information_show.htm?doc_id=77358. Accessed January 10, 2005.

17. U.S. Department of Health and Human Services, Centers for Disease Control and Prevention. Health United States, 2003. DHHS publication no. 2003-1232, 2003: table 19.

18. U.S. Department of Health and Human Services, Centers for Disease Control and Prevention. Health United States, 2003. DHHS publication no. 2003-1232, 2003: table 13.

19. U.S. Department of Health and Human Services, Centers for Disease Control and Prevention. Health United States, 2003. DHHS publication no. 2003-1232, 2003: table 71.

20. U.S. Department of Health and Human Services, Centers for Disease Control and Prevention. Health United States, 2003. DHHS publication no. 2003-1232, 2003: table 74.

21. Szilagyi P. Care of children with special health care needs, the future of children: health insurance for children, 13:1, Spring 2003:137–153. Available at: http://www.futureofchildren.org/information2827/information_show.htm?doc_id=175466. Accessed February 21, 2005.

22. U.S. Department of Health and Human Services, Centers for Disease Control and Prevention. Health United States, 2003. Department of Health and Human Services publication No. 2003-1232, 2003: table 57.

23. Children's Defense Fund. The state of America's children: 2001 yearbook. Washington, D.C., 2001:37.

24. Halfon N, Regalado M, McLearn KT, et al. Building a bridge from birth to school: improving developmental and behavioral services for young children. New York, N.Y.: Commonwealth Fund. Available at: http://www.cmwf.org/publications/publications_show.htm?doc_id=221307. Accessed February 21, 2005.

25. National Center for Children in Poverty. Low income children in the United States. New York, N.Y.: Columbia University, 2003. Available at: http://www.nccp.org/pub_cpf03.html. Accessed January 10, 2005.

26. U.S. Census Bureau. Poverty in the United States: 2000. Washington, D.C.: U.S. Department of Commerce, 2001: table E.

27. Rowland D. Health challenges facing the nation. Joint Economic Committee, United States Congress, Oct. 1, 2003.

28. Epstein H. Enough to make you sick? *New York Times,* Oct. 12, 2003 (magazine). Available at: http://www.nytimes.com/2003/10/12/magazine/12HEALTH.html. Accessed January 10, 2005.

29. Center for Children's Health and the Environment. Children's Unique Vulnerability to Environmental Toxins. New York, N.Y.: Mt Sinai School of Medicine. Available at: http://childenvironment.org/factsheets/childrens_vulnerability.htm. Accessed January 10, 2005.

30. Center for Children's Health and the Environment. The coming of age of environmental pediatrics. New York, N.Y.: Mt Sinai School of Medicine. Available at: http://childenvironment.org/factsheets/environmental_pediatrics.htm. Accessed January 10, 2005.

31. National Center for Environmental Health, Centers for Disease Control and Prevention. What every parent should know about lead poisoning in children. Atlanta, Ga.: CDC. Available at: htttp://www.cdc.gov/nceh/lead/fac/cdc97a.htm. Accessed January 10, 2005.

32. Low lead levels, below those once thought safe, pose risk to children's cognitive functioning, Cornell scientists report. *Cornell News*, April 14, 2003. Available at: http://www.news.cornell.edu/releases/April03/lowlead.kids.ssl.html. Accessed January 10, 2005.

33. U.S. Census Bureau. Current population survey, 2003 Annual social and economic supplement, single-year of age poverty status: 2002 below 100% of poverty—all races. Washington, D.C., U.S. Government Printing Office. Available at: http://ferret.bls. census.gov/macro/032003/pov/new34_100_01.htm [Table POV 34]. Accessed January 10, 2005.

34. U.S. Environmental Protection Agency. America's children and the environment: measure E9: hazardous waste sites. Washington, D.C., U.S. Government Printing Office. Available at: http://www.epa.gov/envirohealth/children/contaminants/e9.htm. Accessed January 10, 2005.

35. Agency for Toxic Substances and Disease Registry, Centers for Disease Control and Prevention. Children's health. Atlanta, Ga.: CDC. Available at: http://www.atsdr. cdc.gov/child/. Accessed January 10, 2005.

36. U.S. Environmental Protection Agency. America's children and the environment (ACE)—environmental contaminants. Washington, D.C., U.S. Government Printing Office. Available at: http://www.epa.gov/envirohealth/children/contaminants/index.htm. Accessed January 10, 2005.

37. U.S. Environmental Protection Agency. America's children and the environment (ACE)—environmental contaminants: data tables. Washington, D.C., U.S. Government Printing Office. Available at: http://www.epa.gov/envirohealth/children/contaminants/ tables.htm. Accessed January 10, 2005.

38. National Center for Health Statistics, Centers for Disease Control and Prevention. Asthma prevalence, health care use and mortality, 2000–2001. Atlanta, Ga.: CDC. Available at: http://www.cdc.gov/nchs/products/pubs/pubd/hestats/asthma/asthma.htm. Accessed January 10, 2005.

39. American Lung Association. Trends in asthma morbidity and mortality. 2001. Available at: http://www.lungusa.org/data/asthma/asthmach_1.html. Accessed January 10, 2005.

40. Shore M. Out of control and close to home: mercury pollution from power plants. 2003. Available at: http://www.environmentaldefense.org/documents/3370_MercuryPower Plants.df. Accessed January 10, 2005.

41. U.S. Environmental Protection Agency. Measure E8: pesticide residue on foods frequently consumed by children. Washington, D.C., U.S. Government Printing Office. Available at: http://www.epa.gov/envirohealth/children/contaminants/e8.htm. Accessed January 10, 2005.

42. U.S. Environmental Protection Agency. Pesticides and food: why children may be especially sensitive to pesticides. Washington, D.C.: U.S. Government Printing Office. Available at: http://www.epa.gov/pesticides/food/pest.htm. Accessed January 10, 2005.

43. Children's Defense Fund. Child health: general health facts. Available at: http://www.childrensdefense.org/childhealth/generalhealthfacts.asp. Accessed January 10, 2005.

44. Annie E. Casey Foundation. Kids Count 2003 data book online. Available at: http://www.aecf.org/kidscount/databook/summary/summary12.htm. Accessed January 10, 2005.

45. National Center for Children in Poverty. Low income children in the United States. New York, N.Y.: Columbia University, 2003. Available at: http://www.nccp.org/pub_cpf03.html. Accessed January 10, 2005.

46. Johnson N, Zahradnik B, Llobrera J. State income tax burdens on low income families in 2002. Washington, D.C.: Center on Budget and Policy Priorities, 2003. Available at: http://www.cbpp.org/4-11-03sfp.pdf. Accessed January 10, 2005.

47. Cohen Ross D, Cox L. Preserving recent progress on health coverage for children and families: new tensions emerge. Washington, D.C.: Kaiser Commission on Medicaid and the Uninsured, 2003. Available at: http://www.kff.org/content/2003/20030729/4125exec.pdf. Accessed January 10, 2005.

48. U.S. Census Bureau. Health insurance coverage in the United States: 2002 U.S. Department of Commerce, current population reports P60-223. September 2003, figure 4.

49. Clemenson L. Poor workers finding modest housing unaffordable study says. *New York Times*, September 9, 2003:A15.

50. Personal Responsibility and Work Opportunity Reconciliation Act of 1996 (Public Law 104-193, 104th Congress, 2nd Session).

51. Chin K, Dean S, Patchan K. How have states responded to the eligibility restrictions on legal immigrants in Medicaid and SCHIP? Washington, D.C.: Kaiser Family Foundation, 2002. Available at: http://www.kff.org/medicaid/upload/13988_1.pdf. Accessed January 10, 2005.

52. Children's Defense Fund Action Council. What you need to know and do to truly leave no child behind. Washington, D.C., 2003.

6

OLDER PEOPLE

Carroll L. Estes and Steven P. Wallace

Introduction

Despite the growing academic and political interest in health equity and in social justice in health care, little attention has been paid to these issues as they relate to older people.

In the United States, *Healthy People 2010* has two central goals—one focusing on equity, to eliminate health disparities, and the other linked to aging, to increase the quality and years of healthy life. Although many of the *Healthy People 2010* targets focus on issues of concern to older persons, disparities among age groups are not included. This omission occurred while the United Nations was declaring 1999 the International Year of Older Persons and developing a program on "Building a Society for all Ages"[1] that links the status of older people to that of others in society. There is a burgeoning literature on disparities within the older population,[2,3] but there has been a decline during the past 30 years in attention given to ageism and inequities based on age. The growing popularity of trends such as "antiaging" medicine and the continuing efforts to blame the elderly for projected deficits in Medicare and Social Security suggest that older people are likely to face less equitable treatment because of their age in the future unless social policies and political ideologies change. Thus, it is important to consider both the inequities within the older population and between the older and younger populations.

Eliminating inequities in the determinants of health care and health status for older people is an ethical imperative. However, it is also in society's social and material interest to promote conditions in which older people can be healthy. Many older people continue to contribute to their families and communities through very old age,[4] and as the "baby-boom" generation ages, an even larger pool of older people with valuable skills and experiences will become important resources. If older people are not healthy, their ability to contribute to their communities declines, and the costs of their debilitating illnesses are borne by society.

The Global Challenge

Population aging is often thought of as a phenomenon of developed countries, but it marks developing countries as well. The number of elderly people (aged 60 and above) exceeded 600 million worldwide in 2000 and is projected to reach 2 billion by 2050.[5] The older population is growing fastest in developing countries, where currently almost two-thirds of all older people (355 million) now live. By 2025, 75 percent of all elderly people are expected to be residing in developing countries. In developed countries, the fastest growing age group is 80 and older. In 1996, almost half (43 percent) of people aged 75 and older lived in four countries: China, the United States, India, and Japan. Life expectancy remains below 50 in more than 10 developing countries, and since 1970, it has fallen or barely risen, in several African countries.[6] Both the AIDS pandemic and development loans requiring the privatization of health care have lowered life expectancy in many developing countries.[7]

Increasing life expectancy is usually viewed as a societal achievement, but it is also seen as a socioeconomic burden of crisis proportions by adherents of "apocalyptic demography."[8] This view, common in the United States and elsewhere, assumes that aging populations will burden public policies to the point of creating disastrous social consequences. Dire warnings of impending national bankruptcy, underinvestment in children, and the overwhelming of available family support stem have been voiced.[9] This scapegoats the elderly for political problems such as budget deficits that reflect tax cuts and rising military spending.[10,11] Internationally, aging is not distinct from social integration, gender advancement, economic stability, or issues of poverty, and societies need to recognize the potential benefits from ongoing contributions of older people.[12]

The aging of societies is mainly an issue of older women.[13] In all societies, women outlive men; by very old age, the female-to-male ratio is generally 2:1.[5] This is a formidable challenge because women are caregivers for people of all ages, especially children and, increasingly, grandchildren. For example, in places where HIV/AIDS prevalence is high, older women are essential caregivers of their adult children and their orphaned grandchildren. Although unpaid, women's caregiving work generally ceases only when they are physically and mentally unable to provide it and in need of care themselves. As a result, older women worldwide experience more economic deprivation and insecurity than do older men.[14] Older women are highly vulnerable to the government upheavals and restrictions of safety-net policies, especially in developing countries.

"Building a Society for All Ages," the theme of the Second World Assembly on Ageing (2002), developed a framework for economic development and poverty reduction that emphasized the importance of active aging, intergenerational solidarity, and the necessity of developed countries helping developing countries.[1] Participants at this conference discussed principles of justice that are used to legitimate social policies. The United States and other developed countries have been supporting free-market–oriented policies that embody an individualistic principle of justice, based on a utilitarian philosophy where maximizing the sum of individuals' health and wealth has been the primary goal—as reflected in regularly reported data on life expectancy and gross domestic product (GDP). These measures ignore the distribution of health and wealth, making them inadequate—even detrimental—to ensuring equal opportunities for all.[1]

One example of implementing increased attention to equity is the recent framework of the World Health Organization (WHO) for evaluating health systems. Its two health objectives—the best attainable level (goodness) and the smallest feasible differences among individuals and groups (fairness)— are applied across three key dimensions of health systems: (a) health outcomes, such as mortality and morbidity; (b) the responsiveness of the health care system, such as being treated with dignity and technically competent care; and (c) the financing of the system. Although not incorporated in the current United Nations documents on aging, such performance measures need to be applied to older people.[2]

The Impact of Social Injustice on the Health of Older People

Injustice among the elderly is well documented. Health status varies by race, ethnicity, income, and gender among older persons. Older African-Americans have worse health than do older whites across all measures of health status, including disease, disability, and self-assessed health.[15] Older Latinos have lower rates than do non-Latino whites of some diseases, most notably heart disease and stroke, but higher rates of diabetes and of disability.[2] Poverty is

TABLE 6-1   Percentage of Self-Assessed Health Status of Persons Aged 65 and Over by Income, Race/Ethnicity, and Gender, United States, 1999

	Fair/Poor Self-Assessed Health
Income	
Below poverty level	36.0
Low: 100–199% poverty level	31.9
Middle: 200–399% poverty level	22.4
High: ≥400% poverty level	16.4
Race/Ethnicity	
Non-Latino African-American	37.7
Non-Latino white	23.0
Latino	34.0
Gender	
Women	25.1
Men	23.7

Modified from Agency for Healthcare Research and Quality, Household Component Analytical Tool (MEPSnet/HC). Rockville, Md.: AHRQ, 2003.

strongly associated with all measures of poor health in old age. And women have more chronic conditions and disability than do men, despite their greater life expectancy.

Self-assessed health status, a good predictor of death and disability as well as current health status,[16] follows social categories of inequality. Older people with the lowest income are more than twice as likely as older people with high incomes to report reduced health status (table 6-1). Both Latinos and non-Latino African-Americans are about 50 percent more likely to report reduced health status as are non-Latino whites. Women are somewhat more likely to report reduced health status than are men.

With the substantial reduction in deaths from acute infectious diseases during the past century, mortality is increasingly due to chronic conditions that are most common in old age. With aging, the disease profile shifts from predominantly infectious diseases to predominantly chronic and degenerative noncommunicable diseases, such as arthritis, hypertension, coronary artery disease, cerebrovascular disease, and cancer. This "epidemiological transition" has occurred in developed countries and is occurring in developing countries.[17] Many chronic diseases could be prevented or delayed through health promotion and disease prevention strategies. Older African-Americans have more chronic conditions than do older whites, and older women have more than do older men (table 6-2).

TABLE 6-2   Percentage of Older People (Aged 65 or Older) With Chronic Conditions, by Race, Ethnicity, and Gender, United States, 2000

	Stroke	Diabetes	Mobility Limitation	Incontinence	Two or More Chronic Conditions*
Non-Latino whites	11.3	16.0	47.3	27.6	71.6
African-Americans	13.3	28.3	56.6	24.0	76.9
Latinos	9.9	23.3	47.6	21.4	67.9
Women	11.1	16.9	53.7	34.6	76.1
Men	11.7	18.8	40.1	15.9	65.6

*Hypertension, diabetes, arthritis, osteoporosis/broken hip, pulmonary disease, stroke, Alzheimer's disease, Parkinson's disease, skin cancer, other cancer.

From Center for Medicare and Medicaid Services (CMS). The characteristics and perceptions of the Medicare population: data from the 2000 Medicare Current Beneficiary Survey. Baltimore, Md.: CMS, 2003.

Elderly people in the United States, where disability rates have declined in recent years, are projected to have healthier lifestyles and better health than comparably aged people in the past.[18] The global generalizability of this trend, however, remains to be established; instead, there may be increasing "population frailty,"[19] longer life but worsening health, and increased morbidity as people live longer, placing greater demands on the health care system.[20]

Inequities also exist in the access to health services by different population groups of older persons. The same social and economic characteristics that are associated with worse health outcomes account for documented differences in the level of use of health services. Unmet medical needs are more common among older African-Americans, those with incomes below the poverty line, and older women (table 6-3). Although most older people have a

TABLE 6-3   Percentage Reporting Access to Health Care Problems, Persons Aged 65 and Over, by Race, Poverty, and Gender, United States, 1993

	Unmet Medical Needs	No Regular Source of Care	Regular Source of Care Not a Private Physician
Whites	9.9	6.1	7.2
African-Americans	18.4	6.6	22.1
Income at or above poverty level	8.8	5.6	7.8
Income below poverty level	27.2	8.2	15.5
Older men	8.7	6.7	10.9
Older women	12.0	5.7	7.0

From Cohen RA, et al. Access to health care, part 3: older adults (series 10, volume 198). Hyattsville, Md.: Vital Health Statistics, National Center for Health Statistics, 1997.

regular site for health care, older African-Americans and those with incomes below the poverty line are less like to have a private physician as their regular source of care; they are more likely to seek care at clinics with reduced continuity of care and limited services.

In addition to differences in receiving any health care, there are disparities among older people in the quality of care they receive. The Institute of Medicine has determined that racial and ethnic disparities in health care are independent of economic status, health insurance, and other factors.[21] Some of the differences in quality of care among older people are reflected in measures of satisfaction with care. Older African-Americans have the lowest satisfaction rates; Latinos, intermediate rates; and whites, the highest rates (table 6-4).

In sum, inequities exist in health status, access to health care, and the quality of care received among different groups of older people based on their social characteristics.

In addition to the inequities that exist within the older population, there is a continuing bias against older people as a group in several health-related dimensions. For example, there is much devaluing of older people by health professionals[22,23] and social-policymakers. Treatment decisions for older people are often influenced by the person's age, rather than a consideration of the costs and benefits of treatment. Older people, for example, are less likely to receive recommendations for cancer treatments that could extend their lives than younger people, even when there is no medical reason to avoid those treatments. The pattern of undertreatment is exacerbated by the underrepresentation of older people in most clinical trials.[24] Some even suggest that older people, such as those over age 80, should receive no curative treatments, regardless of their prognosis, because they have lived out their "natural" lives.[25,26]

Older people are often devalued in discussions of the costs of health and social programs that they use.[11] Some policymakers blame the rising costs of

TABLE 6-4   Percentage of People Aged 65 to 74 Who Are Very Satisfied With Care, United States, 2000

	Follow-up Care	Ease of Access to Physician	Information From Physician	Physician's Concern for Overall Health
White, non-Latinos	22.6	25.1	22.9	23.6
African-American, non-Latinos	11.5	11.4	11.2	11.9
Latinos	18.2	20.2	18.8	17.6
Men	21.1	23.5	21.7	21.8
Women	21.4	23.1	21.2	22.4

From Center for Medicare and Medicaid Services (CMS). The characteristics and perceptions of the Medicare population: data from the 2000 Medicare Current Beneficiary Survey. Baltimore, Md.: CMS, 2003.

Medicare on older people, even though much medical treatment is driven by physician referral, not patient demand. In addition, the rapidly rising costs of prescription medications appear to be largely a function of manufacturer-induced demand (especially by direct advertising to consumers) for high-cost drugs, rather than use of new drugs that improve treatment of disease.[27]

Furthermore, our technology-intensive medical care system is increasingly inappropriate for the chronic disease challenges of older people, including hearing problems, falls, incontinence, and social isolation, as well as polypharmacy and the need for end-of-life care.[28–30] These challenges do not usually require expensive tests, surgical interventions, or state-of-the-art technology. An example is the current treatment pattern of older people with incontinence—a socially embarrassing condition that contributes to social isolation and increases the risk for deconditioning, falls, and institutionalization. It is often erroneously seen as a "normal" part of growing old.[31] Although behavioral therapy, including pelvic exercises, is the most effective treatment of urinary incontinence,[32] drug therapy, surgery, and the use of adult diapers continue to be the most common forms of treatments. An estimated 8 percent of women aged 60 and older have ever had surgery for incontinence.[33] Among men and women over age 50 with incontinence, 20 percent use pads or other absorbent supplies.[34] Adult diapers and drugs produce significant profits for their manufacturers, creating incentives to promote those products; in contrast, behavioral therapy is time-consuming and not very profitable. As a result, many older people with incontinence do not receive adequate treatment for this condition.

Roots and Underlying Causes

Among the underlying causes of social injustice affecting the health of older people are (a) poverty and inequalities associated with differences in socioeconomic status (SES) over the life course (the "graying" of the SES gradient), (b) the biomedicalization of aging, and (c) globalization.

The Graying of the Socioeconomic Status–Health Gradient

The association between health and poverty in all age groups also affects older people. The poor have reduced life expectancy, lower self-rated health status, increased morbidity and disability, and worse functional status.[19] SES, whether defined by income, education, employment, poverty, or wealth, is inversely associated with mortality in virtually all countries studied.[35,36] In addition, socioeconomic inequality, independent of economic status, is related to health status.[37]

The inequitable circumstances of older women and older people of color can be explained by cumulative disadvantage across the life span.[38–40] Health is a life course phenomenon. There is a crucial connection among late-life health, one's early health status, and health events across the life span. Thus, where social injustice early in life affects one's health, health care, and life chances, it is likely to be mirrored later in life.[5] Over the life course, three different types of resources convert early-life inequities into later-life inequities in health: (a) human capital—knowledge and skills of individuals that influence employment, job satisfaction, and income; (b) social capital—the types and density of ties among people that enhance social integration and support; and (c) personal capital—in lifestyle, sense of efficacy, and personal control, which has mainly developed during younger adult years.[38]

Health is influenced throughout the life course by the interactive effects of racism, sexism, social class, and ageism on human, social, and personal capital.[41–44] These inequalities are significantly influenced by the institutional effects of race, government, the market, gender, and family structures.[42,45] Poverty in older women stems partly from "the family care penalty"—the economic and health costs to female caregivers for their substantial unpaid caregiving throughout their life course that affects their ability to develop this human capital.[46] Older women's dependence on the government, including the public health system, increases with aging, widowhood, divorce, and declining economic and health status.[47] Privatization of core public services and reduction of public pensions compound the gender disadvantages of earlier life and place older women at a higher risk for adverse health consequences.[48] Social class and gender inequalities are reproduced by the government through retirement policies that allow the extreme disparities of wealth in adulthood to continue into old age.[39] And housing, employment, and other markets that discriminate against persons of color in early life continue their patterns into old age.

The Biomedicalization of Aging

In Western countries, especially the United States, during the past century and the start of this century, old age has often been equated with specific diseases or a general pathological state. The cultural aversion to aging and veneration of youth has spawned negative attitudes toward older people that are sometimes internalized and manifested in personal low self-esteem, low self-efficacy, and low sense of control—all of which are risk factors for dependency, depression, and illness.[49] The response to this trend has been to define the problems that face older people as rooted in biology and to place the treatment of these problems in the realm of medicine. This biomedicalization of aging[50] has facilitated the "commodification" of the needs of older people, which has, in turn, produced a costly and highly profitable "aging enterprise" and enlarged the medical-industrial complex.[51,52] As a result, the goal of producing medical goods and services has shifted from fulfilling human needs (basic shelter and nutrition) to monetary exchange and private profit—and, with it, increasing social inequality.

The biomedicalization of aging obscures the extent to which the health of older people can be improved by modifying social, economic, political, and environmental factors. Biological and genetic factors account for only 30 percent of successful aging, while behavioral, social, and environmental factors account for 70 percent.[53] Therefore, public health approaches are more likely to support population-level interventions than are approaches that focus on individual behaviors and personal responsibility.[54] Nonbiomedical, population approaches to improving the health of older persons include (a) making a more-equal distribution of wealth; (b) increasing education opportunities; (c) providing adequate housing for all; (d) enhancing the opportunities for meaningful human connections; (e) offering public guarantees of universal access to health care, including long-term care and rehabilitation; and (f) creating policies and community environments that promote healthful behaviors, such as diet and exercise.[55]

Globalization

Growing old is increasingly viewed in a transnational context of international organizations and cross-border migration that creates new conditions and challenges for older people and their families. There is a growing tension between an individual country's policies on aging and those formulated by global organizations and institutions. Aging can no longer be viewed solely as a national issue.[7]

International financial institutions that would gain enormous wealth through privatization claim that no country can afford to support older people through publicly guaranteed retirement and health programs.[48] These institutions use the aging of the population as a reason to pressure governments to privatize pension and health systems—moving away from systems based on social solidarity (where all citizens share financial risk) to systems of individual capitation (where each person is at individual risk).[48]

In developing countries, the marginalization of women occurs when government no longer protects subsistence activities. Women's economic participation is restricted with the (a) increase of self-regulating markets and privatization of farm land for cash crops, creating food insecurity; (b) increase in out-of-pocket costs that accompanies privatization of health services; and (c) decrease in government support for other vital services.[56] These forces encourage some women from developing countries to move to developed countries, where they find work as caregivers for other's children and older people, even as they rely on female relatives back home to care for their own children and aging parents.

What Needs to Be Done

Given the cumulative lifetime disadvantage underlying much of the social injustice that affects the health of older people, measures need to be taken to improve the distribution of health and health services among both the current generation of older people and people who are now young and represent future generations of older people. Today's older people cannot easily change their lifetime history of employment earnings, living conditions, or other resources. Addressing social injustice among older people requires intervention with social policies that reduce inequities—by race, ethnicity, income, and gender—in retirement income, quality of medical care, and community integration.

To promote policy change, it is necessary to raise political awareness.[57] Because older people of color, older poor people, and older women tend to be disenfranchised from the political process,[58] it is important to increase understanding about the health status, process of care, and financial burdens of these groups of older people. Organizations that focus on race and ethnicity, poverty, and women's health need to join those that focus on aging to support this work.

Health policies that focus on structural factors, such as the organization and financing of medical care and the social environment where older people live, affect the entire population. Population-based interventions that potentially affect all older people, such as ensuring access to health care, have the potential political advantage of drawing support from others, including middle-class and politically influential people. Improving the health of older people in the United States therefore requires changing the health care system so that all older people receive appropriate care.

Public policy can influence other important changes in the health care system, including changes in the composition of the health care workforce and the financial incentives within the system. Because patients' satisfaction with physicians is higher when they can choose physicians of the same ethnicity,[59] equity in medical care depends, in part, on the racial and ethnic composition of the physician workforce. Members of racial and ethnic minority groups need to be provided the tools and incentives to pursue careers in health care.

There are also important community level changes that do not involve the medical care system that promote health. Building large supermarkets in inner cities, for example, can increase the consumption of fruits and vegetables by low-income older people.[60] Policies that encourage such construction—usually thought of as economic-development or zoning policies—are also important health policies that may help reduce disparities in nutrition and health. In general, providing older people with financial resources to obtain adequate housing, nutrition, and medical care would contribute to reducing many of the financing, process-of-care, and health-status inequities that they experience.

All of these types of policy changes will require broad coalitions of advocates. Policies that substantially improve the distribution of resources to older people, such as Social Security and Medicare, have been adopted when there has been a broad coalition of advocates, including organized labor, citizen's groups, and health professionals.[61]

To improve equity and justice for the coming generations of older persons, it is most effective if we address earlier phases of the life course. Public policy should encourage the payment of a living wage so that lifetime earnings can lead to Social Security and pension benefits that provide a reasonable income. Recent federal tax reductions, which cut inheritance and unearned-income taxes, have exacerbated inequality by lowering taxes on income that the wealthy rely on while maintaining or increasing payroll taxes paid mainly by lower- and middle-income workers. Racial and gender inequities in wages also need to be addressed because these disparities generate lifelong disadvantages.

Incentives are needed in the U.S. medical care system that promote the most efficacious and least invasive ways of improving the health and quality of life of older people. This will require reimbursement mechanisms and practice settings that prioritize chronic conditions and palliative care.

The United Nations publication *World Ageing Situation*[62] calls for revolutionary thinking in which aging is viewed as a lifelong and society-wide phenomenon that permeates all social, economic, and cultural spheres, compelling "policy interventions that include social and human, as well as economic, investments." Regrettably, neither the WHO nor the United Nations as a whole appears poised to implement either revolutionary thinking or action. Heavily influenced by health and aging research in the developed countries and the U.S. paradigm of "successful" and "productive" aging,[63-65] both the WHO and the United Nations have adopted an overarching general objective of "active aging"—enhancing the quality of life of older people through activities and efforts that increase health, participation, and security.[66]

According to the WHO publication *Towards Policy for Health and Ageing*, there is a dual challenge: first, applying public health measures to achieve healthy aging, and, second, increasing access to affordable medical care.[66] From a public health perspective, more than medical interventions are needed to improve the health of the elderly, especially in developing countries.[67] A healthy life course depends on the safety and security of family and home, housing, sanitation, food and economic security, and a health strategy built on the principles of primary care and supportive social and rehabilitative care.

From a public health perspective, the overall focus on active aging reflects a scientifically proscribed area of emphasis to improve the health of "couch potatoes" in developed countries. The calls for age-friendly services and institutions and long-term care are appropriate. However, even in developed countries, there is a valid critique of an overemphasis on "active aging" insofar as it draws attention and resources away from efforts to overcome the pervasive inequalities and formidable structural barriers of class, race, and gender across the life course[68] that, cumulatively, produce serious health disparities.[40,69] The active aging mantra risks blaming the victim while elevating productivity as the only acceptable metaphor for a good old age.[70] For older women, the message appears to be that there is no end to one's responsibility for unpaid caregiving—now recast as "productive," if rendered during old age.

From a public health perspective, the international documents do not reflect and inculcate strategies that link health services and health improvements with wider fields of intersectoral action, including adequate sanitation, housing, and potable water.[71] In the context of globalization, pressures for privatization, the power of international financial markets and medical-pharmaceutical markets, and the biomedicalization of aging, it is likely that the demography of aging will become an excuse to impose on the world's poor "prefabricated, selectively chosen, market- and technology-driven, externally monitored, and dependency-producing programs."[71]

Although social injustice is inherent in the denial of the means to health, in developing countries the key health issues and best means for addressing them are not likely to be the same as in developed countries. In the poorest developing countries, obtaining the basic necessities of survival precede all other needs and the consequences of injustice against the elderly, the poor, and women are likely to be life-threatening. Inequities between rich and poor countries in the terms of trade and impact of globalization serve to exacerbate the internal inequities. (See chapter 21.)

Fighting Back: Reclaiming Public Health and the State

Older people, women, minorities, and the poor have been largely absent from influential debates of the World Bank—against public pensions—and the World Trade Organization (WTO)—for the commercialization of care services. The major participants in these debates have been governments from rich countries, wishing to deregulate government provision of services, and corporations, wanting to expand into lucrative areas of work worldwide.[7,72,73] Major players in the international trade of health services include health insurance companies, drug companies, and medical equipment suppliers.

Opponents of globalization have been mobilized in areas of human rights, ecology, women's rights, race and ethnic justice, and worker rights. (See box 19-2 on p. 348.) Elder rights advocates are invisible, except for the largely uncritical formal positions articulated in United Nations and WHO documents that offer little guidance or evidence of commitment to the goals of universal, collective, and social obligations enacted through government programs. Although not "wrong" in their entirety, current United Nations and WHO efforts are no match for the active efforts of the WTO, the International Monetary Fund, and the World Bank to privatize government provision of social care and support for the aged. The privatization of those services is now commonly inserted as a condition of development loans and debt relief to developing countries, known as structural adjustment.

Organizations representing older people need to link with larger organizations and forums working on a global justice agenda. The recent upsurge of political activity among pensioners in a number of countries[74] offers a potentially important platform upon which to build age-integrated social movement for social change. The joining of the movements of opposition to the worst abuses of globalization is essential and the role of older-people's organizations is pivotal because older people have much to lose should there be widespread privatization of public health and retirement programs.

An example of positive networking is in the actions of eastern European and Third-World women networking in struggles that define women's rights as human rights as a key principle of citizenship. These efforts have occurred through collaborations, such as Women's EDGE, the Association for Women in Development, the Center for Economic Justice, InterAction/Commission on the Advancement of Women (2000), and the Open Society Institute's Network Women's Program (2002). Declining female political participation and relegation to traditional women's work inspired the first independent Women's Forum in the former Soviet Union in 1991 that adopted the platform that "democracy without women is no democracy." Forms of resistance and collective action are also emerging in submerged networks (those without defined organizational structures), such as the Internet, and everyday forms of resistance, such as boycotts of certain products and business entities.[56] Globalization does not inexorably lead to minimal levels of social protection.[75,76] The road map for the work ahead consists of actions and activities that install pro-welfare, social-protection, and full-employment policies.[77]

Conclusion

Rights for older people must be defined as basic human rights. Social justice for older people must begin with the assertion of the human right to health, as established in the Universal Declaration of Human Rights and other international agreements. This includes the human rights of older people as a group, as well as subgroups of older people who have suffered lifelong injustice. Working to reduce the socioeconomic-health gradient at all ages promotes justice for both current and future cohorts of older people. Promoting public health approaches to aging will reduce the biomedicalization of old age. And activists must denounce macroeconomic adjustment policies and militarization of relationships among nations for their devastating effects on people's health and quality of life; they must demand ethical principles in politics and economics that work to satisfy people's needs.[78]

References

1. United Nations. Second World Assembly on Ageing adopts Madrid Plan of Action and Political Declaration. Madrid, Spain: Second World Assembly on Ageing, 2002.
2. Wallace SP, Villa VM. Equitable health systems: cultural and structural issues for Latino elders. Am J Law Med 2003;29:247–67.
3. Dunlop DD, Manheim LM, Song J, Chang RW. Gender and ethnic/racial disparities in health care utilization among older adults. J Gerontol Soc Sci 2002;57B:S221–33.
4. Wallace SP. Community formation as an activity of daily living: the case of Nicaraguan immigrant elderly. J Aging Stud 1992;6:365–84.
5. Kinsella K, Velkoff VA. An aging world: 2001. U.S. Census Bureau, Series P95/01-1. Washington, D.C.: U.S. Government Printing Office, 2001.
6. United Nations. Human development report. New York, N.Y.: Oxford University Press, 1999.
7. Estes CL, Biggs S, Phillipson C. Globalization and ageing: social theory, social policy and ageing. London, England: Open University Press, 2003.
8. Robertson A. Beyond apocalyptic demography: toward a moral economy of interdependence. In: Minkler M, Estes CL, eds. Critical gerontology: perspectives from political and moral economy. Amityville, N.Y.: Baywood Publishing Company, 1999, pp 75–90.
9. Lamm RD. The moral imperative of limiting elderly health expenditures. In: Altman SH, Shactman DI, eds. Policies for an aging society. Baltimore, Md.: Johns Hopkins University Press, 2002, pp 199–216.
10. Quadagno J. Social Security and the myth of the entitlement "crisis." In: Williamson JB, Watts-Roy DM, Kingson ER, eds. The generational equity debate. New York, N.Y.: Columbia University Press, 1999, pp 140–56.
11. Binstock RH. Scapegoating the old: intergenerational equity and age-based health care rationing. In: Williamson JB, Watts-Roy DM, Kingson ER, eds. The generational equity debate. New York, N.Y.: Columbia University Press, 1999, pp 157–84.
12. Desai N. The world ageing situation. New York, N.Y.: United Nations, 2000.
13. Calasanti TM, Slenin KF. Gender, social inequalities and aging. Walnut Creek, Calif.: Alta Mira, 2001.
14. Estes CL. Social policy and aging: a critical perspective. Thousand Oaks, Calif.: Sage, 2001.

15. Clark DO, Gibson RC. Race, age, chronic disease, and disability. In: Markides KS, Miranda MR, eds. Minorities, aging and health. Newbury Park, Calif.: Sage, 1997, pp 107–26.
16. Idler EL, Kasl SV. Self-ratings of health: do they also predict change in functional ability? J Gerontol Ser B Psychol Sci Soc Sci 1995;50:S344–53.
17. Kinsella K, Velkoff VA. An aging world: 2001. Series P95/01-1. Washington, D.C.: U.S. Government Printing Office, 2001.
18. Manton K, Corder L, Stallard E. Chronic disability trends in elderly in the US. Proc Natl Acad Sci USA 1997;94:2593–8.
19. Verbrugge LM. The dynamics of population aging and health. In: Lewis SJ, ed. Aging and health: linking research and public policy. Chelsea, Mich.: Lewis, 1989, pp 23–40.
20. Olshansky SJ, Rudberg MA, Carnes BA, et al. Trading off longer life for worsening health: the expansion of morbidity hypothesis. J Aging Health 1991;3:194–216.
21. Smedley BD, Stith AY, Nelson AR, eds. Unequal treatment: confronting racial and ethnic disparities in health care. Washington, D.C.: Institute of Medicine, National Academy Press, 2003.
22. Reuben DB, Fullerton JT, Tschann JM, Croughan-Minihane M. Attitudes of beginning medical students toward older persons: a five-campus study. J Am Geriatr Soc 1995;43:1430–6.
23. Kane RL. The future history of geriatrics: geriatrics at the crossroads. J Gerontol A Biol Sci Med Sci 2002;57:M803–5.
24. Muss HB. Older age—not a barrier to cancer treatment. N Engl J Med 2001;345:1128–9.
25. Callahan D. Setting limits: medical goals in an aging society. New York, N.Y.: Simon and Schuster, 1987.
26. Callahan D. Aged based rationing of medical care. In: Williamson JB, Watts-Roy DM, Kingson ER, eds. The intergenerational equity debate. New York, N.Y.: Columbia University Press, 1999.
27. Mintzes B, Barer ML, Kravitz RL, et al. How does direct-to-consumer advertising (DTCA) affect prescribing? A survey in primary care environments with and without legal DTCA. CMAJ 2003;169:405–12.
28. Tinetti ME, Inouye SK, Gill TM, Doucette JT. Shared risk factors for falls, incontinence, and functional dependence. Unifying the approach to geriatric syndromes. JAMA 1995;273:1348–53.
29. Hanlon JT, Schmader KE, Ruby CM, Weinberger M. Suboptimal prescribing in older inpatients and outpatients. J Am Geriatr Soc 2001;49:200–9.
30. Miller SC, Mor V, Wu N, et al. Does receipt of hospice care in nursing homes improve the management of pain at the end of life? J Am Geriatr Soc 2002;50:507–15.
31. Mitteness LS, Barker JC. Stigmatizing a "normal" condition: urinary incontinence in late life. Med Anthropol Q 1995;9:188–210.
32. Burgio KL, Locher JL, Goode TS, et al. Behavioral vs drug treatment for urge urinary incontinence in older women: a randomized controlled trial. JAMA 1998;280:1995–2000.
33. Diokno AC, Burgio K, Fultz H, et al. Prevalence and outcomes of continence surgery in community dwelling women. J Urol 2003;170:507–11.
34. Schulman C, Claes H, Matthijs J. Urinary incontinence in Belgium: a population-based epidemiological survey. Eur Urol 1997;32:315–20.
35. Sen A. Why health equity? Health Economics 2002;11:659–66.
36. Crystal S. America's old age crisis. New York, N.Y.: Basic Books, 1982.

37. Crystal S, Shea D. Cumulative advantage, cumulative disadvantage, and inequality among elderly people. Gerontologist 1990;30:437–43.
38. O'Rand A. Cumulative advantage theory in life course research. Annu Rev Gerontol Geriatr 2002;22:14–30.
39. Williams DR. Socioeconomic differentials in health: a review and redirection. Soc Psychol Q 1990;53:81–99.
40. Collins CA, Williams DR. Segregation and mortality: the deadly effects of racism? Sociol Forum 1999;14:495–523.
41. Robert SA. Socioeconomic position and health: the independent contribution of community socioeconomic context. Annu Rev Sociol 1999;25:489–516.
42. Dressel P, Minkler M, Yen I. Gender, race, class, and aging: advances and opportunities. Int J Health Serv 1997;27:579–600.
43. Williams DR, Mourney RL, Warren RC. The concept of race and health status in America. Public Health Rep 1994;109:26–41.
44. Folbre N. The invisible heart: economics and family values. New York, N.Y.: New York Press, 2001.
45. Estes CL. From gender to the political economy of ageing. Eur J Soc Qual 2000;2.
46. Estes CL, Phillipson C. The globalization of capital, the welfare state and old age policy. Int J Health Serv 2002;32:279–97.
47. Adler N, Boyce WT, Chesney MA, et al. Socio-economic inequalities in health: no easy solution. N Engl J Med 1993;269:3140–5.
48. Adler N, Boyce T, Chesney MA, et al. Socio-economic status and health: the challenge of the gradient. Am Psychol 1994;49:15–24.
49. Rodin J, Langer E. Long-term effects of a control-relevant intervention with the institutionalized aged. J Personal Soc Psychol 1977;35:897–902.
50. Estes CL, Binney EA. The biomedicalization of aging. Gerontologist 1989;29:587–96.
51. Estes CL. The aging enterprise. San Francisco, Calif.: Jossey-Bass, 1979.
52. Estes CL, Harrington C, Pellow D. The medical-industrial complex and the aging enterprise. In: Estes CL, ed. Social policy and aging. Thousand Oaks, Calif.: Sage, 2001.
53. Rowe JW, Kahn RL. Successful aging. New York, NY: Pantheon Books, 1998.
54. Wallace SP. American health promotion: where individualism rules. Gerontologist 2000;40:373–7.
55. Poland B, Coburn D, Robertson A, Eakin J. Wealth, equity and health care: a critique of a "population health" perspective on the determinants of health. Soc Sci Med 1998;46:785–98.
56. Mittelman JH, Tambe A. Global poverty and gender. In: Mittelman JH, ed. The globalization syndrome. Princeton, N.J.: Princeton University Press, 2000.
57. Weissert CS, Weissert WG. Governing health: the politics of health policy. 2nd ed. Baltimore, Md.: Johns Hopkins University Press, 2002.
58. Wallace SP, Villa V. Caught in hostile cross-fire: public policy and minority elderly in the United States. In: Minkler M, Estes CL, eds. Critical gerontology: perspectives from political and moral economy. Farmingdale, N.Y.: Baywood, 1998.
59. Laveist TA, Nuru-Jeter A. Is doctor-patient race concordance associated with greater satisfaction with care? J Health Soc Behav 2002;43:296–306.
60. Wrigley N, Warm D, Margetts B, Whelan A. Assessing the impact of improved retail access on diet in a 'food desert': a preliminary report. Urban Studies 2002;39:2061–82.
61. Wallace SP, Williamson JB. The senior movement in historical perspective. In: The senior movement: references and resources. New York, N.Y.: G. K. Hall, 1992, pp vii–xxxvi.

62. United Nations. UN world ageing situation. New York, N.Y.: United Nations, 2000.
63. Butler R, Brody JA, eds. Strategies to delay dysfunction in later life. New York, N.Y.: Springer, 1995.
64. Rowe JW, Kahn RL. Human aging: usual and successful. Science 1987;237:143–9.
65. World Health Organization. The Perth framework for age-friendly community-based care. Geneva, Switzerland: WHO, 2002.
66. World Health Organization. Towards policy for health and ageing. Geneva, Switzerland: WHO, 2001.
67. World Health Organization and Milbank Memorial Fund. Towards an international consensus on policy for long-term care of the ageing. New York, N.Y.: Milbank Memorial Fund, 2000.
68. Estes CL, Mahakian J, Weitz T. A political economy critique of productive aging. In: Estes C, ed. Social policy and aging: a critical perspective. Newbury Park, Calif.: Sage, 2001.
69. Crystal S, Shea D. Prospects for retirement resources in an aging society. Annu Rev Gerontol Geriatr 2002;22:271–81.
70. Holstein M. Women and productive aging: troubling implications. In: Minkler M, Estes CL, eds. Critical gerontology: perspectives from political and moral economy. Amityville, N.Y.: Baywood, 1999, pp 37–49.
71. Banerji D. Report of the WHO Commission on Macroeconomics and Health: a critique. Int J Health Serv 2002;32:733–54.
72. Vincent J. Politics, power, and old age. Buckingham, England: Open University Press, 1999.
73. Vincent J, Patterson G, Wale K. Politics and old age. Aldershot, Hampshire, England: Ashgate Books, 2002.
74. Walker A, Maltby A. Ageing Europe. Buckinghamshire, England: Open University Press, 1997.
75. Navarro V. Health and equity in the world in the era of globalization. Int J Health Serv 1999;29:215–26.
76. Navarro V. Are pro-welfare state and full employment policies possible in the era of globalization? Int J Health Serv 2000;30:231–51.
77. Kagarlitsky B. The challenge for the left: reclaiming the state. In: Pantich L, Leys C, eds. Global capitalism versus democracy. Woodbridge, Suffolk, England / New York, N.Y.: Merlin Press/Monthly Review Press, 1999, pp 294–313.
78. International Forum for the Defense of the Health of the People. Health as an essential human need, a right of citizenship, and public good: health is possible and necessary. Int J Health Serv 2002;32:601–6.

7

LESBIAN, GAY, BISEXUAL, AND TRANSGENDER/TRANSSEXUAL INDIVIDUALS

Emilia Lombardi and Talia Bettcher

Introduction

"Liberty protects the person from unwarranted government intrusions into a dwelling or other private places. In our tradition the state is not omnipresent in the home. And there are other spheres of our lives and existence, outside the home, where the state should not be a dominant presence. Freedom extends beyond spatial bounds. Liberty presumes an autonomy of self that includes freedom of thought, belief, expression, and certain intimate conduct."[1]

With those words written by Justice Anthony M. Kennedy in 2003, the U.S. Supreme Court removed legislation criminalizing same-gender sexual relations throughout the country—a major event in the history of lesbian, gay, bisexual, and transgender/transsexual (LGBT) men and women. This event makes clear that consensual sexual relationships between adult, same-gender couples are not to be prohibited. Previous legislation was a major barrier for LGBT men and women. While it was not used directly against them very often, it restricted their activities in other situations, such as adoption and employment protections. The removal of legislation criminalizing same-gender sexual activity leads the way toward granting the lives of LGBT men and women greater legitimacy, and hence better health outcomes. However, there is still much to be done.

In general, LGBT people continue to be stigmatized and marginalized both legally and culturally. This can affect their health in various ways:

1. Stigma can impair health through direct acts of violence—even murder.
2. It may affect an individual's psychology. For example, increased stress from stigma, as well as internalized homophobia, may lead to such behaviors as substance use or high-risk sex.
3. Access to health and social services may be constrained. For example, organizations may fail to provide LGBT men and women specific services, may fail to demonstrate adequate LGBT sensitivity, or may even be overtly hostile to them.

While the Supreme Court ruling was clearly an important event, it masks complex issues found within LGBT populations. The ruling focuses specifically on sexual behavior among consenting adults. Transgender and transsexual people often experience discrimination based on gender presentation and identities rather than sexual/affectional orientations. Bisexual individuals continue to be represented, if at all, as indecisive and promiscuous, and bisexual men are often identified only as an STD/HIV bridge between gay men and heterosexual women. Both gay men and lesbians experience discrimination based on their sexual orientation, such as lack of partner benefits, but lesbians must also deal with sexism as well, such as lack of access to economic resources. Moreover, many LGBT people also experience race- and/or class-based injustice that intertwines with LGBT-based injustice in complicated ways. Although progress has been made, these considerations make the promotion of social justice difficult because the failure to address the specific and multiple needs within LGBT communities may actually lead to the promotion of further injustice.

The Impact of Social Injustice on the Health of LGBT Men and Women

Violence

Stigma-based violence and the threat of violence can undermine the health and well-being of LGBT people. This situation is aggravated by the use of "blame-shifting" rhetoric to justify or excuse such violence. In the first 11 months of 2003, for example, more than 30 murders of transgender people were reported worldwide—15 of them occurred in the United States.[2–6] Most of these people were murdered because of their "non-normative" gender presentations. Most of these murder victims were transgender women of color.

Transphobia (the hatred and intolerance people feel toward those who do not conform to traditional gender norms)—and perhaps LGBT phobia more generally—may not always be easily separable from race- and class-based injustice. One of the authors (E.L.), for example, found that African-American men and women reported higher levels of transphobic life events than did others in the study.[3]

Domestic violence among LGBT couples is also much more a problem than some might suppose.[7] Domestic violence in LGBT relationships appears to occur as often as in heterosexual relationships. However, the myth of egalitarian same-gender relationships creates a barrier for those who experience domestic violence. Helping professionals often may not be able to distinguish victim from batterer. Most domestic violence workers assume that there is a heterosexual relationship and that the wife is the victim and the husband, the batterer. As such, many do not know how to respond to reports of same-gender domestic violence.[8] Most shelters admit only women, which leaves men with fewer resources.[9] In addition, many shelters do not acknowledge the gender of transsexual women and refuse services to them. Batterers might also use LGBT-based prejudice to control their victims or to further harass them by informing others about their LGBT identity.

HIV/AIDS

HIV/AIDS remains a major health issue for many LGBT men and women. There has been a resurgence of HIV infection among men who have sex with men, especially among men of color.[10–13] In addition, the rate of HIV infection is high among transgender women (people who are assigned male at birth but who have the gender identity and expression of women).[14–17] Research on the health of LGBT individuals in areas other than HIV/AIDS is limited.[18,19] Mental health and substance use issues are especially important and have been found to be linked to HIV infection.[20,21]

Mental Health and Alcohol, Tobacco, and Other Drugs

Gay men and lesbians generally have higher rates of substance use and mental health disorders, which may be linked to societal discrimination.[22–24] Experiences of violence, harassment, and discriminatory events can significantly affect the mental health of gay men and lesbians.[25,26] Furthermore, factors relating to the hiding and concealment of identities, expectations of rejection, and internalized homophobia are specific stressors that LGB men and women experience.[27] The internalization of negative attitudes about their identity can also weigh heavily on their lives and cause them much distress.[28]

Focus groups conducted with lesbian, gay, bisexual, and two-spirit people (LGBT persons of Native American origin) indicate that hiding one's identity is unhealthy, especially when one hides his or her identity from health care providers.[29] Internalized homophobia can interfere with HIV prevention efforts.[30] Many LGBT people live under the assumption that they will experience negative sanctions if other people find out about them, and as a result many constantly evaluate whether actions or words may identify them as being LGBT.

Transgenderism and transsexuality, unlike homosexuality or bisexuality, are still listed in diagnostic manuals of the American Psychiatric Association as mental illnesses (referred to as "gender identity disorder" and "transvestic fetishism" in the current and recent editions of the *Diagnostic and Statistical Manual of Mental Disorders*).[31] Furthermore, many clinicians conceptualize transsexualism among the psychotic disorders, such as schizophrenia,[32,33] even though transsexuals as a population are not more likely to have mental disorders than are nontranssexual men and women.[34] This problem is augmented by the existence of social policies that require individuals to obtain medical services before allowing them to change/amend their legal documents (such as driver's licenses, passports, and birth certificates) and, therefore, require transgender/transsexual people to seek mental health services and be diagnosed with a mental disorder.

The psychological impact of LGBT-related social injustice can directly influence people's health. Gay men who conceal their identities may have worse health outcomes. Gay men who conceal their homosexual identity have increased incidence of cancer and infectious diseases, and, for those who are positive for HIV infection, concealment is associated with their infection advancing faster than for those who do not conceal their homosexual identity.[35,36] Furthermore, gay men who are sensitive to rejection generally have a greater decrease in CD4 count and a longer time to AIDS diagnosis, in comparison to gay men who conceal their identities and are protected, hiding their identity from others and shielding themselves from possible rejection.[37] This is the dilemma that many LGBT people face: being "out" reduces the amount of internal stress that hiding one's identity creates, but it may sever important social connections that people rely on for support and resources.[38,39]

The levels of alcohol, tobacco, and illicit substance use among gay men and lesbians are higher than those of the general population. One study found that young gay or bisexual men were twice as likely, and lesbian and bisexual women four times as likely, to have used marijuana in the previous year.[40] In the same study, gay and bisexual men were three times more likely, and lesbian and bisexual women four times more likely, to have used the street drug ecstasy in the previous year. Lesbian and bisexual women were also three-and-a-half times more likely to have smoked in the previous month. Other studies have linked LGBT people's substance use to their experiences of discrimination.[23,39,41–43] While smoking in the general adult population is decreasing, gay men and lesbians are still more likely to smoke than the general adult population.[44–46] Preliminary comparisons between young gay men and lesbians have found that lesbians actually smoke more than their gay male counterparts.[47] It is important to note the difficulty of making assessments regarding rates of use because few studies include measures of sexuality and gender identity.

Cardiovascular Disease and Cancer

LGBT men and women are at increased risk for cardiovascular disease.[48–50] Lesbians smoke more and have, on average, a higher body mass index than heterosexual women, which may place them at higher risks of cardiovascular disease.[51–53] Tobacco use of lesbian and bisexual women influences their cancer risks. Because lesbian and bisexual women tend to smoke more, use alcohol more, are less likely to report routine Pap smears, and have more sexual partners, they are at a greater risk of lung, cervical, and other forms of cancer.[54–60]

LGBT men and women experience many problems with access to health care.[24] For example, a transsexual man died of cervical cancer because he could not get a physician to treat him until it was too late.[61] A "masculine" lesbian discussed her experiences trying to get access to health care for a serious health condition; she was refused treatment, comments were made about her by staff members, and a physician claimed her ill health was a result of her immoral lifestyle.[62] In general, many LGBT people are afraid to disclose their lives for fear of being discriminated against. Moreover, health care providers likely fail to collect important information by assuming a person's sex/gender or sexuality. For example, transsexual patients may need medical assistance for problems that members of their identified gender may not be expected to have, such as transsexual men needing gynecological examinations and transsexual women needing prostate examinations.

Additionally, many partners of LGBT men and women experience problems when taking care of their sick or hurt loved ones that do not exist for heterosexual men and women. Some of the issues include:

1. Inability to visit their partners in hospitals
2. Inability to make legal decisions for incapacitated partners
3. Lack of access to health insurance for one's partner and partner's children
4. Lack of coverage for medical expenses by their health insurance
5. Denial of the right to make funeral arrangements and to address other end-of-life issues, such as child custody
6. Denial of many fiscal rights, including Social Security, property ownership, and taxation.[63]

These problems create an added burden for LGBT people in addition to the stress and worry related to having a sick or injured partner. Not only could LGBT persons lose the persons whom they have loved, but also they could lose their homes and custody of their children and have to pay huge health care bills not covered by insurance.

At a deeper level, class status may play a significant role in preventing access to health services through lack of adequate health coverage. In this respect, LGBT (as well as racial) stigmatization and discrimination in schools, universities, and employment may undermine the potential of LGBT people to secure the sort of incomes or jobs that would make health service more affordable. For example, the Los Angeles Transgender Health Study found that 69 percent of the participants did not have postsecondary education, 50 percent earned less than $12,000 annually, 50 percent reported that commercial sex work was a major source of income, and 64 percent reported lacking any health insurance coverage. These findings suggest that class, race, and LGBT disadvantage in education and employment act together in complex ways to prevent adequate access to health services.

Underlying Factors and Roots of This Social Injustice

One needs to recognize not only the existence of stigmatizing views about LGBT people but also the role of simplistic categorization in the promotion of social injustice. The diversity found among LGBT people affects research and access to health care resources. Failure to appreciate this complexity may promote social injustice.

The category "LGBT" contains considerable diversity within it, making it difficult to provide a unified account of the social injustice that confronts LGBT people. Unsophisticated or reductive accounts that attempt to address LGBT social injustice may fail to address all of the problems, and may even leave some individuals out of the solution by failing to address specific issues. For example, some transgender people may seek various bodily-altering medical technologies, such as hormones and surgeries; these technologies, when accessed through "black markets," raise specific health concerns that are easily ignored in a simplistic description of LGBT health, especially those that emphasize sexual orientation.

More generally, the tense relationship between gender-based and sexuality-based social injustice points to the complexity of LGBT issues.[64] For while it may be initially tempting to draw a clear distinction between gender-based and sexuality-based social injustice, the diversity within the category "LGBT" makes it difficult to draw this distinction. For example, "lesbian," "gay," and "bisexual" are categories of sexual orientation, but "transgender" and "transsexual" are categories of gender and gender identity. This diversity makes more difficult attempts to explain (a) LGBT discrimination and stigmatization in terms of the oppression of non-normative sexualities alone, and (b) social injustice only in terms of the enforcement of strict gender norms.[65]

More deeply, it is difficult to distinguish between being assaulted because of one's gender presentation and one's perceived sexual orientation.[66] Gay bashing in public space, for example, may be facilitated by non-normative gender cues. Stigma against gay men, lesbians, and bisexual people may often be gender based; for example, gay men may be represented as "feminine"—"not real men."[65] Moreover, gender presentation and gender identity may be important in some gay and lesbian relationships, such as "butch" and "femme" identities. By contrast, transgender and transsexual individuals may find themselves subject to reductive representations—such as "really a gay man" or "really a lesbian"—and subject to violence on the basis of perceived sexual orientation.[66] Hence, gender and gender identity may be implicated in social injustice against LGB individuals, and sexuality implicated in social injustice against transgender individuals.

The social injustice faced by LGBT people lies in the complex intersections of gender-based and sexuality-based oppressions, where deep cultural views about gender and sexually appropriate conduct are enmeshed. It is useful to distinguish between different forms of stigma and the background assumptions that ground them. For example, one might distinguish LGBT stigmas that are grounded in religious perspectives (LGBT individuals seen as "sinful") from those that flow from more "scientific" or "medical" discourses (LGBT sexualities and identities seen as "pathological"). One might also identify prevalent cultural views about gender, such as "the natural attitude about gender," and distinguish them from higher-order theoretical legal, medical, or other discourses that also promote stigmatizing views in different, albeit related, ways.[67–69]

In addition, such social injustice is often linked with other forms of injustice, making it difficult to separate LGBT injustice from other forms of injustice. For example, lesbians may face discrimination not only on the basis of sexuality but also as women. The existence of hybrid forms of discrimination is especially important with respect to the intersections between race- and class-based injustice and LGBT injustice and the possibility of complex, hybrid forms of social injustice. There are many LGBT people of color who also experience hybrid forms of discrimination. In addition, LGBT discrimination and stigma may take on distinctive forms in culturally specific contexts. For example, within some Latino cultural contexts, religion plays an important role in promoting negative views about LGBT people.[70] The very way in which "LGBT" identities are negotiated may vary considerably depending on cultural context. For example, homosexuality may be conceptualized differently in Latin America and North America, suggesting different sexual identifications of Latinos and Latinas who live in different places.[71]

Moreover, it is not clear that language and culturally specific terms may be easily translated or assimilated into Anglo "LGBT" terms without significant distortion.[72] For example, the Chicano colloquial term *jota* may be roughly translated "dyke" or "lesbian," but such translations cannot easily capture the roles that such terms play in the culturally specific ways of life within which such terms are actually deployed and negotiated. Related to this, mainstream U.S. "LGBT" identifications can be seen from certain vantage points as distinctively "white Anglo," and consequently any identification with such terms may also take on connotations of cultural betrayal.[73] Finally, it may be difficult to discuss the ways in which homosexuality has been viewed as "aberrant" without also discussing the ways in which racialized sexualities have been stereotyped and devalued. For example, African-American sexuality has been historically represented in mainstream white American discourse as "degenerate" or "dirty."[74] Given this, it is unclear to what extent one may seriously discuss representations of homosexuality as "sick" or "degenerate" without also appreciating the possible connections with racial representations and the role that both sorts of stigma may have on African-American homosexuals and lesbians.[75]

An analysis of the social injustice faced by LGBT people, therefore, should consider its race and class stratification as well as the specific gender and sexuality differences among LGBT people. For example, discrimination against LGBT people may be more likely in lower-paying jobs; thus race and class could interact with gender and sexuality to a create a context that is far more problematic for people than either would be separately. Internalized LGBT stigmatization and its impact on self-esteem may not always be easily separated from internalized racial stigmatization. And the ability of medical and social service organizations to provide services to LGBT people may be impaired by failures to accommodate culturally specific issues—indeed, by their "white" specificity.

What Needs to Be Done

Legislative and Other Policies

Legislative and other policies that explicitly prohibit discrimination and violence against LGBT people may reduce the social injustice experienced by LGBT individuals and thereby improve their health. Such policies can also reduce their own internalized prejudice against LGBT people and themselves, thereby improving their mental health. This strategy may also decrease discrimination at school and work so that LGBT people can afford and access adequate medical care. Nevertheless, such policies need to be thoroughly examined for possible racist or classist assumptions and/or consequences that provide advantage to particular groups within LGBT communities while harming others.

Domestic partner legislation that gives partners of LGBT men and women many of the same benefits as married, heterosexual couples has been a welcome development for many LGBT families. The legal recognition of same-gender relationships in a manner similar to heterosexual relationships will have major implications toward improving the lives of LGBT people.

Transgender/transsexual individuals also need legislation and policies that legitimize their lives and identities.[76–78] The ability of transgender/transsexual men and women to change important legal documents varies by document and locality. In some localities, little to no medical intervention is required to change one's legal sex or name, while in others, surgery is required. However, in many instances, even this may not be sufficient, as many places do not allow people to change their legal sex designations on documents or to be able to live their lives fully. There have been recent court cases with mixed responses to opposite-gender marriages of transsexual individuals, and all cases involved people who underwent some operative procedure as a requirement for changing legal sex designation.

Transgender/transsexual men and women need affordable and more reliable access to medical care that will enable them to better embody their gender identity. As such, legislative and other policies must prevent denial of public and private insurance coverage for such procedures, because doing so restricts people's ability to interact in society in their identified gender. Many transgender men and women are considered to be one gender in some instances and another gender in others. The process of changing one's gender must be made easier so that people do not need to guess what to do next and whether they can afford access to medical services necessary to change one's legal gender.

Roles of Health Care Facilities and Organizations

Health care facilities and organizations need to have policies that protect the dignity of those accessing care and prohibit discrimination or harassment based on people's LGBT status. Organizations must allow domestic partners and all children being raised by same-gender couples to have the same rights as those in opposite-gender relationships. As such, they must respect the existence of domestic partners and treat them as they would any other partner in a committed relationship—including end-of-life activities.

In addition to policies and procedures that do not discriminate against LGBT men and women, personnel within these organizations need training about issues relating to LGBT health. Training needs to inform people about the diversity found among LGBT people and not focus on specific stereotypes or media images. Although HIV/AIDS is important, especially for gay men, it should not be seen as the only health risk faced by LGBT people. Diversity among LGBT people needs to be recognized and understood, especially the relevance of race, culture, and class. Health care workers need to know how to promote sensitivity and to provide culturally relevant care.

Educational Measures

Because access to educational resources affects employment opportunities, which, in turn, affects access to adequate health insurance and overall health and well-being, teachers and school administrators need to be trained to treat LGBT youth without discrimination and to educate students about LGBT issues. Such measures help provide LGBT students with a safe place to learn and promote supportive cultural attitudes. These educational approaches should be sensitive to race, class, and culture. In addition, programs are needed that enable disenfranchised LGBT people to access educational resources.

Research Issues

There is a need to ensure that measures are included to identify LGBT people within health care research. Most studies of LGBT people use relatively small convenience samples that greatly limit their generalizability to the larger population. To be inclusive, survey instruments should:

1. Differentiate between sexual orientation and gender (transgender and bisexual individuals should not be assimilated into lesbian or gay categories).
2. Allow people to self-identify as lesbian, gay, or bisexual, and allow transgender/transsexual individuals to self-report their gender identity and sexual orientation—rather than having interviewers or staff members decide. Instruments should also be sensitive to language- and culture-specific identifications.
3. Allow people to identify unmarried domestic partners, rather than forcing categorization as "single" or "married."
4. Be aware of and allow for the diversity of attitudes and behaviors found among LGBT people.
5. Be cognizant of—and sufficiently sophisticated to investigate—other forms of social injustice and the impact that this might have on some LGBT people. For example, studies that examine possible correlations between LGBT stigma and health outcomes ought to be sufficiently sophisticated to measure the role of race and race stigma in promoting lower health outcomes among LGBT people of color.

6. Recognize that terminology—including "LGBT," "gay," "lesbian," "transgender," and "queer"—may have white/Anglo cultural connotations that can undermine efforts at promoting social justice.

Conclusion

There has been improvement in the status of LGBT people in the United States, as evidenced by the 2003 Supreme Court decision regarding laws criminalizing same-gender sexual relationships, but much remains to be done. Changes in legislation and social policies are needed to provide LGBT people with adequate resources and benefits. Health care providers need to be informed about LGBT issues in culturally sensitive ways to address inadequacies in health care. And researchers need to be sufficiently sophisticated to investigate the complexity of LGBT issues and their intersection with other forms of injustice.

Most of all, there needs to be a change in the social environment that creates social injustice against LGBT people—a change that can only be brought about through education and by addressing multiple forms of social injustice. To foster greater change, coalitions need to be developed and nurtured, not only among the diverse groups found within the LGBT population but also with other groups that experience social injustice.

References

1. John Geddes Lawrence and Tyron Garner, Petitioners, v. Texas. 539 U.S. 558 (2003).
2. Smith GA. Remembering our dead. 2003. Available at: http://www.rememberingour dead.org. Accessed January 8, 2005.
3. Lombardi E. Understanding genderism and transphobia. In review.
4. Lombardi EL, Wilchins RA, Priesing D, et al. Gender violence: transgender experiences with violence and discrimination. J Homosex 2001;42:89–101.
5. Clements K. The Transgender Community Health Project: descriptive results. San Francisco, Calif.: San Francisco Department of Public Health, 1999.
6. Reback CJ, Simon, Paul A, et al. The Los Angeles Transgender Health Study: community report. Los Angeles, Calif.: Van Ness Recovery House, Prevention Division, 2001.
7. Burke LK, Follingstad DR. Violence in lesbian and gay relationships: theory, prevalence, and correlational factors. Clin Psychol Rev 1999;19:487–512.
8. Ristock JL. Exploring dynamics of abusive lesbian relationships: preliminary analysis of a multisite, qualitative study. Am J Commun Psychol 2003;31:329–41.
9. Merrill GS, Wolfe VA. Battered gay men: an exploration of abuse, help seeking, and why they stay. J Homosex 2000;39:1–30.
10. Malebranche DJ. Black men who have sex with men and the HIV epidemic: next steps for public health. Am J Public Health 2003;93:862–5.

11. Clifton CE. A black gay man's call to action to the black community. Positively Aware 2003;14:7.
12. Leslie NS, Deiriggi P, Gross S, et al. Knowledge, attitudes, and practices surrounding breast cancer screening in educated Appalachian women. Oncol Nursing Forum 2003;30:659–67.
13. Gross M. When plagues don't end. Am J Public Health 2003;93:861–2.
14. Clements-Nolle K, Marx R, Guzman R, et al. HIV prevalence, risk behaviors, health care use, and mental health status of transgender persons: implications for public health intervention. Am J Public Health 2001;91:915–21.
15. Simon PA, Reback CJ, Bemis CC. HIV prevalence and incidence among male-to-female transsexuals receiving HIV prevention services in Los Angeles County. AIDS 2000;14:2953–5.
16. Sykes DL. Transgendered people: an "invisible" population. California HIV/AIDS Update 1999;12:80–5.
17. Nemoto T, Luke D, Mamo L, et al. HIV risk behaviours among male-to-female transgenders in comparison with homosexual or bisexual males and heterosexual females. AIDS Care 1999;11:297–312.
18. Boehmer U. Twenty years of public health research: inclusion of lesbian, gay, bisexual, and transgender populations. Am J Public Health 2002;92:1125–30.
19. Dean L, Meyer IH, Robinston K, et al. Lesbian, gay, bisexual, and transgender health: findings and concerns. J Gay Lesbian Med Assoc 2000;4:102–51.
20. Strathdee SA, Hogg RS, Martindale SL, et al. Determinants of sexual risk-taking among young HIV-negative gay and bisexual men. J Acquir Immune Defic Syndr Hum Retrovirol 1998;19:61–6.
21. Greenwood GL, White EW, Page-Shafer K, et al. Correlates of heavy substance use among young gay and bisexual men: the San Francisco Young Men's Health Study. Drug Alcohol Depend 2001;61:105–12.
22. Herek GM, Gillis JR, Cogan JC. Psychological sequelae of hate-crime victimization among lesbian, gay, and bisexual adults. J Consult Clin Psychol 1999;67:945–51.
23. Skinner WF. The prevalence and demographic predictors of illicit and licit drug use. Am J Public Health 1994;84:1307–10.
24. Lee R. Health care problems of lesbian, gay, bisexual, and transgender patients. West J Med 2000;172:403–8.
25. Meyer IH. Minority stress and mental health in gay men. J Health Soc Behav 1995;36:38–56.
26. Garnets L, Herek GM, Levy B. Violence and victimization of lesbians and gay men: mental health consequences. In: Herek GM, Berrill KT, eds. Hate crimes: confronting violence against lesbians and gay men. Newbury Park, Calif.: Sage, 1992, pp 207–26.
27. Meyer IH. Prejudice, social stress, and mental health in lesbian, gay, and bisexual populations: conceptual issues and research evidence. Psychol Bull 2003;129:674–97.
28. Williamson IR. Internalized homophobia and health issues affecting lesbians and gay men. Health Educ Res 2000;15:97–107.
29. Brotman S, Ryan B, Jalbert Y, et al. The impact of coming out on health and health care access: the experiences of gay, lesbian, bisexual and two-spirit people. J Health Soc Policy 2002;15:1–29.
30. Huebner DM, Davis MC, Nemeroff CJ, et al. The impact of internalized homophobia on HIV preventive interventions. Am J Commun Psychol 2002;30:327–48.

31. American Psychiatric Association. Diagnostic and Statistical Manual of Mental Disorders: DSM-IV-TR (Text Revision) (4th ed.). Washington, D.C.: American Psychiatric Associaiton, 2000.
32. Campo J, Nijman H, Merckelbach H, et al. Psychiatric comorbidity of gender identity disorders: a survey among Dutch psychiatrists. Am J Psychiatry 2003;160:1332–6.
33. Habermeyer E, Kamps I, Kawohl W. A case of bipolar psychosis and transsexualism. Psychopathology 2003;36:168–70.
34. Haraldsen I, Dahl A. Symptom profiles of gender dysphoric patients of transsexual type compared to patients with personality disorders and healthy adults. Acta Psychiatr Scand 2000;102:276–81.
35. Cole SW, Kemeny ME, Taylor SE, et al. Accelerated course of human immunodeficiency virus infection in gay men who conceal their homosexual identity. Psychosom Med 1996;58:219–31.
36. Cole SW, Kemeny ME, Taylor SE, et al. Elevated physical health risk among gay men who conceal their homosexual identity. Health Psychol 1996;15:243–51.
37. Cole SW, Kemeny ME, Taylor SE. Social identity and physical health: accelerated HIV progression in rejection-sensitive gay men. J Personal Soc Psychol 1997;72:320–35.
38. Meyer IH. Prejudice, social stress, and mental health in lesbian, gay, and bisexual populations: conceptual issues and research evidence. Psychol Bull 2003;129:674–97.
39. Stall R, Wiley J. A comparison of alcohol and drug use patterns of homosexual and heterosexual men: the San Francisco Men's Health Study. Drug Alcohol Depend 1988;22:63–73.
40. McCabe SE, Boyd C, Hughes TL, et al. Sexual identity and substance use among undergraduate students. Substance Abuse 2003;24:77–91.
41. Stall R, Paul JP, Greenwood G, et al. Alcohol use, drug use and alcohol-related problems among men who have sex. Addiction 2001;96:1589–601.
42. McKirnan DJ, Peterson PL. Psychosocial and cultural factors in alcohol and drug abuse: an analysis. Addict Behav 1989;14:555–63.
43. Hughes TL, Eliason M. Lesbian, gay, bisexual, and transgender issues in substance abuse. J Prim Prev 2002;22:263–98.
44. Emery S, Gilpin EA, Ake C, et al. Characterizing and identifying "hard-core" smokers: implications for further reducing smoking prevalence. Am J Public Health 2000; 90:387–94.
45. Ryan H, Wortley PM, Easton A, et al. Smoking among lesbians, gays, and bisexuals: a review of the literature. Am J Prev Med 2001;21:142–9.
46. Stall RD, Greenwood GL, Acree M, et al. Cigarette smoking among gay and bisexual men. Am J Public Health 1999;89:1875–8.
47. Skinner W, Otis MD. Drug and alcohol use among lesbian and gay people in a southern U.S. sample: epidemiological, comparative, and methodological findings from the Trilogy Project. J Homosex 1996;30:59–92.
48. Roberts SA, Dibble SL, Nussey B, et al. Cardiovascular disease risk in lesbian women. Womens Health Issues 2003;13:167–74.
49. Ungvarski PJ, Grossman AH. Health problems of gay and bisexual men. Nursing Clin North Am 1999;34:313–31.
50. Valanis BG, Bowen DJ, Bassford T, et al. Sexual orientation and health: comparisons in the women's health initiative sample. Arch Fam Med 2000;9:843–53.
51. Bradford J, Ryan C, Honnold J, et al. Expanding the research infrastructure for lesbian health. Am J Public Health 2001;91:1029–32.
52. Moran N. Lesbian health care needs. Can Family Physician 1996;42:879–84.

53. White J, Dull VT. Health risk factors and health-seeking behavior in lesbians. J Womens Health 1997;6:103–12.
54. Burnett CB, Steakley CS, Slack R, et al. Patterns of breast cancer screening among lesbians at increased risk for breast cancer. Women Health 1999;29:35–55.
55. Dibble SL, Roberts SA, Robertson PA, et al. Risk factors for ovarian cancer: lesbian and heterosexual women. Oncol Nursing Forum 2002;29:E1–7.
56. Matthews AK, Brandenburg DL, Johnson TP, et al. Correlates of underutilization of gynecological cancer screening among lesbian and heterosexual women. Prev Med 2004;38:105–13.
57. Rankow EJ, Tessaro I. Cervical cancer risk and Papanicolaou screening in a sample of lesbian and bisexual women. J Fam Pract 1998;47:139–43.
58. Cochran SD. Emerging issues in research on lesbians' and gay men's mental health: does sexual orientation really matter? Am Psychol 2001;56:931–47.
59. Horn-Ross PL, Canchola AJ, West DW, et al. Patterns of alcohol consumption and breast cancer risk in the California Teachers Study cohort. Cancer Epidemiol Biomarkers Prevent 2004;13:405–11.
60. Hamajima N, Hirose K, Tajima K, et al. Alcohol, tobacco and breast cancer—collaborative reanalysis of individual data from 53 epidemiological studies, including 58,515 women with breast cancer and 95,067 women without the disease. Br J Cancer 2002;87:1234–5.
61. Davis K. Southern comfort [documentary]. HBO Theatrical Documentary, 2001.
62. Feinberg L. Trans health crisis: for us it's life or death. Am J Public Health 2001;91: 897–900.
63. Cahill S, Mitra E, Tobias S. Family policy: issues affecting gay, lesbian, bisexual and transgender families. Washington, D.C.: National Gay and Lesbian Task Force, January 22, 2003.
64. Rubin G. Thinking sex: Notes towards a radical theory of the politics of sexuality. In: Vance C, ed. Pleasure and danger: exploring female sexuality. Boston, Mass.: Routledge and Kegan Paul, 1984, pp 267–319.
65. Namaste VK. Genderbashing. In: Namaste VK, ed. Invisible lives: the erasure of transsexual and transgendered people. Chicago, Ill.: University of Chicago Press, 2000.
66. Butler J. Against proper objects. In: Weed E, Schor N, eds. Feminism meets queer theory. Indianapolis, Ind.: Indiana University Press, 1997, pp 1–30.
67. Garfinkel H. Studies in ethnomethodology. Englewood Cliffs, N.J.: Prentice-Hall, 1967.
68. Bornstein K. Gender outlaw: on men, women, and the rest of us. New York, N.Y.: Routledge, 1994.
69. Kessler SJ, McKenna W. Gender: an ethnomethodological approach. New York, N.Y.: John Wiley and Sons, 1978.
70. Trujillo C. Chicana lesbians: the girls our mothers warned us about. Berkeley, Calif.: Third Woman Press, 1991.
71. Almaguer T. Chicano men: a cartography of homosexual identity and behavior. Differences: A Journal of Feminist Cultural Studies 1991;3:75–100.
72. Lugones M. El pasar discontínuo de la cachapera/tortillera del barrio a la barra al movimiento [The discontinuous passing of the cachapera/tortillera from the barrio to the bar to the movement]. In: Lugones M, ed. Pilgrimages/peregrinajes: theorizing coalition against multiple oppressions. New York, N.Y.: Rowman & Littlefield, 2003, pp 167–180.
73. Moraga C. Loving in the war years: lo que nunco pasó por sus labios. Boston, Mass.: South End, 1983.

74. West C. Black sexuality: the taboo subject. In: West C, ed. Race matters. Boston, Mass.: Beacon Press, 1994, pp 81–91.

75. Collins PH. The sexual politics of black womanhood. In: Collins PH, ed. Black feminist thought: knowledge, consciousness, and the politics of empowerment. 2nd ed. New York, N.Y.: Routledge, 2000, pp 123–48.

76. Swartz L. Updated look at legal responses to transsexualism: especially three marriage cases in U.K., U.S. and New Zealand. Int J Transgenderism 1997;1(2). Available at: http://www.symposion.com/ijt/ijtc0201.htm. Accessed January 8, 2005.

77. Dasti JL. Advocating a broader understanding of the necessity of sex-reassignment surgery under Medicaid. N Y Univ Law Rev 2002;77:1738–75.

78. Frye PR. The International Bill of Gender Rights vs. The Cider House Rules: transgenders struggle with the courts over what clothing they are allowed to wear on the job, which restroom they are allowed to use on the job, their right to marry, and the very definition of their sex. William Mary J Women Law 2000;7:133.

8

PEOPLE WITH DISABILITIES

Nora Ellen Groce

Introduction

The image of the little boy in the polio prevention poster was arresting. Perhaps 4 or 5 years of age, he had obviously responded to the photographer's request by pulling himself up on his crutches, looking straight into the camera, and beaming his most winning smile. The caption, however, was what caught one's attention. "Let's make him the last," it told the reader, pleading for more active commitment to the local polio immunization campaign.

Preventing polio is an admirable public health goal, but it is not the only one.* What will become of the little boy in the poster? Certainly, his life should be worth more than simply encouraging public health professionals to redouble their efforts. Yet research clearly shows that compared with his peers, this boy will be far less likely to receive adequate health care or

---

*While many types of disability may be preventable, some individuals and families with certain hereditary disorders, such as deafness and dwarfism, have made a strong case for continuing to have children with these traits, who can share their family's genetic heritage and social legacy. The assumption that all types of disability should be prevented is not, therefore, as straightforward as it is sometimes presented.

education and far less likely to participate in the social, economic, or religious life of his community.

Six hundred million people, 10 percent of the world's population, live with a physical, sensory, intellectual, or mental health impairment significant enough to make a difference in their daily lives. Eighty percent of these people live in developing countries[1] (fig. 8-1). Social justice cannot be achieved unless these people with disabilities—among the poorest and the most marginalized—are fully included (box 8-1).

Disability as a Social Justice Issue

The primary issues faced by disabled individuals are not only their specific impairments but also the social stigma, reduced access to resources, and poverty that limit their full potential. For example, in many countries, people with disabilities are still denied the right to decide when, where, and with whom they

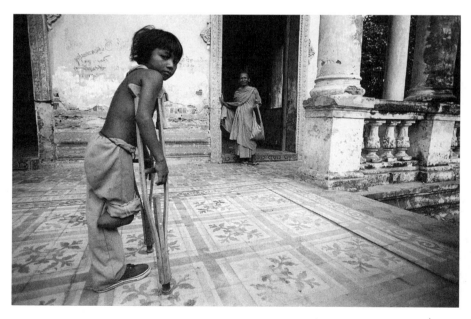

Figure 8-1 A boy disabled by a landmine stands in a courtyard of a UNICEF-assisted rehabilitation center in Cambodia. This boy is one of the fortune few. Most disabled people in both developing and developed countries have inadequate access to necessary services and reduced opportunities in education, employment, and other aspects of life. (Photograph: UNICEF/HQ92-0629/Roger Lemoyne.)

BOX 8-1 Terminology

Much attention has been devoted to getting away from pejorative terms and phrases. Older terms such as "cripple" have given way to more politically neutral terms. To say that someone is a "wheelchair user" rather than "confined to a wheelchair" shifts the emphasis to an individual making use of an appliance rather than being a victim imprisoned in an object.

Some issues of terminology are of more relevance in one language than are others. For example, the term *handicap* ("cap in hand" or "beggar") has a more pejorative connotation in English than in French, where the term *handicap* carries a more neutral connotation.

At its best, this debate over proper language fosters rethinking and re-evaluation of basic assumptions by members of society—and, as such, is analogous to the shifts in many languages brought about by women's rights movement. (This is particularly true in languages where general terms about those with a disability include concepts like "the unfortunates" and "the cursed.") At its worst, controversy over the proper language about disability has taken much time and energy, which could more fruitfully be directed at more substantive issues facing disabled populations. It has also led to the generation of a number of terms (usually by people who are not themselves disabled) that are politically correct but unlikely to enter common speech, such as "the differently-abled." A good rule of thumb is to ask members of the local disability community what terms they prefer be used. Another solution to this ongoing debate over terminology was offered by a mother at a meeting of parents of young children with severe intellectually disabilities in Canada. The mother turned to the audience, composed largely of human rights lawyers and physicians, and said, "Please promise me you will tell the professionals you work with that there is one term that applies to everyone with a disability, no matter what type of disability they have. Tell them the term is 'citizen.'"

will live. They have no say over how they will support themselves and may be denied the right to marry and have a family.[2] Gender and ethnic or minority status can compound these inequities.[3] Hundreds of thousands continue to be institutionalized against their will, although community-based inclusionary models provide far better and more cost-effective services.[4,5] The literacy rate for people with disabilities worldwide may be as low as 3 percent, and for women, as low as 1 percent.[6] Unemployment rates for people with disabilities are often 80 percent or higher.[7] The most common form of employment for disabled individuals outside of their households remains begging.[3]

Worldwide, one family in four has a member with a significant disability, and this ratio is growing.[1,8] Injury and violence, as well as lack of access to adequate health care, continue to disable millions of people. Many other types of disabilities are not currently preventable. In addition, improved health care, particularly for critically ill newborns and those who are seriously injured or chronically ill, means that many people who previously would have died, now survive—often for decades—with a disability.

Although there is extensive literature on disability, the vast bulk of it addresses clinical, rehabilitative, or vocational issues rather than public health. Outside of specific data sets from developed countries, where income-maintenance schemes and general health care initiatives have prompted officials to keep statistics for rehabilitative or educational services, there is a lack of epidemiological or demographic data on disabled populations.[1,8] Little attention has been paid to how people with disabilities can and should be incorporated into broader public health initiatives or social justice campaigns.

Yet people with disabilities are often at increased risk for many chronic and infectious diseases, from Alzheimer's disease to malaria, and for social and behavioral problems, such as malnutrition, domestic violence, and substance abuse.[3,9] They are also more likely to be denied legal, social, and political rights, largely because, in many countries, they continue to face severe stigma and discrimination.[6,10]

Disability is often assumed to be evidence of bad blood or incest, divine displeasure, or punishment for sins. Too often, people with disabilities and their families are relegated to the margins of society. Such social interpretation of disability is important because disability cannot be understood outside of a cultural matrix. Within every society, attitudes and inclusionary or exclusionary practices are, in part, shaped by beliefs about why a disability occurs and what the anticipated adult roles are for people with disabilities.[11] Differences in socioeconomic status, class, caste, and educational level also make a significant difference in the quality of life for people with disabilities.[3,6]

Where disability is stigmatized, a common corollary is that people with disabilities are deprived of the resources of that society. In such societies, people with disabilities often contend with a "charity model." That gives them no inherent right to the resources of a community. In poorer societies, the unmet needs of people with disabilities are sought through individualized appeals for charity—begging on a street corner or the steps of a church. In more industrialized societies, such unmet needs are often addressed by more organized appeals, such as telethons and public fundraisers. These kinds of charitable appeals, whether done by individuals or organizations, differ significantly from how needs could be addressed through a "rights-based" model, in which all individuals are believed to be entitled to an equitable share of the community's resources.

Disability, Poverty, and Inequality

People with disabilities may account for as many as one in five of the poorest people in the world. Even among the very poor, people with disabilities are recognized to be the poorest members of the community. Disability rates can be used as a socioeconomic indicator to help assess poverty and development.[1] Not all disability is associated with poverty, but there is a heightened chance that once a disability occurs, those who lived above the poverty line will be driven into poverty. Those who were poor before the disability are more likely to become destitute.[3]

Disability disproportionately affects the poor.[7,8] Those who are poor are likely to live and work in more physically dangerous environments, have less to eat, and receive poorer quality medical care or none at all. This feedback loop between disability and poverty places people with disabilities at a marked disadvantage at every stage of their lives.[6]

Disabled children, particularly those with more visible disabilities, are frequently assumed to be in frail health and unlikely to survive into adulthood. Indeed, in many countries, a significantly disabled child is referred to as "an innocent" or a "little angel."[9] From this perspective, sending such children to school, including them in social interactions, or preparing them for participation in the adult world seems unnecessary. Families with disabled children have often anticipated their early death, but not their possible survival (box 8-2).

Disabled adolescents and young adults are rarely allowed to learn marketable skills or participate in the formal and informal "rites of passage"— such as learning to drive, playing sports, and dating—that prepare all other young people for their transition to adulthood. Where no services exist, such young people usually must either continue to live as "children" in their parents' households, face institutionalization, or find themselves on the street. One-third of all street children are disabled.[9]

As adults, people with disabilities are often denied the right to work outside the home. They are also often forbidden to marry or have children or to participate in those religious, social, and recreational activities that mark their status as adult members of society. They often have no political voice and frequently are barred from taking oaths or giving testimony in court, which severely restricts their ability to call upon protection from the legal system or to question legal decisions made for them by family or society.

To be female and disabled is frequently referred to as being doubly disabled. Survival itself is often at issue.[12] For example, a poor family may delay buying medicine for a disabled daughter, hoping that the condition will clear on its own. An indication of the extent of this problem can be seen in the survival figures of individuals who have had polio from Nepal, where the survival rate for males is 12 percent compared 6 percent for females. As polio affects males and females

BOX 8-2 Disability and Education

Sara had looked forward to school for years. Third in a family of five children, Sara, age 8, has waited an additional 2 years to start school because of her parent's reluctance to let her venture beyond their rural homestead. Born with a withered right arm, Sara's parents feared that she would be the object of ridicule by local children and a sign to other parents that their family had been cursed. But she was bright and inquisitive, and a full season of pestering on her part had finally led her parents to relent. Taking her seat in the classroom, the surrounding students looked at her uneasily. Many were playmates, who already knew her from home. It was the teacher who would decide her fate, however, and the teacher's reaction was swift and uncompromising. "You would be a distraction to other children," the teacher told her. "And besides, I do not know how to teach crippled children. There is a special school for your kind in the city if you want to go." Sara dissolved into tears and returned home. Twelve years later, her eyes still fill with tears as she recounts the incident.

Sara's experience in her West African village school is hardly unique. However, inclusion into general classroom settings is not unknown. For example, up to 40 percent of disabled children in rural northwest Pakistan have attended school in general classrooms.[1] Yet, in many countries children with disabilities are simply turned away even through their specific disability would not preclude them being able to function within a general classroom. In other cases, minor adaptations—allowing a child with poor eyesight to sit closer to the board, or moving a class from the second to the first floor of a building to allow a child who has mobility problems to attend—is all that is required. In cases where special adaptations are needed, such as sign language interpretation or instruction for children who are deaf or special adaptations for children with intellectual disabilities, more resources are needed.

Unfortunately, many countries have only one or two schools for special education, often located in capital cities, that tend to serve children from more affluent families. While such schools are helpful for those who attend or for teachers who can receive some training through them, the capacity of these schools is limited. They are usually underfunded and short of staff and facilities; they can rarely educate more than several hundred children at a time. In many countries, this means that there are "waiting lists" for such schools that, in theory, number in the tens of thousands.

Some countries are beginning to respond. Uganda, for example, has now established a nationwide program to serve every disabled school-aged child. Each district has an office of special needs education, integrated with the district's education office. Within each district, three specially trained teachers are appointed as assistant inspectors of schools to oversee services related to special needs education and to provide training and support for

(continued)

teachers, communities, local leaders, and parents on issues of education and inclusion. In addition, all 13,000 schools in Uganda have been grouped into clusters of 15 to 20, with a special needs education coordinator available for each cluster to make educational plans for each disabled child.

Regrettably, however, in many countries, education for disabled children is still a low priority. Adult education and literacy programs designed specifically for adults with disabilities are all but unknown. Any attempt to bring these millions of individuals with disability into the economic, social, and political mainstream or to reach them effectively in public health campaigns will not occur unless their educational needs are seriously considered.

Reference

1. Milas M. Children with disability in ordinary schools: an action study of non-designed educational integration in Pakistan. Peshwar National Council of Social Welfare, 1986.

in equal numbers, the gender imbalance reflects higher mortality rates in females.[6] A study in six Asian-Pacific nations found that the incidence of disability was higher for women than for men, making the higher survival rate for men with disabilities in these countries even more strikingly unequal.[12]

Women with disability often receive significantly less education, are less likely to marry, and have much more difficulty finding employment than do disabled males or nondisabled women.[6] With little ability to support themselves and few prospects for marriage, millions of women with disability live in abject poverty and at increased risk of physical and psychological abuse.[13]

People with disabilities who are members of ethnic and minority populations are also at increased risk. Coming from traditions that differ from that of the majority population, they are less likely to be included in available services and programs. Women with disability from ethnic or minority communities often find themselves contending with forces that exclude them on the basis of gender as well as disability and heritage.[3]

The Impact of Social Injustice on People With Disabilities

Public health work is frequently framed in terms of disability prevention. However, the need to ensure that people with disabilities maintain good health is all too often overlooked. This lack of attention is perhaps not surprising, because few schools of public health or medicine integrate issues of disability into the curriculum. When addressed at all, information on disability is usually offered in electives taken only by those students with an already-established interest in the subject.

In health services and programs in the community, the question of whether people with disabilities are being reached and served is rarely raised—whether the focus is breast cancer screening, dental care, or reproductive health. Research on the distribution of chronic and infectious diseases among disabled people and on their knowledge, attitudes, and practices concerning various health and social-welfare issues—research that is frequently performed on other vulnerable subgroups, such as women and racial/ethnic minorities—is rarely pursued.

Access to non–disability-related medical care is also limited.[14] Health care facilities frequently are simply inaccessible. Stairs block access for wheelchair users. Medical equipment that requires patients to transfer from a wheelchair or to stand—from examining tables to dental chairs to x-ray machines—are difficult to locate. A lack of sign language interpreters makes medical consultation difficult for many deaf people. Access to clinics, testing sites, and counseling programs may require more organization and planning than individuals with mental health problems or intellectual impairments are capable of providing (box 8-3).

Problems go beyond accessibility. In both developed and developing countries, those who seek care for conditions not related to their disability report that clinicians seem fixated on their disabilities no matter what the condition is for which they seek help.[3,13] Clinicians often refuse to provide basic vaccinations, reproductive health information, or chemotherapy to people with disabilities because they assume that people with disabilities do not have need for these services or do not have the right to use scarce resources.[3,9] During times of disaster and political upheaval, disabled people face additional challenges (box 8-4).

Disability-Specific Resources

Issues of unmet rehabilitative needs for some also lessen the ability of people with disabilities to fully participate in society. Not all people with disabilities need rehabilitative care; some never need it and many more need it for limited amounts of time or intermittently throughout the lifecycle. Therefore, one can be both disabled and healthy.[2]

The availability of rehabilitative care and prosthetic devices, such as artificial limbs, wheelchairs, hearing aids, and eyeglasses, however, must be specifically addressed because it is usually accorded a low priority by health professionals and policy-makers. Lack of such resources often restricts people with disabilities far more than does their specific impairment.

Worldwide, an estimated 3 percent of those who need rehabilitation services receive any care.[6,8] Rehabilitative services tend to be concentrated in urban areas and are prohibitively expensive. Programs that require long-term

BOX 8-3 Similarities and Differences Among People With Disabilities

People with different types of disability often face markedly different sets of problems. For example, an individual with a physical impairment who needs assistance with activities of daily living, such as dressing, toileting, and feeding, may benefit significantly from environmental adaptations such as ramps, grab bars, and automated doors. An individual who is deaf may have no physical restrictions but will need a sign language interpreter in order to communicate effectively with the surrounding hearing world. An individual who is intellectually impaired may be physically fit and fully able to communicate but may need help in organizing and carrying out daily responsibilities. An individual with a mental health problem may be fully able to meet both physical and intellectual challenges but need support and appropriate medication in order to continue to function successfully in the community.

Historically, disabled individuals, on the basis of their specific disabilities, have been divided into distinct constituencies. The concept of "disability" as a politically viable category developed in the late 1960s when people with a broad range of disabilities started to join together in an emerging Disability Rights Movement. They argued that, no matter what types of disabilities they had, most faced common challenges. Their lives were structured and their options determined by (a) complex medical, legal, and educational bureaucracies; (b) a social security system not designed to serve those people with disabilities who wanted some measure of independence and self-determination; and (c) the broader society where prejudice and stereotypes were still widespread.

Because resources for people with disabilities are extremely limited, disability advocacy and service organizations are frequently forced to compete with each other for these limited resources. Organizations working on behalf of those who are blind or physically disabled, for example, must often justify why funding for their projects or programs will yield greater benefits or why their constituents are more worthy of support than are individuals with other types of disabilities.

care are unavailable to many, especially women in those societies where they are not allowed to travel or live away from home unescorted. Globally, women and children receive less than 20 percent of all rehabilitation services.[12] In developing countries, community-based rehabilitation (CBR), in which services and expertise is offered at the community level with a triage system in place to access greater expertise, offers some promise. However, CBR programs are chronically underfunded, rarely brought to the necessary scale, and usually the first programs cut when funding is reduced.

BOX 8-4 Disability During Times of Disaster and Political Upheaval

During times of natural disasters and political upheaval, individuals with disability often face a complex set of problems. For example, a recent study by the Center for Services and Information on Disability (CSID) examined the fate of individuals with physical mobility problems during times of natural disasters in 10 coastal districts in Bangladesh.[1] Only 17 percent of individuals with mobility impairments had been taken to cyclone shelters; 55 percent of them remained at home while their families went to shelters. The remaining 28 percent either sought safer shelter in a built structure nearby or were forced to cling to a tree or other permanent structures. Following the disaster, individuals with mobility problems were much less likely to be able to access relief supplies—largely because, in order to get emergency food rations, building materials, or medicines, people were required to travel to central distribution sites and stand in line for long hours—difficult or impossible for many of those with mobility impairments. Only 2 percent of the families with a disabled individual in the CSID study had received any special attention during the rehabilitation phase following the disaster.

Such problems are compounded when families are forced to flee their homes. Individuals with disability are often left behind in times of war and famine when families flee; in particular, when they are forced to flee on foot. Being left behind in times of emergency is not related solely to the physical inability of individuals with some types of disabilities to keep up. In many disaster situations, families who anticipate becoming refugees and seeking asylum in another country may fear that all members of the family will be denied asylum if one in the family is disabled. (This is a realistic fear, as many countries, including the United States, have routinely denied asylum because of disability status—arguing that the new immigrants would be unlikely to become self-supporting.) Social and political unrest often leads to the closure of health care institutions, schools, and other resources that have been responsible for providing support and advocacy. In such situations, individuals with disability are often left behind, with only the thinnest of social support systems in place—the neighbor down the street who promises to look in once in a while or distant relatives.

Although there has been increasing attention to the fate of people disabled during political upheaval and natural disasters, most disaster relief organizations still do not anticipate how to reach and serve these people, within either communities or refugee camps. Some relief organizations have responded to queries about serving individuals with disability by stating that they actually see few individuals with disabilities. The troubling question is: "Then where are they?"

Reference

1. Rahman N. Disasters and disability: service delivery or rights? Dhaka, Bangladesh: National Forum of Organizations Working with Disability, 2004.

HIV/AIDS and Disability

A study that this author pursued on the impact of HIV/AIDS and the global disability community helps to illustrate the interlocking problems faced by people with disabilities.

Although AIDS researchers have studied the disabling effects of HIV/AIDS on previously healthy people, almost no attention has been given to the risk of HIV/AIDS for people with existing disabilities. A review of both the published literature and resources on the Internet yields only a few articles on the risk posed by HIV to people with disabilities, with most attention directed to people affected by both mental illness and drug addiction.[15]

Why have people with disabilities not been included? It appears to be because it is commonly assumed that people with disabilities are not at risk. They are incorrectly thought to be sexually inactive, unlikely to use drugs, and at less risk for violence or rape than their nondisabled peers. Yet they actually have equal or increased risks for all known risk factors for HIV/AIDS compared with their nondisabled peers.

For example, extreme poverty and social sanctions against marrying an individual with a disability mean that people with disabilities, especially women with disabilities, are likely to become involved in a series of unstable relationships and have less ability to negotiate safer sex within these relationships.[12] Factors such as increased physical vulnerability, the need for attendant care, life in institutions, and the almost universal belief that disabled people cannot be a reliable witness on their own behalf places many disabled males and females at risk of being victims of sexual abuse and rape at rates up to three times as high as their nondisabled peers.[13] In cultures in which it is believed that HIV-positive individuals can rid themselves of the virus by having sex with virgins, there has been a significant rise in the rape of disabled children and adults, who have been specifically targeted because they are assumed to be virgins.[16] Bisexuality and homosexuality have been reported within disabled populations at rates comparable to that of the general population.[17] People with disabilities are at increased risk of substance abuse and less likely to have access to interventions. Disabled adolescents in particular are rarely reached by safer sex campaigns.[3]

Educating disabled populations about AIDS is also difficult. Lack of access to education has resulted in extremely low literacy rates, which makes communication of messages about HIV/AIDS even more difficult. This lack of access is reflected in significantly lower rates of knowledge about HIV prevention in several studies among deaf people and adolescents with intellectual impairments.[3,18] Sex education programs for those with disabilities are rare.[18–20] Few HIV/AIDS educational campaigns target, and fewer include, disabled populations.[15] Indeed, where HIV/AIDS educational campaigns are on radio or television, groups such as the deaf and the blind are at a distinct disadvantage.

People with disabilities who become HIV positive are equally disadvantaged, having far less access to general health services than do nondisabled people.[11,21] Indeed, care is often both too expensive for impoverished people with disabilities and physically inaccessible.[22] A growing number of reports from disability advocates worldwide point to significant unreported rates of infection, disease, and death due to HIV/AIDS.[22]

Despite these risk factors, our global survey identified only a few HIV/AIDS pilot programs and interventions for disabled populations.[15,22] While a number of these projects are innovative, almost all are small and underfunded. HIV/AIDS campaigns that specifically target people with disabilities as members of the general public are rarer still.[23] There is a pressing need to understand the impact of HIV/AIDS on disabled populations and to design and implement programs and policy for them in a more coherent and comprehensive manner. And AIDS is only one of a number of public health issues in which such exclusion has occurred.

Roots and Underlying Issues

How could such a large and vulnerable population be so significantly overlooked? The answer in part is that "experts" and "policymakers" are also the product of the societies in which they are raised and, thus, accept commonly held assumptions about people with disabilities as scientific "fact." Just as in earlier eras, assumptions about women or members of ethnic or minority groups went unchallenged, much of what we think we know about people disabilities reflects our cultural biases, not biological fact. This is compounded by the common assumption—not proven fact—that the needs of those with disability are invariably too expensive or too complex to be addressed immediately.

What Needs to Be Done

What is needed most is awareness that people with disabilities must be included—and the commitment to do so (fig. 8-2). In many cases, people with disabilities can be included in health programs at little or no additional costs. For example, in many countries, ramps into clinics can be made of pounded sand, stone, or bamboo. General AIDS prevention campaigns and smoking cessation messages for the general public can easily be designed to be simple and straightforward to enable individuals with intellectual impairments to understand them.

Arguments for the need to improve public health and social justice for people with disabilities increasingly meet with positive responses. At professional

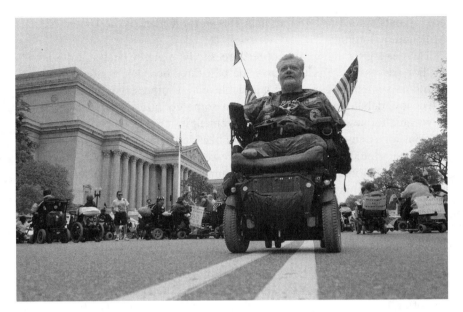

Figure 8-2 Disabled man demonstrating at the Justice Department in Washington, D.C., advocating for better Medicare and Medicaid benefits for long-term care for disabled people. (AP Wide World Photos.)

conferences, nongovernmental organization (NGO) meetings, and United Nations forums, discussions of the needs of disabled populations now often bring warm responses from colleagues. However, problems remain. "I would very much like to help disabled children in my community," a colleague recently confided after I had given a talk on social injustice and disabled adolescents. "But I can't even get services to nondisabled children."

The problem, of course, is that there is no reason why people with disabilities should be listed last on a long list of social problems—to be addressed after other problems are solved. For one thing, the lives of people with disabilities are no less valuable than the lives of anyone else. Moreover, many public health and social justice issues will never completely disappear. If disabled populations must wait until all other inequalities are solved, they will wait forever.

More important, other problems will not themselves be solved unless people with disabilities are part of the common solutions. Global poverty, for example, will never be fully eradicated unless people with disabilities are included in all international health and development schemes. As former World Bank President James Wolfensohn has noted, "Unless disabled people are brought into the development mainstream, it will be impossible to cut poverty in half by 2015 or to give every girl and boy the chance to achieve a primary education by the same date—goals agreed to by more than 180 world leaders at the United Nations Millennium Summit."[24]

There is a growing number of resources to help public health professionals as they address these issues. Over the past three decades, a global disability rights movement has emerged and achieved an impressive record of public advocacy, debate, and involvement. In some countries, it has successfully advocated for new legislation. The movement is currently pressing the United Nations for a convention on the rights of disabled people. Disability advocates can—and should—serve as a major resource for public health and social justice professionals. Indeed, growing numbers of people with disabilities are also seeking training in public health, law, medicine, and political science and can now serve as both advocates and experts.

The involvement of people with disabilities in helping to identify and define the needs and concerns of disabled populations is particularly important to note, because all too often public health professionals and organizations interested in disability issues continue to call upon only nondisabled experts in rehabilitation or medicine for guidance. These experts often have much they can offer, but decisions on behalf of people with disabilities can no longer be made without their input at all stages of policy and program planning.

Those who are concerned with social justice issues in pubic health can also make a significant contribution by ensuring that disability issues are included in all phases of public health education and practice. The example of women in health and development provides a useful model. Thirty years ago, there was little in public health that specifically addressed women beyond the arena of maternal and child health. Today, few public health or social justice issues can be raised without careful consideration of how women are affected, both as members of the general population and as a specific group. In the same way, people with disabilities must routinely be included in all public health activities.

Conclusion

Advocates in public health and social justice must rethink many basic assumptions about disability. The issue is not disability prevention or disability services but recognition that disability is—and will continue to be—an inevitable part of life. Although disability is inevitable, denial of human rights to people with disabilities, their lack of equitable access to public health and social services resources, and their disproportionate rates of poverty should not be. These threats to social justice are socially determined and, as such, can be socially redefined. The public health and social justice needs of people with disabilities are strikingly similar to those of their nondisabled peers. What distinguishes people with disabilities are not their common needs but the fact that these needs continue to go so largely unmet.

The expectation that an individual with a disability will either recover or die does not fit current reality. People with disabilities will often survive whether or not they receive an education, are provided medical and rehabilitative care, or are included in the social, religious, and economic affairs of their communities. Their existence and our own, however, will be much richer if they are allowed to develop to their full potential.

References

1. Department of International Economic and Social Affairs, Statistical Office, United Nations. Disability statistics compendium: statistics on special population groups (series y, no. 4). New York, N.Y.: United Nations, 1990.
2. United Nations. Standard rules on the equalization of opportunities for persons with disabilities (General Assembly resolution 48/96). New York, N.Y.: United Nations, December 1993.
3. World Bank. Adolescents and youth with disability: issues and challenges. Working paper. Washington, D.C.: The World Bank.
4. Mental Disability Rights International. Not on the agenda: human rights of people with mental disabilities in Kosovo. Washington, D.C.: Mental Disability Rights International, 2002.
5. Crossmaker M. Behind locked doors: institutional sexual abuse. Sexuality and Disability 1991;7:201–19.
6. Helander E. Prejudice and dignity: an introduction to community-based rehabilitation. New York, N.Y.: United Nations Development Program, 1998.
7. Brock K. A review of participatory work on poverty and ill being: consultations with the poor. Prepared for Global Synthesis Workshop, September 22–3, 1999. Washington, D.C.: Poverty Group, PREM, World Bank, 1999.
8. Elwan A. Poverty and disability: a survey of the literature. Washington, D.C.: Social Protection Unit, Human Development Network, The World Bank, 1999.
9. UNICEF. An overview of young people living with disabilities: their needs and their rights. New York, N.Y.: UNICEF Inter-Divisional Working Group on Young Peoples Programme Division, 1999.
10. Ingstad B, Whyte S, eds. Disability and culture. Berkeley, Calif.: University of California Press, 1995.
11. Groce N, Zola I. Disability in ethnic and minority populations. Pediatrics 1993;91;5: 1048–55.
12. Economic and Social Commission for Asia and the Pacific. Hidden sisters: women and girls with disabilities in the Asian and Pacific region. New York, N.Y.: United Nations, 1995.
13. Nosek M, Howland C, Hughes R. The investigation of abuse and women with disabilities: going beyond assumptions. Violence Against Women 2001;7:477–99.
14. Altman BM. Does access to acute medical care imply access to preventive care? A comparison of women with and without disabilities. J Disability Policy Stud 1997; 8:99–128.

15. Groce N. HIV/AIDS and people with disability. Lancet 2003;361:1401–2.
16. Groce N, Trasi R. Rape of individuals with disabililty: AIDS and the folk belief of virgin cleansing. Lancet 2004;363:1663–64.
17. Cambridge P. How far to gay? The politics of HIV in learning disability. Disability Society 1997;12:427–43.
18. Gaskins S. Special population: HIV/AIDS among the deaf and hard of hearing. J Assoc Nurses AIDS Care 1999;35:75–8.
19. Collins P, Geller P, Miller S, et al. Ourselves, our bodies, our realities: an HIV prevention intervention for women with severe mental illness. J Urban Health 2001;78:162–75.
20. McGillivray J. Level of knowledge and risk of contracting HIV/AIDS amongst young adults with mild/moderate intellectual disability. J Appl Res Intellectual Disabilities 1999;12:113–26.
21. Lisher D, Richardson M, Levine P, et al. Access to primary health care among persons with disabilities in rural areas: a summary of the literature. Rural J Health 1996;12:45–53.
22. Groce N. HIV/AIDS and disability: capturing hidden voices. Washington, D.C.: The World Bank, 2004. Available at: http://cira.med.yale.edu/globalsurvey. Accessed June 14, 2005.
23. Yousafzai A, Edwards K, Groce N, Wirz S. Knowledge, personal risk and experiences of HIV/AIDS among people with disabilities in Swaziland. Int J Rehab Research 2004;27:247–51.
24. Wolfensohn J. Poor, disabled and shut out. *The Washington Post,* December 3, 2002:A25.

9

INCARCERATED PEOPLE

Ernest M. Drucker

Introduction

Over the past 30 years, high levels of imprisonment have become a driving force of social injustice in the United States. While largely unrecognized as a public health issue, mass incarceration derails the lives of millions by damaging opportunities for work, education, housing, and a stable family life, undermining many of the foundations of personal health and well-being and community cohesion—the principal safeguards against crime in any society.[1] When incarceration occurs at very high rates and with great disparities in its application, it becomes an important way of relating social injustice to public health.

Studying patterns of mass incarceration and its consequences helps us understand the most persistent health and social problems of this society because of (a) the magnitude of the population affected; (b) the huge disparities in the racial and ethnic composition of prison populations (relative to the population as a whole); and (c) the direct effects of incarceration for the individuals imprisoned and collateral damages for the families and communities affected. Incarceration policies and practices in the United States are the modern heir to our long legacy of state mechanisms that perpetuate social and racial injustice in the tradition of slavery; segregation; and discriminatory immigration, trade union, and social welfare policies that isolate, stigmatize, and marginalize the most economically disadvantaged.[2]

The contrast of U.S. incarceration policies to those of other developed societies is astonishing. While the United States has only 5 percent of the world's population, it has 25 percent of its prisoners. Today more than 6.5 million Americans—almost 4 percent of the adult population—are under the control of the criminal justice system (table 9-1). In 2004, over 2 million people were in federal, state, and local prisons and jails, and another 4.6 million were on probation and parole.[2] Since 1975, over 25 million individuals have been incarcerated—more than the total imprisoned in the previous 100 years. New York State, with more than 100,000 inmates in 2000, had the highest incarceration rate in the 120 years that state records were kept, a trend that holds nationally.[3]

The U.S. imprisonment rate is now at the highest level in its history: nearly 700 per 100,000 people. Most other countries have substantially lower rates (fig. 9-1). European countries average less than one fifth the U.S. incarceration rate, and many average only one tenth of it.[4,5]

Prison budgets in the United States are also at an unprecedented level, averaging over $25,000 per inmate or about $50 billion annually—most of it coming from state budgets needed for social and health services. With $100 billion used to build new prisons since 1980, the United States has created a prison industrial complex—a vast system of over 5,000 federal, state, and local prisons and jails housing millions of inmates and employing an equal number of law enforcement and correctional workers.

This corrections "industry" has a huge economy of prison construction, health and mental health services, and food and equipment sales. In addition, the operation of private, "for-profit" prisons has become a significant feature of the U.S. correctional system. By 2001, over 6 percent of the entire system and 12 percent of the federal system (142,521 beds in total) were being run privately—with 75 percent of the business going to two publicly traded international security firms; one of these had $147 million in contracts in 2002.[6-9]

TABLE 9-1 U.S. Prison Rates in State and Federal Prisons and Local Jails, per 100,000 Adults Aged 18 to 29, by Race, Gender, and Age Group, 2000

Age Group	Male			Female		
	White	Black	Hispanic	White	Black	Hispanic
18–24	649	4,180	1,710	68	349	137
25–29	1,615	12,877	4,339	170	752	314

From U.S. Department of Justice, Bureau of Prison Statistics. April 2002, NCJ No. 198877 p. 11.

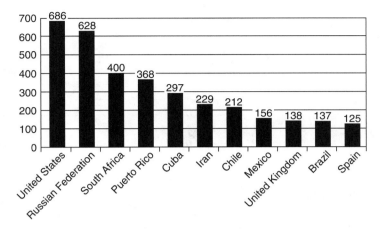

Figure 9-1 Incarceration rates per 100,000 people for United States and selected other countries in 2000. (From Incarceration rates by country [selected countries]. Available at: http://www.kcl.ac.uk. In 2003 [before expansion], the EU incarceration rate averaged 150 per 100,000.)

Mass Incarceration and Race

A hallmark of incarceration in the United States is the striking economic, ethnic, and racial disparity in its application. While representing only about 12 percent of the total U.S. population, African-Americans comprise nearly 50 percent of the prison population. Worldwide, over 10 percent of all prisoners are African-American males.[2]

Incarceration is now becoming the norm for a substantial proportion of African-American men. Over one-third of all black men aged 20 to 29 in the United States are now in prison or jail, or on parole and probation. More black males go to jail than to college. In Washington, D.C., more than 75 percent of all black men can expect to be incarcerated at some point in their lives.[10] A random telephone survey conducted in central Harlem in 2002 found that 9 percent of all those responding had been in jail in the previous year and between 35 and 40 percent knew of someone who had been released from prison in the previous year.[11]

This pattern is not entirely new. A large racial disparity in prison rates has always existed in the United States and was an important feature of the post–Civil War era of reconstruction, when freed slaves were converted to prisoners and put back on the plantation under vagrancy laws.[12] Outside of the South, however, the current magnitude of black–white disparities in incarceration is unprecedented. In the late nineteenth century in New York State,

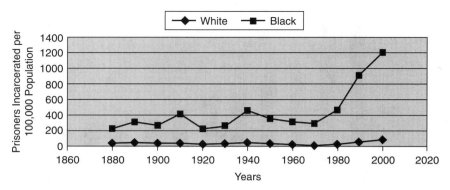

Figure 9-2 Incarceration rates by race for 1880–2000 in New York State. (From U.S. Census; and Hupart JH, unpublished report on New York State historical data on prison rates. Based on New York State Department of Prisons [1880–1960], New York State Department of Correctional Services [1961–2000].)

for example, about four blacks were locked up for every white; today that ratio is 12:1.[3] For nonviolent drug offenses (about 30 percent of all New York State cases), that ratio is 40:1, and for Hispanics, it is 30:1, relative to whites (fig. 9-2).[13] Drug incarcerations are at the heart of the huge growth of racial and ethnic disparities seen in our prisons. Yet there is no evidence of any great difference in the rates of illicit drug use by these groups: in New York State, for example, drug overdose rates for blacks, whites, and Hispanics are within 20 percent of each other.[14] Compounding the adverse effects of welfare policies, unemployment, and broken families, incarceration for drug offenses predicts future criminal involvement and subsequent more-serious crimes.

Collateral Damages of Incarceration

The impact of incarceration extends well beyond the massive populations in prisons. It has profound consequences for the families and communities who are its principal targets—the black and Hispanic urban communities, which account for more than 80 percent of all inmates in the United States. Over 2.5 million school-aged children currently have an incarcerated parent. This has important adverse effects on the mental health of these children and families, both when the family member is put behind bars and after release. Over 600,000 prisoners in the United States reenter the community each year, with powerful consequences for urban community life due to their social, political, and economic disenfranchisement.[15]

How Social Injustice Affects the Incarcerated

Any effort to understand the health impact of incarceration must reckon with its huge scale and its role in the specific communities and populations most affected, beginning with the effects on prisoners themselves—both while under the control of the criminal justice system and after release.

The Health of Prisoners

Others have documented the many serious health problems of the incarcerated.[16] Not surprisingly, these are the same problems seen among low-income people in the community who are overrepresented in prisons: poor access to health care, drug addiction, alcoholism, and infectious diseases—especially sexually transmitted diseases (STDs), viral hepatitis, and HIV/AIDS. The conditions of prison life serve to amplify all of these problems, such as the transmission of HIV/AIDS, other STDs, and hepatitis B and C virus infection through rape and through the sharing of contraband drug–injecting equipment.

Beyond the high levels of pathology among incarcerated populations in the United States, poor inmate health services persist in many of the nation's prison systems. Despite the constitutional entitlement to "decent medical care" (under the 8th Amendment barring "cruel and unusual punishment") and frequent court mandates to provide it, there remain persistent failures to fulfill this obligation.[16]

Ultimately, however, incarcerated people do not represent a distinct population. They are overwhelmingly drawn from the same populations that inhabit the poor and minority communities of the United States, as is true in many other nations. The particular risks and disparities in health care that are the norm in prisons mirror faithfully those to which these same populations are exposed when in their home community. Further, many of the specific health risks and patterns of social injustice faced by incarcerated people persist after their release. This is due to the socially disabling effects of multiple periods of incarceration that poor African-American and Hispanic men routinely face, such as the loss for drug offenders of eligibility for many jobs and many federal health entitlements. In the United States, where incarceration has become "normative for these groups" (p. 181),[17] repeated periods of incarceration must be understood as a major determinant of the health of those populations subject to the highest rates of imprisonment.

While in some circumstances, such as court-ordered care, prisoners may receive better medical care in prison than they receive outside of prison, the norm is inadequate health care for the incarcerated. This too often mirrors and worsens the inadequate health care of the poor outside of prison, especially in the case of mental illness. In combination with the ill health that these populations bring with them into the prisons, the result is a pattern of health problems not seen in any other institutional population in the United States. More than 80 percent of U.S. prison inmates enter prison with problems of drug abuse or dependency, and drug use often continues throughout prison stays— often with more dangerous injecting. After release, inmates face an increased risk of acquiring bloodborne diseases, STDs, and (by 10-fold) dying of an overdose.[18,19] The violence and stresses of prison life and the poor quality of diet and medical care all increase the risks of complications of diabetes, hypertension, and other chronic diseases, which are so prevalent among the incarcerated, especially black and Hispanic inmates and those with histories of tobacco and/or alcohol abuse.

Mental health problems are another hallmark of U.S. prison populations. Following deinstitutionalization in the 1970s, the strong association of drug use and mental illness led the criminal justice system to become the default system for the chronic mentally ill in the United States—most dramatically, among the poor. Today, approximately 500,000 inmates have a major psychiatric disorder. Serious psychiatric cases are recurrent in the prison system. Over 40 percent of those in solitary confinement—which is widely used to discipline prisoners—have major psychiatric disorders.[20] While those in solitary represent only 5 percent of the prison population, they account for almost half of the suicides. Homelessness before and after incarceration is widespread; almost 25 percent of those released from prison will end up in a shelter or on the street within the first 6 months after release.[21]

The psychological trauma of being incarcerated under brutal circumstances and the routine abuse, humiliation, and disregard of fundamental human rights that go along with mass incarceration in the United States are similar to the widely publicized accounts of abuse by U.S. prison guards in the war in Iraq—and in Afghanistan and at Guantanamo.

These apparently criminal offenses by U.S. servicemen and servicewomen abroad may be understood in the context of (a) the harsh conditions and racial disparities of mass incarceration in the United States (box 9-1), and (b) the daily portrayals of the prison world in the U.S. news media in ways that desensitize the American public to their true nature. As incarceration becomes commonplace, it engenders a callous disregard of the damaging effects on individuals and their families, and denial of any political responsibility for all of its social consequences—often shifting the blame to the victims, their families, and their communities.

BOX 9-1 Prisoner Abuse and Torture in the United States and Iraq

There are some clear lines between the abuses of mass incarceration in the United States and the treatment of prisoners in the Iraq war. Many of the military personnel in Iraq were reservists who were formerly prison guards in the United States, influenced by that system's values and practices. Accustomed to processing many inmates at home, these recruits were poorly trained to serve the military police function—especially in the midst of a conflict like the Iraq occupation and insurgency, where friends are hard to distinguish from foes and fellow soldiers are randomly killed or wounded daily. This is a classic formula for dehumanization of the enemy, the abuse of prisoners, and the commission of war crimes.

The *New York Times* columnist Bob Herbert has described U.S. prisons where "inmates are viewed as less than human, routinely treated like animals," brutalized and degraded "in ways remarkably similar to the abuses at Abu Ghraib" (p. 17).[1] He recounted that, in 1996, officers from the Tactical Squad of the Georgia Department of Corrections raided Dooly State Prison, in Unadilla, Georgia, where

> officers opened cell doors and ordered the inmates, all males, to run outside and strip. With female prison staff members looking on, and at times laughing, several inmates were subjected to extensive and wholly unnecessary body cavity searches. The inmates were ordered to lift their genitals, to squat, (and) to bend over and display themselves.
>
> One inmate who was suspected of being gay was told that if he ever said anything about the way he was being treated, he would be locked up and beaten until he wouldn't "want to be gay anymore." An officer who was staring at another naked inmate said, "I bet you can tap dance." The inmate was forced to dance, and then had his body cavities searched (while another) was slapped in the face and ordered to bend over and show himself to his cellmate. The raiding party apparently found that to be hilarious.

As in Iraq, these abuses appear to have been sanctioned by prison leadership and committed with impunity—the commissioner of the Georgia Department of Corrections was present at the Dooly State Prison raid. And governmental accountability for these crimes is limited—a law passed by Congress in 1996 bars most inmates from receiving any financial compensation for such abuse. A lawsuit filed by the Southern Center for Human Rights, representing several prisoners in Georgia who sought compensation in the late 1990s for treatment that was remarkably similar to the abuses at Abu Ghraib, was denied. Herbert concluded, "The treatment of the detainees in Iraq was far from an aberration. They, too, were treated like animals, which was simply a logical extension of the way we treat prisoners here at home."

(continued)

BOX 9-1 (*continued*)

Ultimately, the systematic abuse and humiliation of prisoners in both U.S. and Iraqi prisons is torture—a human rights violation and crime that should be subject to protection under international law.

Reference

1. Herbert B. America's Abu Ghraibs. The *New York Times*, May 31, 2004.

Collateral Damage: Effects on Prisoners' Families and Communities

"Collateral damage" is the military term for unintended effects of wartime violence on noncombatants—bystanders caught in the line of fire. The same phrase applies to U.S. incarceration policies where, in addition to the crime victims, there are many other "innocent" casualties—not of crime, but of punishment.

Most significant, more than half of incarcerated men have children under age 18 and more than half of these men were living with their children at the time they were sent to prison. (For women, the percentage in both instances is greater than 80 percent.) A recent Human Rights Watch report estimated that in New York State, which had 70,000 prisoners in 2001, there were 23,537 children who had a parent in prison as a result of drug charges and an estimated 124,496 children who had at least one parent imprisoned as a result of the state's "Rockefeller drug laws," which were enacted three decades ago and mandate long sentences for nonviolent drug offenses.[15] Nationally, there are more than 2 million minor children of current inmates (in prison for all offenses), and more than 20 million children have had a parent incarcerated since the early 1970s.

The incarceration of a parent—often repeatedly—disrupts these children's social environment and the financial stability of their families, weakening parental bonds and placing severe stress on the caregivers left behind to fend for themselves. This often leads to a loss of discipline in the household and to feelings of shame and anger for the children, which are manifested in behavioral problems. Poor school performance, unsupervised free time, financial strain, decreased contact with adults, and suppressed anger are all precursors of delinquency.[22] Despite widespread awareness of this problem, there is no systematic effort to minimize the impact of parental incarceration on children.

Drug-enforcement policies are particularly important for understanding mass incarceration. They account for the most racially disparate incarceration rates during the past 25 years. More prisoners are incarcerated for drug offenses in the United States today—more than 450,000—than the number of prisoners incarcerated for all offenses in the European Union, which has a population 25 percent larger than the United States. Most of the growth of incarceration in the United States in the past three decades has been driven by public policies on drugs.[23] Beginning in 1973, the "Rockefeller drug laws" in New York State (initiated by Governor Nelson Rockefeller) mandated long prison sentences for nonviolent drug offenders. Soon after, they became a model for state and federal drug enforcement. Between 1975 and 2000, the rate of drug incarcerations in New York State increased from 8 percent of the prison population to more than 30 percent.[13]

Since 1974, more than 150,000 people have been incarcerated in New York State, where over 110,000 person-years of life have been lost to imprisonment for drug offenses alone in this time.[24] About 90 percent of the prisoners have been male, with a median age (in 2000) of 35; 78 percent have been New York City residents, 94 percent black or Hispanic, and 70 percent have come from just six New York City neighborhoods.

In the United States, there are now more than 450,000 individuals incarcerated for nonviolent drug offenses. To this number must be added almost 2 million drug offenders on parole or probation—lives greatly diminished by incarceration and control by the criminal justice system. With the chronic inadequacies of addiction treatment in the United States, positive drug tests are a leading cause of reincarceration for drug offenders violating their probation and parole.

Economic Disenfranchisement

As one inmate put it, "My sentence really began the day I was released." Extensions of the impact of incarceration into the postsentence life of felons also increase the burden on their families beyond the time of prison terms. Specifically, felony conviction usually means a greatly reduced chance of gainful employment. In most states, 75 to 95 percent of jobs requiring a state license are barred to those with felony records. They are disqualified for many professional careers, such as those for beauticians and barbers, taxi drivers, or U.S. Postal Service employees. Many felons lose their driver's licenses and the job opportunities that require one. They lose eligibility for military service. Felons with drug offenses are also temporarily or permanently barred from visits to their families in public housing and from getting important federal benefits, such as home and school loans that might help them pursue lives without crime.

Civic Death: Felony Disenfranchisement

Intensifying the damage done to family and community structure, felony convictions also mean the loss of the right to vote—in prison, while on parole, and, in some states, while on probation. In 7 states, convicted felons are barred from voting for life. Currently, an estimated 4.4 million Americans are barred from participating in the most meaningful expression of civic life—even after they have "paid their debt" to society. Almost half of these disenfranchised people (about 2 million) are black.

At any given time, 30 to 40 percent of all black men aged 18 to 30 are thus disenfranchised.[25] The usual voting rate of this age group, regardless of race, is about 25 percent, meaning that for young black young men in those areas with high incarceration rates, more people may be disenfranchised than those who vote.[26] As the 2000 presidential elections in Florida demonstrated, this is political disempowerment writ large—affecting not just individuals but entire communities.

Roots and Underlying Issues

To understand the political roots of mass incarceration as social injustice, one must understand the "war on drugs" (p. 16).[23] The arrest and incarceration of nonviolent drug offenders have led to a 10-fold increase in the prison population over the past three decades. U.S. government surveys make clear that the prevalence of illicit drug use differs only slightly by race and ethnicity.[27] Why, then, are so many African-Americans imprisoned for drugs?

It is largely the result of (a) the huge illegal drug industry, which is a major part of the economy and operates openly in most minority communities; and (b) the vulnerability of the low-level user-dealers in these communities to police "buy and bust" operations—low-risk methods that stoke police arrest rates and prosecutors' conviction rates (95 percent are plea-bargained without trial). These drug laws and prosecution practices are by now deeply embedded in our criminal justice system.[17] Their restrictions of judicial discretion by mandatory sentencing policies represent the triumph of political forces of the right and the acquiescence by more liberal political forces for fear of being dubbed "soft on crime." Governor Rockefeller of New York, seen as a moderate Republican by many in the early 1970s, promoted these laws to distinguish himself from the liberal wing of his party. In appearing to address the burgeoning heroin epidemic of the time by this tough stance, he succeeded in undermining the newly successful methadone programs of that era, which were just beginning to establish their efficacy.[28]

This unprecedented use of incarceration in the United States represents an ominous sea change in the American criminal justice system. It is creating an imbalance of power in the judicial system and a move away from earlier notions of rehabilitation, toward a "more punitive approach of incapacitation and retribution" (p. 61).[29] It is deforming the entire legal apparatus by increasing prosecutorial powers, minimizing and weakening the defense function, and decreasing judicial discretion and power—especially in drug enforcement, where harsh mandatory sentences account for much of the national growth in incarceration since 1975. Incarceration has now become the "presumptive method of punishing lawbreakers" (p. 67).[29] Incarceration is the default position of the criminal justice system instead of alternative punishments that leave offenders in the community, such as drug treatment, probation, work programs, and restorative justice strategies, which attempt to compensate and heal victims' families.

All societies need to deal with crime and punishment, to establish and enforce laws, and to expend resources to restrain and sometimes imprison those who transgress. However, mass incarceration is another matter. Mass incarceration systematically undermines black family and community life on a scale not seen since slavery, by destroying the very social capital needed to prevent crime.[30–32] And it may contribute to the persistent deficits seen in the physical and psychological health and well-being of the entire black population.[33–35]

What Needs to Be Done

Clearly, we must recognize that incarceration should be used sparingly, especially for nonviolent offenders who are the parents of minor children—to recognize that our "cure" is worse than the "disease." But how may we get to this point? Approaches are now being developed to reverse these trends and limit the damage they have done by addressing the specific social injustices affecting the incarcerated, their families, and their communities.

Improve Community Services

Involvement of youth in drug use and the local drug trade can be addressed by improved alternative activities for youth, better schools, and support for families in poor communities. Offering nonjudgmental and accessible health care, with better diagnostic, therapeutic, and preventive services in those communities (including counseling, education, and screening for mental health problems, drug abuse, and HIV and STDs), can significantly reduce the chronic health problems that often become evident in prisons.

Provide Better Health Services to Those Incarcerated

This is the subject of constant litigation, but it remains a persistent challenge as states cut budgets and privatize prison health services. There is also a great need to improve programs and services available to those just released from prison and those on probation or parole.

Reform Drug Laws

Marijuana laws account for more than 300,000 people in prison and over 800,000 arrests annually. Reform of these laws has significant public support. Medical use of marijuana should be legalized and possession of small amounts of marijuana for personal use should be decriminalized, as has been done in the United Kingdom and Australia, and is now being considered in Canada.

Repeal Mandatory Sentencing Laws

Mandatory sentencing laws need to repealed, especially those for nonviolent drug offenses. While some headway is being made through the use of "drug courts" that order treatment of nonviolent drug offenders instead of their incarceration, the real need is to replace the old drug laws with new ones that allow judges discretion to discriminate between dangerous criminals and the vast number of defendants with drug-dependency problems.

Assist Family Members

We must work to reduce the collateral damage to the children, families, and communities most affected by implementing policies and programs to help them when their family members are sent to prison—and when they are discharged. There are some preliminary efforts now under way to limit these collateral harms of incarceration for families and children. On New York's Lower East Side, Family Justice, Inc./La Bodega de la Familia, begun under the sponsorship of the Vera Institute of Justice, provides intensive support to drug offenders' families when they are released from prison in order to reduce the risk that they will return to criminal activity. To reduce the impact on children when a parent is incarcerated, several programs of the Osborne Association and the Fortune Society supporting families of inmates in New York now offer the most basic supports to children aged 4 to 14: counseling, educational tutoring, and helping children write letters to incarcerated parents. More than 80 percent of children with parents in prison never get to visit them, so these programs organize visits to the often-remote prisons where their parents are incarcerated. Some programs are using videotechnology to enable "tele-visiting" between inmates and their families at home.

Address Voting Disenfranchisement

Disenfranchisement has become a major focus of political activity since the 2002 election, in which over 2 million blacks were unable to vote due to these laws. Some preliminary work is under way to re-register former inmates and restore their voting rights, such as the Jeht Foundation programs for ex-offenders to reinvolve them in the society in positive ways. (See http://www.jehtfoundation.org.) But many more such programs are desperately needed. In addition, the National Association for the Advancement of Colored People (NAACP) Legal Defense Fund and the Brennan Center for Constitutional Rights at New York University School of Law are litigating felony disenfranchisement on the basis of racial disparities in the application of criminal penalties.

Conclusion

The unprecedented rate and racial disparity of incarceration in the United States have their roots in the application of drug laws and their disproportionately harsh mandatory-sentencing policies. Although there is no evidence of any significant differences in the use of illicit drugs by minority populations, the specific conditions of their purchase and use in poor communities—such as at shooting-gallery and street-drug markets—expose minority users to arrest and prosecution, and then to a series of plea bargains and establishment of criminal records that lead to very long mandatory sentences for subsequent (and predictable) drug violations. About one-third of incarcerated people are nonviolent drug offenders, and another third are drug-dependent individuals prosecuted for acquisitive crimes associated with their drug use. In addition, the increasingly normative nature of incarceration of minority men in urban centers feeds the growth of gangs and greater involvement in drugs and criminal culture.

We, as a society, must learn how to limit our use of incarceration—especially in response to youthful drug use—and find other means to enforce many other laws. This means setting lower incarceration rates as targets and holding political leaders accountable for meeting them. We should reduce the number of prisoners to levels that other democratic states have achieved through the use of more-effective and less-damaging social policies.

The principal reforms needed are (a) changes in drug policies to reduce criminalization of drug use, and (b) application of a public health model to address drug problems worldwide, replacing prosecution with effective treatment, education, and prevention efforts. We must abolish laws that are patently unjust and counterproductive—especially antiquated and discredited drug laws, which have led us to make imprisonment "normal" for so many Americans. We should direct much of the huge resources expended in the criminal justice system—more than $100 billion annually—to housing, health care, education, and social supports in those communities now most heavily affected by mass incarceration policies.

Acknowledgments The author's work has been supported by The Jeht Foundation and The Soros Justice Fellowship program of the Open Society Institute; he acknowledges the seminal work and encouragement of Nils Christie and the research and helpful conversations about these issues with Ricardo Barreras, Marc Mauer, Jacob Hupart, Bob Gangi, and Jamie Fellner.

References

1. Christie N. Crime control as industry. 3rd ed. London, U.K.: Routledge, 2002; and Garland D. Mass imprisonment: social causes and consequences. Thousand Oaks, Calif.: Sage, 2001.
2. Mauer M. Race to incarcerate. 2nd ed. New York, N.Y.: The New Press, 2000.
3. New York State Department of Prisons (1880–1960), New York State Department of Corrections (1961–2000), US Census (1880–2000). Washington, D.C.: U.S. Department of Commerce, Bureau of the Census.
4. Walmsley R. World prison population list, 4th ed. Available at: http://www.kcl.ac .uk/depsta/rel/icps/downloads.html. Accessed May 2, 2005.
5. Walmsley R. World prison population list, 3rd ed. Research infdings No. 166. Available at: http://www.ad.vscr.cz/news_files/03_Walmsley.doc. Accessed February 2005.
6. U.S. Department of Justice, Bureau of Justice Statistics. Private adult correctional facility census, 2001. Washington, D.C.: Bureau of Justice Statistics, 2001.
7. Greene J. Bailing out private jails. *The American Prospect*, September 2001.
8. Greene J. Entrepreneurial corrections: incarceration as a business opportunity. In: Mauer M, Chesney-Lind M, eds. Invisible punishment: the collateral consequences of mass imprisonment. New York, N.Y.: The New Press, 2002.
9. Huling T. Building a prison economy in rural America. In: Mauer M, Chesney-Lind M, eds. Invisible punishment: the collateral consequences of mass imprisonment. New York, N.Y.: The New Press, 2002.
10. Braman D. Families and incarceration. In Marc M, Chesney-Lind M, eds. Invisible punishment: the collateral consequences of mass imprisonment. New York, N.Y.: The New Press, 2002.
11. Galea S. New York Academy of Medicine, personal communication, April 2003.
12. Oshinsky DM. Worse than slavery: Parchman Farm and the ordeal of Jim Crow justice, paper edition. Glencoe, Ill.: Free Press, 1997.
13. New York State Dept of Corrections. Department of Correction reports to The Corrections Association of New York. Unpublished report, 2003.
14. Annual Mortality Reports, New York State DOH (2002), Annual CDC Mortality Data. Available at: http://wonder.cdc.gov. Accessed April 2, 2005.
15. Fellner J. Collateral damage: children of inmates incarcerated in NY State under Rockefeller drug laws. New York, N.Y.: Human Rights Watch, June 2002.
16. Farmer P. The house of the dead: tuberculosis and incarceration. In: Marc M, Chesney-Lind M, eds. Invisible punishment: the collateral consequences of mass imprisonment. New York, N.Y.: The New Press, 2002.
17. Clear T. The problem with addition by subtraction: the prison-crime relationship in low income communities. In: Mauer M, Chesny-Lind M, eds. Invisible punishment: the collateral consequences of mass imprisonment. New York, N.Y.: The New Press, 2002.

18. Singleton N, et al. Drug related mortality among newly released offenders. Findings #187, London, U.K.: UK Home Office, 2003.

19. Graham A. Post-prison mortality: unnatural death among people released from Victorian prisons between January 1990 and December 1999. Aust N Z J Criminol 2003; 36:94–108.

20. The health status of soon to be released inmates: a report to Congress. Washington, D.C.: National Commission on Correctional Health, 2003.

21. Metraux S, Culhane D. The intersection of corrections services and shelter use: findings from New York City. Unpublished manuscript, University of Pennsylvania, 2004.

22. Gabel K, Johnstone E, eds. Children of incarcerated parents. Lanham, Md.: Lexington Books, 1995.

23. Drucker E. Drug prohibition and public health: 25 years of evidence. Public Health Rep 1999;114:14–29.

24. Drucker E. Population impact of mass incarceration under New York's Rockefeller drug laws: an analysis of years of life lost. J Urban Health Bull N Y Acad Med 2002;79. (Full text of article accessed at NYAM/JUH Website: www.jurban.oupjournals.org.)

25. The Sentencing Project (Washington, D.C.) and Human Rights Watch (New York, N.Y.). Losing the vote: the impact of felony disenfranchisement laws in the United States. New York: Human Rights Watch, October 1998.

26. Mauer M, Chesney-Lind M, eds. Invisible punishment: the collateral consequences of mass imprisonment. New York, N.Y.: The New Press, 2002.

27. National Institute of Drug Abuse. Monitoring the future: Racial and ethnic disparities report. Washington, D.C.: NIDA, 2004.

28. Massing M. The fix. Berkeley, Calif.: University of California, 1998.

29. Davis AJ. Incarceration and the imbalance of power. In: Mauer M, Chesney-Lind M, eds. Invisible punishment: the collateral consequences of mass imprisonment. New York, N.Y.: The New Press, 2002.

30. Rose DR, Clear TR. Incarceration, social capital, and crime: examining the unintended consequences of incarceration. Criminology 1998;36:441–79.

31. Wilson WJ. There goes the neighborhood. *New York Times*, OpEd, Sunday, June 16, 2003.

32. Putnam DR. Bowling alone. Carmichael, Calif.: Touchstone Books, 2001.

33. Geiger HJ. Racial and ethnic disparities in diagnosis and treatment: a review of the evidence and a consideration of causes. Washington, D.C.: Institute of Medicine, August 2002.

34. Byrd MW, Clayton LA. National Center for Health Statistics, report of the Secretary's Task Force on Black and Minority Health. USDHHS, 1994.

35. Treadwell HM. Poverty, race, and the invisible men. Am J Public Health 2003;5: 705–6.

10

HOMELESS PEOPLE

Lillian Gelberg and Lisa Arangua

Introduction

Homelessness is a focus of increasing social and public health concern worldwide, even in countries with superior safety nets. The United Nations Committee on Human Rights defines absolute homelessness as the condition of those without any physical shelter who sleep outdoors, in vehicles, or in abandoned buildings or other places not intended for human habitation, as well as those people staying in temporary forms of shelter, such as emergency shelters or in transition houses.[1] An estimated 100 million people worldwide fit this definition of absolute homelessness.[2] The estimated number of homeless people in the United States is 3.5 million,[3] in England and in France, at least 500,000,[4–6] and in Canada, tens of thousands.[7]

The demographic characteristics of homeless people vary from country to country. In developed countries, 60 to 95 percent of homeless people are male (fig. 10-1). Single men account for most chronically homeless individuals (those with a current homeless episode of 1 year or longer). Homeless families are frequently reported in the United States but only rarely in other countries. The median age of homeless people in the United States is 32 years; in most European countries, it is 40. Minority and indigenous persons are overrepresented in the homeless population.

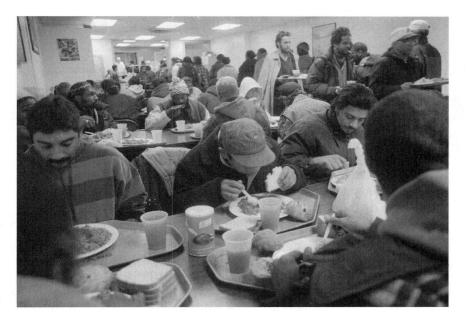

Figure 10-1 Homeless people eating dinner at the Bowery Mission in New York, which serves 500 to 600 meals a day. (AP Wide World Photos.)

Mortality and disease severity of homeless people far exceed those of the general population and the housed poor population and are due to factors such as extreme poverty, delays in seeking care, nonadherence to therapy, substance-use disorders, and psychological impairment. Homeless people in their 30s and 40s develop severe disabilities and seek hospital care at rates that are seen in people decades older. The homeless condition itself is a powerful contributor to adverse health outcomes; for example, street-dwelling homeless people have significantly worse health outcomes than do homeless-shelter residents.

The multitude of social and health problems that homeless people endure reflects a variety of social injustice issues. The homeless condition itself represents the convergence of multiple factors, including poverty, high housing costs, and a shortage of subsidized public housing units. The exposure to substandard environmental conditions that affects the health of homeless people is related to urban development failures. The complex health, social, and psychological problems commonly experienced by homeless people as a result of these factors present a therapeutic challenge. Many health care providers lack the time or necessary training to treat homeless persons. Even in countries with socialized medicine, general primary care physicians often fail to fully register homeless people who seek to register at a practice because of associated social problems, complex health problems, substance abuse, and lack of medical records.

How Social Injustice Affects the Health of Homeless People

Homeless people, as a group, are exposed to among the highest levels of virtually all social and environmental risk factors for adverse health effects and thus pose serious public health challenges. The impact of homelessness on health can be profound for the newly homeless, long-term homeless, formerly homeless, or episodically homeless. Even relatively short bouts of homelessness expose individuals to deprivations such as hunger and poor hygiene and to victimization through robbery, physical assault, or rape.[8] Homeless persons have a very high prevalence of untreated acute and chronic medical, mental health, and substance-abuse problems. Many health problems, such as infections due to overcrowded living conditions in shelters, hypothermia from exposure to extreme cold, and malnutrition due to limited access to food and cooking facilities, are a direct result of homelessness.[9] Homeless persons who have a substance-abuse or mental health problem or a physical disability are at increased risk of remaining homeless.[10] Poor health among the homeless is due to many factors, including extreme poverty, inadequate family and other social supports, the pressing demands of day-to-day survival, delays in seeking care and reduced access to care, nonadherence to therapy, and cognitive impairment.

Health Status

Approximately 35 percent of homeless persons in developed countries report having poor health,[11–14] compared with 21 percent of housed persons of lower socioeconomic status (SES) and 4 percent of housed persons of higher SES.[13–15] Factors such as length of time people are homeless or the condition of living on the streets significantly increase the probability of perceived poor or fair health status.[14,16]

Contagious diseases and infections, such as tuberculosis (TB),[17] HIV infection,[18] hepatitis B virus infection,[19] and hepatitis C virus infection,[20] are more common among the homeless than among housed people. In most developed countries, TB prevalence rates among the homeless are 3 to 20 times greater than in the general population.[21,22] Prevalence of HIV infection among the homeless in developed countries ranges from 2 to 9 percent—3 to 10 times greater than that of the general population.[23,24] Among homeless adults in the United States, 23 to 47 percent have had previous exposure to hepatitis B virus, compared with 5 to 8 percent in the general population, and 1 to 12 percent are currently infected with this virus, compared with 0.1 to 0.5 percent for the general population.[25,26] In developed countries, between 22 and 44 percent of homeless adults and between 5 and 17 percent of homeless adolescents have tested positive for hepatitis C virus infection[27,28]; these rates are 10 to 12 times greater than that of the general population.

Substance Use

Between 69 and 82 percent of homeless people in developed countries currently smoke—more than double the rate of lower SES groups and more than three times the rate in the general population.[29]

Homeless persons describe high rates of alcohol and drug use. The prevalence of alcohol dependence among the homeless ranges from about 25 percent in England, France, and Spain, to 60 percent in the United States and 73 percent in Germany[30–33]—three to five times greater than rates of the general population in these countries. The high rates in the United States and Germany may result from high per-capita alcohol use, easy accessibility, and relatively low cost.

Rates of illicit drug dependence are also high among the homeless. In Germany, England, Spain, and France, the prevalence of drug dependence among the homeless ranges from 9 to 16 percent.[30,31,33,34] Drug dependence is more prevalent in the United States (30 to 49 percent) and the Netherlands (60 percent).[35,36] Rates of drug dependence among the homeless are four to six times greater than those of the general population in these countries. Drugs of choice among the homeless in the United States are cocaine and marijuana, whereas in Spain and the Netherlands they are opioids and heroin. The prevalence of both alcohol and drug abuse is higher among homeless men than among homeless women.

Obesity and Sedentary Lifestyle

The prevalence of obesity in homeless persons ranges from 23 percent in Germany to 39 percent in the United States—almost three times the rate of the general population.[37,38] In contrast, the homeless in Japan do not appear to have any significant problems with obesity.[39] Limited physical activity is significantly more common among homeless persons (47 percent), compared with the general population (15 percent). Heart disease, diabetes, and hypertension are higher among the homeless largely because of their sedentary lifestyles.[40]

Mental Health

Since the 1960s, mental health services have gone through major transitions in developed countries, leaving an increasing number of mentally ill people living on the streets or in shelters or hostels.[41] Over a lifetime, 34 to 45 percent of the homeless in England and almost 60 percent of the homeless in the United States and France experience a serious mental disorder—rates that are two to four times those in the general population.[34,42,43] Lifetime major depression (20 percent) and recent major depression (15 percent) are the most prevalent mental disorders. More than half of homeless persons suffering from a chronic mental health disorder also experience comorbid substance abuse/dependence problems.[35] Rates of schizophrenia among the homeless range from 4 to 9 percent in Germany, Canada, the United States, Spain, and England to 15 percent in France.[30,33,44,45] Rates of mental disorders are higher for men than they are for women, except for rates of lifetime depression and serious mental disorder without associated substance abuse.

Mortality

Homelessness is strongly associated with an increased risk of death in several countries.[46–48] For homeless people in developed countries, the average age at death is between 45 and 50 years.[46–48] The age-adjusted number of years of potential life lost (YPLL) before age 75 is three to four times higher for homeless persons than for the general population.[49,50] Cause of death differs significantly among the homeless in different countries. For example, in the United States, homicide, accidents, substance abuse, liver disease, heart disease, HIV infection, pneumonia, and influenza are the leading causes of death among the homeless.[46,49] In some other countries, leading causes of death are substance abuse, cardiovascular disease, alcoholic liver disease, and suicide.[47,50,51] Homeless persons in other developed countries have much lower mortality rates than those in the United States[48–50]; access to social and health services as well as cultural factors may better explain this difference.

Health Care Access and Utilization

Of homeless persons in Canada and the United States, 75 percent report receiving some form of health care in the past year.[52] However, 25 percent of homeless persons reported that they needed to see a doctor in the past year but were unable to do so.[53] Additionally, most homeless persons seek care at places that do not provide the continuous quality care that can address their complex health problems. Of those homeless persons who sought care in the past year, 32 percent received care at a hospital emergency department, 27 percent at a hospital outpatient clinic, 21 percent at a community health clinic, 20 percent at a hospital as an inpatient, and 19 percent at a private physician's office.[3] High rates of emergency department use among homeless persons represent the substitution of emergency department care for conditions more suitable for outpatient primary care. Having a regular source of care, which is strongly associated with access to health services and use of preventive health services, is very low among homeless persons, with more than half lacking a regular source of care.

In the United States and Canada, about 24 percent of the homeless are hospitalized each year.[52,53] About 75 percent of hospitalized homeless persons are hospitalized for conditions that are often preventable, such as substance abuse, mental illness, trauma, respiratory disorders, skin disorders, and infectious diseases except AIDS—a rate 15 times that in the general population.[54] Following hospital discharge, 40 percent of homeless persons are readmitted to the hospital within 14 months, usually with the same diagnosis. The finding that most homeless inpatients could have been treated less expensively in an outpatient setting highlights the difficulty in sustaining treatment intensity for homeless persons outside the hospital. Despite higher rates of medical hospitalization and higher rates of disease, homeless persons are, in fact, less likely to use medical ambulatory services than other sectors of the population. Homeless persons often delay seeking medical attention at an early stage when illness could be prevented. Homeless adults, given their increased need for care, may benefit from improvement and increased availability of primary and preventive care.

Disparities in Health Status Among the Homeless

The degree of homelessness, as measured by number of homeless episodes, length of time homeless, and living in unsheltered conditions, has profound effects on health status and use of health services. Unsheltered homeless persons are more likely to use illegal drugs, have an acute skin injury, report daily alcohol use, be victimized, experience an accident or injury, and be exposed to TB than are sheltered homeless persons.[55] Unsheltered homeless women are more likely to report fair or poor health status, be engaged in risky sex, have poor pregnancy outcomes, have more gynecological conditions, be forcibly raped, have poor mental health, and use drugs and alcohol, compared with sheltered women.[56–59]

Despite their overwhelming health needs, unsheltered and long-term homeless persons are significantly less likely to use health services. Sheltered homeless persons are more likely to report use of health services than are unsheltered homeless persons.[53,60] Unsheltered and long-term homeless persons are less likely to use nonurgent ambulatory care services or be hospitalized and more likely to have unmet needs for care and use emergency departments than more stably housed homeless persons.[56,61,62] Long-term homeless persons are also less likely to have a regular source of care and to receive substance abuse treatment. Homeless persons with extended homelessness have twice the mortality rates of others, even after controlling for all other factors.[63]

Roots and Underlying Issues

Historically, two competing political and economic models—the social democratic model and the individual rational choice model—have profoundly influenced health and social policies regarding the homeless.

The social democratic model, which stresses the social rights of citizens in society, emphasizes that everyone is entitled to the resources that provide good health. Thus, society should seek to maximize the aggregate health of all. Under this model, the better health enjoyed by the upper classes is evidence that the poor and homeless could enjoy better health. As a result, the population is less healthy than it could be and, with the right policies in place, society could achieve better aggregate health for all. The social democratic model is the foundation of the European health care system and its superior safety net, which emphasizes the social ethic of the principle of solidarity. This model also found its way into the U.S. health care system during the "Great Society" initiative of the Johnson administration in the 1960s, and strains of it have persisted through the public health insurance systems of Medicaid, Medicare, and Social Security Insurance (SSI).

The individual rational choice model, which advocates individual effort and the freedom to exercise individual choice, stresses that people bear some responsibility for their individual risks for illness and death. Differences in health status reflect choices—in lifestyles, social conditions, and health habits—that have a greater influence on health status than medical care. Because individuals bear responsibility for health, this model calls into question whether differences in health can be construed as injustices. The model incorporates a justification for curbing political excesses, controlling administrative costs, and preventing overutilization of resources; hence, the market became the framework through which many rights could be realized. The model of individual rational choice also facilitates a distinction between the "deserving poor" and the "undeserving poor." Advocates harness a public fear that undeserving able-bodied malingerers will "free-ride" on other citizens who contribute compulsorily to the provision of public health benefits. "Deserving homeless" groups, under this model, include veterans, the disabled, the mentally ill, older people, and families with children.

However, neither of these models has clearly addressed a population health perspective that focuses on the social determinants of health in society. The social democratic model has created a system that ultimately increases access to medical care. The persistence in disparities in health among the homeless within countries with universal health care demonstrates that access alone will not eliminate health disparities in society. Many who support this model and its emphasis on medical care cite the super-sophisticated subspecialty system as perpetuating inequities and advocate for a strong primary care network, which will improve health status. Specialty care, which commands more health care resources, is virtually a closed system that worldwide is heavily accessed and used by groups better off socioeconomically.[64–66] However, the emphasis on the role of medical care, especially primary care, as explaining why groups of higher SES are healthier than the homeless overlooks evidence that demonstrates that social and cultural environments and other factors influence morbidity and mortality.

The individual rational choice model relies heavily on the process of economic growth, which is presumed to automatically bring improvements in population health. The Industrial Revolution improved sanitation, food safety, housing conditions, and life expectancy. But the human record shows no necessary direct relationship between economic advance and population health status. In the early modern period, economically advanced towns had the highest mortality rates among the lower classes.[67] Population health can serve as an index for economic strength. In nineteenth-century Britain, the absence of a significant political response to population health during a period of increased economic growth resulted in epidemiological devastation lasting half a century and significantly affecting the economy.[68] Japan and Scandinavia have succeeded in recently transforming economic growth into improved health for most citizens, resulting in the highest life expectancy rates in the world, which, in turn, has heightened these countries' economic potency.

Recently, there has been an overzealous application of the individual rational choice model, even in countries that have espoused the social democratic model. International policy priorities of the late twentieth and early twenty-first century have been marked by suspicion of central government and a heavy emphasis on the promotion of free trade and rapid economic growth, even at the expense of government investment in welfare and health services. Leading economists, including central finance ministers and administrators, have not supported the position that the social determinants of health should be considered in all major government initiatives or further research related to these determinants. The United Kingdom, Canada, and the United States have implemented fiscal policies over the past 15 years that have restricted public spending and increased income inequality through tax benefits for those with higher incomes.[69] Homeless persons and other disadvantaged people will be paying the health price for policies such as these that ultimately support the global market economy's growth. Epidemic-level health problems globally have provoked some governments, such as Canada and England, to begin to seriously examine the merits of the social determinants movement.[70,71]

What Needs to Be Done

A guiding and globally embraced political and social ethic for population health is critically needed to address the complex factors at play that severely affect the health of the homeless. This social ethic needs to address not only the equitable access to health services, but also the quality of care received and other contextual factors that may be affecting health.

Homeless people, even in countries with superior safety nets, report the stigma of being homeless and the prejudice of health care providers as a primary factor in not receiving care. These findings are consistent with emerging research that demonstrates that even at equivalent levels of access to care, impoverished groups experience a lower quality of health care services and are less likely to receive even routine medical procedures than higher income groups. Those delivering health care to homeless persons must carefully consider how their usual procedures and advice will be heard and experienced by those who do not have a home. Appropriate models of care must be developed, taught to clinicians, and replicated in the community. Medical education must perpetuate attitudes and professional paradigms that are attuned to the real and consistently changing needs of homeless people. Because most care provided to homeless people is in emergency departments rather than in special clinics for the homeless, all medical and surgical trainees in medical school, residency, and fellowship programs must be trained to develop an appreciation for and sensitivity to their patients' housing and poverty status.

Worldwide, clinics designated as treating the homeless report that they have difficulty in recruiting physicians. England reports that primary care physicians are not fully registering homeless patients due to the difficulty in treating them. Medical education reform and health care reform could ameliorate some of the major physician-recruitment barriers experienced by these clinics: poor working conditions, inadequate salaries, physician bias against working with homeless patients, and lack of respect that this work now receives from the medical profession.

Health care, however, is only one of many complex factors that explain health disparities among the homeless. Social and environmental factors also play an important role. As seen in our studies, disparities in health behaviors, such as cigarette use, obesity, and communicable disease, are also shaped by social and physical environments where homeless persons live. Most poor neighborhoods where homeless people live are littered with liquor and convenience stores that heavily market cigarettes and sell unhealthy food and drink. In addition, crowded shelters, substandard and unsanitary housing conditions, and social influences, such as drug use and high-risk sexual behaviors, place the homeless at higher risk for socially and environmentally induced health conditions, such as asthma (associated with mold), tuberculosis (associated with crowded living quarters), and infections with HIV, hepatitis A virus (associated with unhygienic and unsanitary living conditions), hepatitis B virus, and hepatitis C virus.

Redevelopment of low-income neighborhoods may be critically important to reduce disparities in health among impoverished groups such as the homeless. Recent studies have shown that countries with equally distributed environmental and social factors concerning sanitation, air quality, food and water safety, housing conditions, nutrition, and exercise have significantly narrowed the socioeconomic gap in health disparities.[72–74] Countries in which these contextual conditions have not been equally distributed would ultimately require redirecting resources, significant government investment, and collective efficacy (the capacity of neighborhood members to improve social and structural development according to collective principles and desires).

One promising model that could influence a guiding social ethic in health is the concept of "institutional" rational choice. According to the institutional rational choice model, social and environmental context facilitates and perpetuates patterns of behavior.[75] This model broadens the focus on solely the individual to include institutions or context, and thus challenges the individual rational choice model. Thus, factors such as the sensitivity of health care providers, the general quality of health care, and the social and physical environments in which homeless people live are included in the model as influencing health and individual behavior. The model ultimately encompasses many of the complex institutional, environmental, and social structures that profoundly influence the health of homeless persons.

The persistent and widening gap in health disparities between the homeless and higher income groups is largely the result of society's acceptance of approaches that focus exclusively on altering individual behavior as a means of improving health. The institutional rational choice model reveals how social justice demands recognition of how economic structures, cultural norms, and health institutions shape decision-making processes to undermine the prospects for self-determination and equality for homeless and poor people. In this sense, the model can take a leading role in setting priorities for social, economic, and health policy to better promote health among society's most vulnerable members, as well as helping to motivate a more clearly defined social ethic in health care.

Conclusion

Consideration of the health of homeless persons globally should not be limited to addressing their physical health, mental health, and substance abuse problems. It should also address attitudes toward and treatment of the poor worldwide, as well as welfare and housing policies. Globally, we have become ever more intimately interdependent on each other and on the consequences of our collective actions. Social justice for homeless people must reflect the collective efforts of local and global political leadership and cross-class alliances. This collective effort requires a thoroughgoing mobilization and participation of the population in a social ethic that focuses on the institutional, social, and physical elements that profoundly influence the health of homeless people in our societies.

References

1. Springer S. Homelessness: a proposal for a global definition and classification. Habitat International 2000;24:475–484.
2. United Nations Centre for Human Settlements (Habitat). Strategies to combat homelessness. HS/599/00 E-. Available at: http://www.unhabitat.org/en/uploadcontent/publication/HS-599.pdf. Accessed January 13, 2005.
3. Burt M, Aron L, Douglas T, et al. Homelessness: programs and the people they serve. Washington, D.C.: Interagency Council on Homelessness, 1999.
4. Leff J. All the homeless people: where do they all come from? BMJ 1993;306: 669–70.
5. Connelly J, Crown J, eds. Homelessness and ill health: report of a Working Party of the Royal College of Physicians. London, England: Royal College of Physicians, 1994.
6. Chauvin P, Mortier E, Carrat F, et al. A new out-patient care facility for HIV-infected destitute populations in Paris, France. AIDS Care 1997;9:451–9.
7. Hwang S. Homelessness and health. Can Med Assoc J 2001;164:229–33.
8. Link B, Susser E, Stueve A, et al. Lifetime and five year prevalence of homelessness in the United States. Am J Public Health 1994;84:1907–12.
9. Fischer P, Breakey W. Homelessness and mental health: an overview. Int J Mental Health 1986;14:6–41.
10. Culhane D, Kuhn R. Patterns and determinants of public shelter utilization among homeless adults in New York City and Philadelphia. J Policy Analysis Manag 1998; 17:23–43.
11. A report on the qualitative exploration for the entrants of winter season's temporary accommodation. Tokyo, Japan: Society of Welfare Office Director of Tokyo's 23 Wards, 1995.
12. Usherwood T, Jones N, Hanover Project Team. Self-perceived health status of hostel residents: use of the SF-36D health survey questionnaire. J Public Health Med 1993; 15:311–4.
13. Gallagher T, Andersen R, Koegel P, et al. Determinants of regular source of care among homeless adults in Los Angeles. Med Care 1997;35:814–30.
14. Nyamathi A, Leake B, Gelberg L. Sheltered vs non-sheltered homeless women: differences in health, behavior, victimization and utilization of care. J Gen Intern Med 2000;15:565–72.
15. National Center for Health Statistics. Health, United States, 1998: with socioeconomic status and health chartbook. Hyattsville, Md.: NCHS, 1998.

16. White MC, Tulsky JP, Dawson C, et al. Association between time homeless and perceived health status among the homeless in San Francisco. J Commun Health 1997;22:271–82.

17. Barnes P, Yang Z, Preston-Martin S, et al. Patterns of tuberculosis transmission in central Los Angeles. JAMA 1997;278:1159–63.

18. Zolopa A, Hahn J, Gorter R, et al. HIV and tuberculosis infection in San Francisco's homeless adults. JAMA 1994;272:455–61.

19. Gelberg L, Robertson M, Leake B, et al. Hepatitis B among homeless and other impoverished US military veterans in residential care in Los Angeles. Public Health 2001; 115:286–91.

20. Beech BM, Myers L, Beech DJ, et al. Human immunodeficiency syndrome and hepatitis B and C infections among homeless adolescents. Semin Pediatr Infect Dis 2003;14:12–9.

21. Yamanaka K, Akashi T, Miyao M, et al. Tuberculosis statistics among the homeless population in Nagaya City from 1991–1995. Kekkaku 1998;73:387–94.

22. Gelberg L, Panarites C, Morgenstern H, et al. Tuberculosis skin testing among homeless adults. J Gen Intern Med 1997;12:25–33.

23. Robertson MJ, Clark RA, Charlebois ED, et al. HIV seroprevalence among homeless and marginally housed adults in San Francisco. Am J Public Health 2004;94:1207–17.

24. Manzon L, Rosario M, Rekart ML. HIV seroprevalence among street involved Canadians in Vancouver. AIDS Educ Prevent 1992;Fall:86–9.

25. Cheung R, Hanson A, Maganti K, et al. Viral hepatitis and other infectious diseases in a homeless population. J Clin Gastroenterol 2002;34:476–80.

26. McQuillan G, Coleman P, Kruszon-Moran D, et al. Prevalence of hepatitis B virus infection in the United States: the National Health and Nutrition Examination surveys, 1976 through 1994. Am J Public Health 1999;89:14–8.

27. Desai R, Rosenheck R, Agnello V. Prevalence and risk factors for hepatitis C virus infection in a sample of homeless veterans. Soc Psychiatry Psychiatric Epidemiol 2003;38:396–401.

28. Nyamathi A, Dixon E, Robbins W, et al. Risk factors for hepatitis C virus infection among homeless adults. J Gen Intern Med 2002;17:134–44.

29. Kermode M, Crofts N, Miller P, et al. Health indicators and risks among people experiencing homelessness in Melbourne, 1995–1996. Aust N Z J Public Health 1998; 22:464–70.

30. Kovess V, Magin-Lazarus C. The prevalence of psychiatric disorders and use of care by homeless people in Paris. Soc Psychiatry Psychiatric Epidemiol 1999;34:580–7.

31. Munoz M, Koegel P, Vazquez C, et al. An empirical comparison of substance and alcohol dependence patterns in the homeless in Madrid (Spain) and Los Angeles (CA, USA). Soc Psychiatry Psychiatric Epidemiol 2002;37:289–98.

32. Vazquez C, Munoz M, Sanz J. Lifetime and 12-month prevalence of DSM-III-R mental disorders among the homeless in Madrid: a European study using CIDI. Acta Psychiatr Scand 1997;95:523–30.

33. Fichter M, Quadflieg N. Prevalence of mental illness in homeless men in Munich, Germany: results from a representative sample. Acta Psychiatr Scand 2001;103: 94–104.

34. Shanks N, George S, Westlake L, et al. Who are the homeless? Public Health 1994; 108:11–9.

35. Koegel P, Sullivan G, Burnam A, et al. Utilization of mental health and substance abuse services among homeless adults in Los Angeles. Med Care 1999;37:306–17.

36. Sleegers J. Similarities and differences in homelessness in Amsterdam and New York City. Psychiatric Serv 2000;51:100–4.
37. Luder E, Ceysens-Okada E, Koren-Roth A, Martinez-Weber C. Health and nutrition survey in a group of urban homeless adults. J Am Diet Assoc. 1990;90:1387–1392.
38. Langnase K, Muller MJ. Nutrition and health in an adult urban homeless population in Germany. Public Health Nutrition 2001;4:805–11.
39. Takano T, Nakamura K, Takeuchi S, et al. Disease patterns of the homeless in Tokyo. J Urban Health 1999;76:73–84.
40. Gelberg L, Linn L. Assessing the physical health of homeless adults. JAMA 1989; 262:1973–9.
41. Koegel P, Burnam A, Farr R. The prevalence of specific psychiatric disorders among homeless individuals in the inner-city of Los Angeles. Arch Gen Psychiatry 1988;45: 1085–92.
42. Victor C. Health status of the temporarily homeless population and residents of North West Thames region. BMJ 1992;15:6850.
43. Tompkins CN, Wright NM, Sheard L, et al. Associations between migrancy, health and homelessness: a cross-sectional study. Health Soc Care Commun 2003;11:446–52.
44. Munoz M, Vazquez C, Koegel P, et al. Differential patterns of mental disorders among the homeless in Madrid (Spain) and Los Angeles (USA). Soc Psychiatry Psychiatric Epidemiol 1998;33:514–20.
45. Geddes J, Newton R, Young G, et al. Comparison of prevalence of schizophrenia among residents of hostels for homeless people in 1966 and 1992. BMJ 1994;308: 816–9.
46. Hwang S, Orav E, O'Connell J, et al. Causes of death in homeless adults in Boston. Ann Intern Med 1997;126:625–8.
47. Ishorst-Witte F, Heinemann A, Puschel J. Morbidity and cause of death in homeless persons. Arch fur Kriminol 2001;208:129–38.
48. Babidge N, Buhrich N, Butler T. Mortality among homeless people with schizophrenia in Sydney, Australia: a 10 year follow-up. Acta Psychiatr Scand 2001;103:105–10.
49. Hibbs J, Benner L, Klugman L, et al. Mortality in a cohort of homeless adults in Philadelphia. N Engl J Med 1994;331:304–9.
50. Hwang S. Mortality among men using homeless shelters in Toronto, Ontario. JAMA 2000;283:2152–7.
51. Nordentoft M, Wandall-Holm N. 10 Year follow-up study of mortality among users of hostels foe homeless people in Copenhagen. BMJ 2003;327:81.
52. Hwang S, Gottlieb J. Drug access among homeless men in Toronto. Can Med Assoc J 1999;160:1021.
53. Kushel M, Vittinghoff E, Haas J. Factors associated with the health care utilization of homeless persons. JAMA 2001;285:200–6.
54. Salit S, Kuhn E, Hartz A, et al. Hospitalization costs associated with homelessness in New York City (special article). N Engl J Med 1998;338:1734–40.
55. Gelberg L, Andersen R, Leake B. The behavioral model for vulnerable populations: application to medical care use and outcomes. Health Serv Res 2000;34:1273–302.
56. Lim Y, Andersen R, Leake B, et al. How accessible is medical care for homeless women? Med Care 2002;40:510–20.
57. Wenzel S, Leake B, Gelberg L. Health of homeless women with recent experience of rape. J Gen Intern Med 2000;15:265–8.
58. Stein J, Lu M, Gelberg L. Severity of homelessness and adverse birth outcomes. Health Psychol 2000;19:524–34.

59. Wenzel S, Andersen R, Gifford D, et al. Homeless women's gynecological symptoms and use of medical care. J Health Care Poor Underserved 2001;12:323–41.

60. O'Toole T, Gibbon J, Hanusa B, et al. Utilization of health care services among subgroups of urban homeless and housed poor. J Health Politics Policy Law 1999; 24:91–114.

61. Lewis J, Andersen R, Gelberg L. Health care for homeless women; unmet needs and barriers to care. J Gen Intern Med 2003;18:921–8.

62. Kushel M, Perry S, Bangsberg D, et al. Emergency department use among homeless and marginally housed: results from a community-based study. Am J Public Health 2002;29:778–84.

63. Barrow S, Herman D, Cordova P, et al. Mortality among homeless shelter residents in New York City. Am J Public Health 1999;89:529–34.

64. Alter D, Iron K, Austin PC, Naylor D. Socioeconomic status, service patterns, and perceptions of care among survivors of acute myocardial infarction in Canada. JAMA 2004;291:1100–7.

65. Goddard M, Smith P. Equity of access to health care services: theory and evidence from the UK. Soc Sci Med 2001;53:1149–62.

66. Van Doorslaer E, Wagstaff A, van der Burg H, et al. Equity in the delivery of health care in Europe and the U.S. J Health Econ 2000;19:553–83.

67. Wrigley EA. A simple model of London's importance in the changing British society and economy, 1650–1750. Past Present 1967;37:44–70.

68. Hamlin C. Public health and social justice in the age of Chadwick: Britain 1800–1854. Cambridge, England: Cambridge University Press, 1998.

69. Carter M. Transient people, transient policies: a study of recent policy initiatives towards single homeless people. London, England: London School of Economics Homeless Group, 1992.

70. Acheson D. Report of independent inquiry into inequalities in health. London, England: Stationary Office, 1998.

71. Robertson A. Shifting discourses on health in Canada: from health promotion to population health. Health Promotion International 1998;13:155–166.

72. Wagstaff A, Van Doorslaer E. Equity in the finance and delivery of health care: concepts and definitions. In E Van Doorslaer, A Wagstaff, F Rutten (eds). Equity in the finance and delivery of health care: an international perspective. Oxford, England: Oxford University Press, 1993, pp 7–19.

73. Wilkinson RG. Unhealthy societies: the afflictions of inequality. London: Routledge, 1996.

74. Wilkinson RG. Socioeconomic determinants of health. Health inequalities: relative or absolute material standards? SMJ 1997;314:591–595.

75. Marlis E, Kannan M (eds). Preferences, institutions and rational choice. Oxford, England: Oxford University Press, 1995.

11

FORCED MIGRANTS: REFUGEES AND INTERNALLY DISPLACED PERSONS

Michael Toole

Introduction

One of the most stark examples of the relationship among social injustice, inequality, and poor health outcomes occurs among populations that are forcibly displaced. The major forced population movements in the past 50 years have been a result of (a) systematic persecution of certain population groups, such as religious or ethnic minorities; (b) widespread human rights abuses, such as torture, imprisonment, deprival of legal rights, and inadequate access to food, health care, education, and other social services; and (c) exposure to systematic violence intended to terrorize communities. Most of these situations have evolved in the context of economic uncertainty, political transition, and the emergence of predatory social formations.

During the Cold War period, civil war, persecution, and forced displacement of civilian populations were often masked by the ideological nature of the parties involved in armed conflict. In the 1970s and early 1980s, millions of refugees fled civil wars, which were mainly between pro- and anti-Communist forces in Central America (Guatemala, El Salvador, and Nicaragua), Asia (Indochina and Afghanistan), and Africa (including Ethiopia and Angola). Even during this period, however, movements that were apparently politically motivated sometimes disguised the underlying oppression of minorities by power elites. As examples, the right-wing Guatemalan government directed military action against indigenous Mayan communities, the new communist Pathet Lao government harassed members of the Hmong ethnic minority group in Laos, and the socialist Ethiopian government (dominated by the Amhara ethnic group) actively oppressed other ethnic groups (such as the Tigrayans). In each case, many refugees from the oppressed ethnic minorities fled into neighboring countries.

After the Cold War ended, most of the factions in armed conflicts ceased to masquerade as ideologically motivated, and civilian populations were increasingly targeted by violence—simply on the basis of their belonging to ethnic or religious minority groups. Many of these conflicts arose during a period of economic uncertainty and political transition; for example, as the former Yugoslavia abandoned communism, a small nationalist elite emerged, which violently resisted independence movements in the various republics and embarked on a massive campaign of "ethnic cleansing."

At the end of 2003, there were approximately 12 million refugees worldwide.[1] These people had crossed international borders, fleeing war or persecution for reasons of race, religion, nationality, or membership in particular social and political groups. Refugees are clearly defined by international legal conventions and, therefore, entitled to protection and assistance by the United Nations High Commissioner for Refugees (UNHCR).

The sources of most of the world's refugees continue to be countries in Asia, Africa, and the Middle East (fig. 11-1). However, at the end of 2003, three Asian countries—Afghanistan, Myanmar (Burma), and Vietnam—were the source of more than 3.5 million refugees. While the global total of

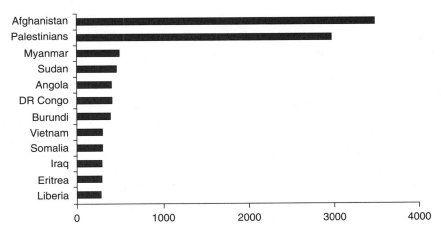

Figure 11-1 Source of the world's 12 largest refugee populations in 2002 (in thousands). (From U.S. Committee for Refugees and Immigrants, 2002.)

refugees declined in the early 1990s, there was a further increase between 1998 and 2001, with major refugee crises in Kosovo, East Timor, and West Africa, followed by another decline.

In addition, there were, at the end of 2003, about 24 million persons who had fled their homes for the same reasons as refugees, but who had remained inside their own countries and did not legally qualify for refugee status.[1] These internally displaced persons have been in especially precarious situations because they often have been beyond the reach of international agencies, which rely on the cooperation of national governments to deliver relief aid.

Effects of Social Injustice on the Health of Refugees

The social injustice experienced by civilians who eventually become refugees, internally displaced persons, or the victims of a siege, such as the inhabitants of Sarajevo, has often had a direct impact on their health status.

The story of Kosovo is revealing. Starting in 1989, when Serbian nationalism was being inflamed by the ruling elite in Belgrade, Kosovar Albanians suffered a gradually escalating gradient of discrimination. Ethnic Albanians found it difficult to obtain land titles, could not access professional employment, and could not enter universities. By 1998, Serbian police imposed severe restrictions on the physical movement of Albanians and frequently intimidated and harassed them.[2] These restrictions extended to access by Albanians to health care. The actual process of traveling to a hospital was restricted by random detention at checkpoints and lengthy identification checks. The general climate of fear meant that travel to a hospital after dark was impossible. Albanians were arbitrarily charged for their treatment, whereas Serbs did not have to pay. By early 1999, heavily armed police patrolled the main hospital in Pristina, snipers operating from the roof terrorized patients, Albanians who had been injured by violence were increasingly denied treatment, and all Albanian employees of the hospital had been fired.[2]

This spiral of human rights abuses culminated in massacres of Albanian civilians in their villages, which led to NATO intervention in March 1999. By the end of May, about 1.4 million Kosovars had been uprooted, including 442,000 in Albania, 250,000 in Macedonia, and more than 600,000 in Kosovo; and more than 67,000 had been displaced into Montenegro.[3] Following the success of the NATO campaign in June, most Kosovars returned to their homes; however, in a tragic irony, this repatriation led to the forced displacement of nearly 250,000 non-Albanian minorities from Kosovo, including Serbs and Roma.

The international community's assistance to Kosovar refugees was generous and effective in preventing disease outbreaks and excess mortality.[4] However, the impact of the forced migration on mental health was significant.

A large study by the U.S. Centers for Disease Control and Prevention in late 1999 found that 17 percent of adult Kosovar Albanians had a psychiatric disorder and, not surprisingly, 90 percent expressed strong feelings of hatred toward Serbs—and half of these Kosovar Albanians reported strong feelings of revenge.[5]

Impact of Violence

In other situations that have led to mass population displacement, the extent to which basic human rights have been denied has varied and included the worst possible types of violation. The systematic discrimination experienced by Kosovar Albanians was also experienced by Muslims in Bosnia, Serbs in Croatia, and Muslims in Chechnya—leading in all three cases to open armed conflict, many civilian casualties (between 25,000 and 60,000 in Bosnia), and millions of refugees and internally displaced persons.

The most dramatic manifestation of this gradient of terror has been genocide. Indisputably, genocide has occurred at least twice since World War II: first in Cambodia from 1975 to 1979 when a fanatical elite (the Khmer Rouge) declared war on its educated urban population, and then in Rwanda in 1994, when Hutu extremist leaders exploited long-standing ethnic animosity to slaughter approximately 1 million ethnic Tutsis. A more recent conflict in Sudan has also led to charges of genocide. Since late 2003, systematic human rights abuses have been perpetrated by the *janjaweed* militia against the Zaghawa, Masaalit, and Fur peoples in the Darfur region. The Sudan government has been accused of supporting the militia. By the end of 2004, more than 30,000 civilians had been killed, 1.5 million had been internally displaced, and 200,000 were living in refugee camps in neighboring Chad.

Organized violence has a major, direct public health impact when it results in such high numbers of civilian casualties. Since World War II, approximately 190 armed conflicts have occurred, affecting 92 countries.[6] Most occurred in Asia, Africa, and Latin America; however, since 1990, four European conflicts—in Chechnya, Azerbaijan, Georgia, and the former Yugoslavia—have caused more than 250,000 deaths. Some wars are still fought primarily between competing armies, such as the Iran-Iraq conflict (1980 to 1988), but most now take place within states. Civilian populations have increasingly been the intentional targets of military actions, as can be seen in the shelling of urban centers during the conflicts in Bosnia and Herzegovina, Chechnya, Angola, Lebanon, and Somalia. In addition, modern weapons such as napalm, cluster bombs, and land mines do not discriminate between combatants and innocent civilians. In Mozambique, the antigovernment forces killed approximately 100,000 civilians in 1986 and 1987 and between 5 million and 6 million people were either internally displaced or fled to neighboring countries.[7]

In addition to deaths and injuries caused by trauma, a further direct effect of armed conflict has been sexual violence. Rape is increasingly recognized as a feature of internal wars. In some conflicts, rape has been used systematically as an attempt to undermine opposing groups; as examples, in the conflicts in Rwanda and in the former Yugoslavia, women were systematically abused. The conflict in the former Yugoslavia, where there are an estimated 10,000 to 60,000 rape survivors,[8] has firmly placed the issue of systematic use of rape on the international agenda. The more extensive development of women's organizations helped to ensure that these events were made more visible and that support for survivors was mobilized. However, some forms of sexual abuse, such as male rape, have been poorly recognized, if at all.

In addition to long-lasting mental health disorders, rapes have resulted in the transmission of HIV. Wars and political conflict present high-risk situations for the transmission of sexually transmitted infections (STIs), including HIV infection.[9] There are various ways in which war predisposes to STI transmission, such as:

- Widespread population movement
- Increased crowding
- Separation of women from partners who otherwise provide a degree of protection
- Abuses and sexual demands by military personnel and others in positions of power
- Weakened social structures, thereby reducing inhibitions on aggressive behavior and violence against women.

Aside from these additional exposures, access to barrier contraceptives, to treatment for STIs, to the prerequisites for maintaining personal hygiene, and to health promotion advice are all compromised in conflict situations.

Immeasurable psychological trauma has been caused by widespread human rights abuses, including detention, torture, and forced displacement. The extent of mental health "trauma" experienced during and in the aftermath of war and conflict is controversial, with some analysts identifying significant proportions of affected populations suffering from posttraumatic stress disorder and others arguing that this term and the response to it medicalize an essentially social phenomenon.[10]

Indirect Effects on Health

Refugees and internally displaced persons have often been exposed to long periods of deprivation and denial of access to food and basic services. This deprivation has in many cases been linked directly to membership in a specific ethnic, religious, or social group, such as southern Sudanese Christians, Bosnian Muslims, Kosovo Albanians, residents of Tigray province in Ethiopia, and East Timorese supporting independence.

Political disturbances, as they evolve in a country, generally have a significant effect on national and local economies. In some cases, such as in Indonesia in 1998, an economic crisis may initiate political turmoil where there have been underlying tensions among political factions, ethnic or religious groups, or disadvantaged geographic areas. In Indonesia, ethnic tensions led to open violent conflict in a number of provinces. In such situations, especially in low-income countries, one of the first health effects is undernutrition in vulnerable groups, which is caused by food scarcity. According to the Food and Agriculture Organization (FAO) of the United Nations, all except 2 of the 15 countries with the highest rate of undernourishment in the world have recently experienced armed conflict (table 11-1).[11]

Local farmers may not plant crops as extensively as usual, or they may decrease the diversity of their crops due to the uncertainty created by the economic and/or political situation. The cost of seeds and fertilizer may increase and government agricultural extension services may be disrupted, resulting in lower yields. Distribution and marketing systems may be adversely affected. Devaluation of the local currency may drive down the price paid for agricultural produce, and the collapse of the local food processing industry may further diminish demand for agricultural products.

If full-scale armed conflict occurs, the fighting may damage irrigation systems, crops might be intentionally destroyed or looted by armed soldiers, distribution systems may completely collapse, and there may be widespread theft and looting of food stores. In countries that do not normally produce agricultural surpluses or that have large pastoral or nomadic communities,

TABLE 11-1   Countries With Prevalence
(Rates) of Undernourishment (Defined by FAO
as Inadequate Dietary Energy Intake) Greater
Than 40% of Their Populations, 1999–2001

Afghanistan	Haiti
Angola	Liberia
Burundi	Mozambique
Central African Republic	Rwanda
Democratic Republic	Sierra Leone
of Congo	Somalia
Eritrea	Tanzania*
Ethiopia	Zambia*

*Not recently affected by armed conflict.

especially in sub-Saharan Africa, the impact of food deficits on the nutritional status of civilians may be severe. If adverse climatic factors intervene, as often happened during the 1980s and 1990s in drought-prone countries, such as Sudan, Somalia, Mozambique, and Ethiopia, the outcome may be catastrophic famine. A study by the International Food Policy Research Institute compared actual mean food production per capita with "peace-adjusted" values for 14 countries. The study found that in 13 countries, food production was lower in war years, with declines ranging from 3.4 percent in Kenya to over 44 percent in Angola, with a mean reduction of 12.3 percent.[12]

When food aid programs are established, there may be inequitable distribution due to political and gender factors, food stores may be damaged or destroyed, food may be stolen or diverted to military forces, and the distribution of food aid may be obstructed.[13] The resulting food shortages may cause prolonged hunger and eventually drive families from their homes in search of relief. There have been many examples of food aid diversion, including in Mozambique and Ethiopia in the 1980s and southern Sudan and the former Yugoslavia in the 1990s. In the Central African Republic (CAR), 40 to 50 percent of the cattle owned by members of the pastoralist federation had been killed during the fighting between progovernment and antigovernment forces from October 2002 to March 2003, which mostly took place in the cattle-rearing north. Many herdsmen had already gone to Cameroon, Chad, and Sudan. Should this continue, it could transform the CAR—once an exporter of meat, with 3.2 million cattle in 2001—into a meat importer.

Since the 1970s, numerous studies have documented the public health impact of population displacement. Among refugees, mortality rates have varied widely from relatively low rates among Kosovar and East Timorese refugees to rates that are 25 times baseline mortality in the country of origin. The highest death rate recorded among refugees has been among those Rwandans who fled to eastern Zaire in 1994.[14]

For refugees in developing countries, the major causes of death have consistently been measles, diarrhea (including outbreaks of cholera and dysentery), malaria, acute respiratory infections, and meningitis, reflecting the crowding, poor water, and sanitation in many refugee camps.[15] Severe malnutrition has characterized a number of refugee populations, exacerbating the high mortality due to infectious diseases. In eastern Europe, the most important public health impact has been death and injury caused by the violence associated with armed conflict. In addition, armed conflict has often included the intentional destruction of medical facilities and the concentration of medical resources to treat military personnel, both of which, in turn, have led to deterioration in other medical services, such as management of chronic diseases, elective surgery, and provision of obstetrical and neonatal services (fig. 11-2).

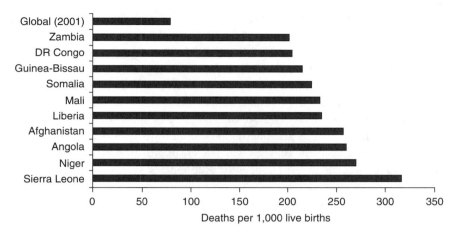

Figure 11-2 The 10 countries with the highest child mortality rates in the world. Seven of them have experienced recent conflict. (Based on data in Black RE, Morris SS, Bryce J. Where and why are 10 million children dying every year? Lancet 2003;361:2226–34.)

Roots and Underlying Issues

The definition of refugees, described in the Convention and Protocol Relating to the Status of Refugees (1951)[16] as people who have crossed international borders "fleeing war or persecution for reasons of race, religion, nationality, or membership in particular social and political groups," implies that they have experienced systematic injustice. However, this definition was developed immediately after World War II in response to the massive movements of refugees within Europe. It suggests a political context in which one government is the oppressor and asylum is being sought under the protection of another government. The situation today is far more complex than the people who drafted the Convention could have envisaged.

Article 25 of the Universal Declaration of Human Rights, proclaimed by the United Nations General Assembly in 1948, states that "everyone has the right to a standard of living adequate for the health and well-being of himself and of his family, including food, clothing, housing and medical care. . . ." In times of war, this declaration and other declarations, laws, covenants, and treaties that constitute the body of human rights law are complemented by international humanitarian law. The latter is "a set of rules aimed at limiting violence and protecting the fundamental rights of the individual in times of armed conflict."[17] (See chapters 1 and 27.)

These legal instruments relate to the obligations of nation-states and their governments. However, recent studies have suggested that many millions of people live in situations where "traditional distinctions between people, army, and government have been blurred, and new ways of projecting power have emerged."[18] Many people can no longer rely on their governments, or even organized resistance groups (once called liberation movements), to protect their basic human rights. They live in areas governed by a variety of warlords, international criminals, and opportunists who have developed and have sustained "shadow" economies that link diamond dealers in the conflict zones of Sierra Leone with members of the Russian Mafia; jade mine owners in northern Burma with army generals and international drug traffickers; leaders of ethnic separatist movements in the Balkans with leaders of prostitution rings in western Europe; and warlords in the Democratic Republic of Congo (DRC) with international money launderers and diamond smugglers. These parallel economies within an increasingly unregulated global economic system have created new elites of wealth and power who live outside the boundaries of international law and the governments of sovereign states. They remain wealthy and powerful by exploiting the poor and powerless, often sustaining their influence by taking advantage of the fears generated by perceived differences among various ethnic and religious groups. The Serbian power elite in Belgrade exploited these fears in the early 1990s, provoking widespread ethnic violence, while enriching themselves by controlling illegal sanctions-busting trade operations. Likewise, Somali warlords exploited traditional differences among familial clans, eventually eroding the authority of the central government and leading to the total collapse of governance. These alternative economies have thrived, in part, because the liberalized international economic system has increasingly marginalized the least developed countries of Africa.

In this lawless environment, social inequalities greatly increase. Not only are people subject to discrimination and terror, but they also have minimal access to basic social services. The DRC is an extreme example of this situation. This country is "ground zero" of what has been called an "African world war."[18] Nearly 20 armed groups—Congolese and foreign—are vying for political advantage or economic gain. Attempts to curb the war, through peace accords signed in Zambia, have been desperately inadequate, as has the small United Nations force meant to keep the "peace." The intractable war comes on the heels of decades of misrule and misappropriation of the country's vast natural wealth. Congo's infrastructure and health system are in ruins. Of the 300 health districts in the country, 79 are more than 62 miles (100 km) from their referral hospitals. The lack of government funds and foreign aid means that 100 districts are left without any external funding. Human resources fare no better: The country's 50 million people have only 2000 Congolese physicians to serve them. Life expectancy is 45 years. One in four children dies before age 5. Large parts of the country are inaccessible to humanitarian assistance. A mortality survey conducted in 2004 was the largest (involving 19,500 households) and the fourth such survey conducted in the country since 2001. The first three surveys found that an estimated 3.3 million people had died as a result of the armed conflict in DRC, which commenced in 1998. The fourth survey, conducted in 2004, found that the national crude mortality rate of 2 deaths per 1,000 per month was 67 percent higher than before the war and that 3.8 million people had died.[19]

The custodian of international humanitarian law is the International Committee of the Red Cross (ICRC). For many decades after the end of World War II, the ICRC was able to negotiate adherence to the Geneva Conventions by the parties involved in internal conflicts. However, since 1990, ICRC and other neutral humanitarian nongovernmental organizations (NGOs) have had increasing difficulty in ensuring the protection of civilians affected by civil wars. Its own staff has often been the targets of violence, despite the sanctity of the Red Cross symbol. The chief delegate of the ICRC in the former Yugoslavia was killed in a vehicle clearly marked with the symbol. A number of delegates were killed in Chechnya, Sudan, and central Africa. In one of the most flagrant acts, the ICRC Iraq headquarters in Baghdad was bombed in 2003. In addition to these incidents, humanitarian agencies have increasingly been forced to compromise their neutrality by negotiating with warlords to ensure safe passage and even paying to have armed guards to protect their staff members, as was the norm in Somalia in 1992 and 1993. This practice has often bestowed legitimacy on armed groups that are little more than criminal gangs, contributing, in turn, to the intimidation by these groups of local communities.

Poor Health as a Risk Factor for Conflict

Recent studies have indicated that poor national health indicators may increase the risk of conflict within a country. Population Action International conducted a study of the relationship between civil conflict in the 1970s, 1980s, and 1990s with demographic and social indicators, using data from 180 countries. The study found that countries in the early stage of the demographic transition (high birth and high child-mortality rates) were at higher risk of armed conflict. The study found that a decline in the annual birth rate of 5 per 1000 corresponded with a 5 percent reduction in risk of civil conflict during the following decade (table 11-2).[20]

International Responses

The vulnerability of populations subjected to these extreme conditions of injustice has often been compounded by the inconsistency of the international community's response to their plight. Inequity has characterized the global response to their needs. Although the impact of these conflicts on populations has varied greatly, the response by the international community—itself a

TABLE 11-2   Relationship Between Infant Mortality, Birth Rate, and Civil Conflict

Birth Rate 1985–1990 (births per 1,000)	Average Infant Mortality Rate, 1985–1990 (infant deaths per 1,000 live births)	Risk of Outbreak of Civil Conflict, 1990–2000 (%)
≥45	125	53
35–44	78	34
25–34	42	24
15–24	20	16
<15	10	5

From FAO. The state of food insecurity in the world 2003. Rome: FAO, 2004.

relatively new concept since 1990—has generally not been based solely on humanitarian needs. The scale of the response has often been determined by (a) media interest, such as the *New York Times* coverage between July 5 and 12, 1992, of the Somalia famine (five stories in eight days); (b) geopolitical concerns, such as in Kuwait, Iraq, Kosovo, and Afghanistan; (c) the domestic agendas of donor nations, such as President George H. W. Bush's support for United Nations intervention in Somalia during the next to the last month of his presidency in December 1992; and (d) the strength of international advocacy groups, such as those in Australia that provided extensive public support for intervention in East Timor. In 1999, President Bill Clinton exhorted the world community to take action in Kosovo ("a moral imperative"), citing Serb atrocities against Kosovar Albanians. No such moral imperative, however, has been cited to mobilize support for similarly oppressed populations in Africa.

A dramatic shift in geopolitical priorities has occurred as a result of the terrorist attacks in the United States in 2001. Among wealthy nations at present, the pressing concerns of ensuring national security overshadow the humanitarian motives that had their brief airing in the 1990s. Afghanistan is but one example of the blurring of humanitarian and military objectives. Humanitarian action depends on (a) concern for humanity, (b) impartiality of assistance, (c) the independence of the organization delivering aid, and (d) neutrality in the relevant conflict. These principles are only adhered to if there is unhindered access to people in danger, independent evaluation of their needs, independent and impartial distribution of aid according to the level of need, and independent impact monitoring. NGOs are concerned that humanitarian action has been severely compromised in recent humanitarian programs taking place in military environments, such as in Kosovo, Afghanistan, East Timor, and Iraq, where military objectives have subsumed humanitarian goals. In addition, grave humanitarian needs of large populations in Liberia, Sierra

Leone, Angola, and the DRC have largely been ignored by major donor governments.

What Needs to Be Done

Social injustice and inequality are most pronounced in those politically unstable and impoverished countries where armed conflict has occurred and where the line between political struggle and organized crime is blurred. These conditions are not confined to those countries where civil wars are widely recognized, such as in Africa (including the long civil war in the DRC, involving troops from seven African countries), central Asia, the Middle East, and eastern Europe. They also exist in Colombia, where right-wing and left-wing guerrilla movements spread terror; in Burma, where government officials and liberation groups sponsor ruthless drug-trafficking armies and suppress the democracy movement; and in Algeria, where Islamic extremists terrorize local communities.

During the 1990s, these situations were referred to as "complex political emergencies" and the response was often to mount complex humanitarian operations that focused on the delivery of food and medicines, while neglecting the underlying causes of conflict. This approach was evident in Bosnia between 1993 and 1995, when United Nations "peacekeepers" averted their eyes to the most widespread abuses of human rights in Europe since World War II. The focus on short-term humanitarian responses has shifted recently to a broader discourse on the relationship among economic and social development, national and international security (and the prevention of terrorism), and humanitarian emergencies.

Professor Mark Duffield, Director of Conflict, Development, and Security Studies at Lancaster University in the United Kingdom, has stated that underdevelopment and the resultant exclusion and destabilization of developing countries are threats to global security.[21] He calls for a coalition of politicians, United Nations agencies, NGOs, military establishments, and private companies to promote a potentially "pro-poor system of global liberal governance" (p. 10).[21] The goals of these global players can be complementary if one accepts that:

1. Poverty reduction can only be achieved through a commitment to equity and substantial investment in access to basic health and education.
2. Poverty alleviation, good health, and education promote economic growth, political stability, and national security.
3. Improvements in the quality of life of the poor will prevent the emergence of extremist movements and reduce international terrorism and the need for counterterrorist military interventions.

The appropriate response to the continued threat of complex emergencies that generate refugees and internally displaced persons is firm commitment to a combination of prevention and preparedness planning. Poorer countries need greatly increased international assistance to reduce poverty and improve health services and education. Population Action International, an independent policy advocacy group based in Washington, D.C., published a report in 2003 that said[20]:

> Progress through the demographic transition helps reduce the risk of civil conflict, and thus contributes to a more peaceful and secure world. Over the past 40 years this progress has been impressive, albeit uneven, in all of the world's regions. Movement in this direction, however, is uneven and in peril. Continuing declines in birthrates and increases in life expectancy in the poorest and worst-governed countries will require much more international collaboration and assistance than are evident today, and greater efforts to improve the lives of women and increase their participation in government and throughout society. (p. 20)

Armed conflicts rarely occur in economically prosperous countries; thus, equitable economic development is an important preventive measure against complex emergencies. And so is the promotion of the commitment made at the United Nations Millennium Summit in 2000 by all United Nations member nations to eight key development goals, three of which relate directly to public health. (See table 21-7 on p. 394 and chapter 28.)

During the past few decades, wealthy countries have become less committed to supporting the development of poorer countries. For example, in 1961, the per-capita income in donor countries was about US$13,300; by 2000, it was about US$30,000. However, between 1961 and 2000, the per-capita amount allocated by wealthy countries to development assistance remained unchanged.[21] In many donor countries, the proportion of gross domestic product (GDP) spent on development assistance has been steadily declining. Only Denmark, Norway, Netherlands, and Sweden currently exceed the United Nations development assistance target of 0.7 percent of GDP; the United States spends only 0.1 percent of its GDP on development assistance. (See fig. 21-1 on p. 384.) The generous pledges made at the Millennium Summit may be an indication of a reversal in that downward trend.

At the same time, a more concerted effort—based on humanitarian need, rather than on political expediency—is needed to ensure a consistent international response to evolving conflict-related emergencies. More work is needed to resolve conflicts using diplomatic initiatives, backed up, when necessary, by proportionate use of force—a contentious and highly emotional issue. There is still no consensus on what should bring about a forceful international response to mass human rights abuses. The whims of public opinion cut two ways: The same public that demands intervention to prevent widespread human rights abuses is as likely to demand withdrawal if the intervention goes sour (as in Somalia) or leads to excessive "collateral damage" (as in Kosovo).[3]

Conclusion

In 2004, more than 37 million people globally were displaced from their homes by the threat of persecution and violence. Many have experienced years of systematic injustice that has limited their freedom of movement and employment and has restricted their access to food, health care, education, and other human needs. Many of these people can no longer rely on their governments to protect their human rights or to provide basic social services. In many cases, they are being exploited by quasi-criminal groups that masquerade as legitimate political movements. These warlords wield increasing power and influence, and amass significant wealth through the exploitation of populations under their control. Many of them collude with government authorities and transnational entities to sustain a parallel economy that thrives in the unregulated environment of a globalized economy. It is the poor and powerless who are eventually faced with no option other than to flee their home—and sometimes their country—to survive. The toll on the health of displaced populations is severe.

The plight of these people can be addressed only if the international community is serious about addressing the root causes of poverty, poor governance, exploitation, and the terrible inequity between the rich and poor countries of the world. The Millennium Summit development goals provide a useful unifying target that requires a multifaceted approach to achieve. Liberal politicians, military leaders concerned with increasing global insecurity, United Nations organizations, NGOs concerned with equity and justice, and private corporations that depend on political stability and global prosperity all have much to gain from a coordinated campaign to resolve conflicts and alleviate poverty and powerlessness. Such a campaign would yield vast gains to the public's health.

References

1. United States Committee for Refugees. World refugee survey 2004. Washington, D.C.: United States Commission for Refugees, 2004.
2. Organization for Security and Co-operation in Europe. Report on Kosovo. Chapter 11: violation of human rights in Kosovo. Available at: www.osce.org. Accessed January 13, 2005.
3. Winter R (ed.). World refugee survey 2000. Washington, D.C.: United States Committee for Refugees, 2001.
4. United Nations Subcommittee on Nutrition. Refugee nutrition information system. Geneva, Switzerland: United Nations, 1999.

5. Lopes CB, Vergara A, Agani F, et al. Mental health, social functioning, and attitudes of Kosovar Albanians following the war in Kosovo. JAMA 2000;284:567–77.

6. World Health Organization. World report on violence and health. Geneva, Switzerland: WHO, 2000.

7. Ugalde A, Zwi A, Richards P. Health consequences of war and political violence. In: Kurtz L, ed. Encyclopaedia of violence. New York, N.Y.: Academic Press, 2002.

8. Swiss S, Giller JE. Rape as a crime of war. JAMA 1993;270:612–5.

9. Zwi AB, Cabral AJ. Identifying "high risk situations" for preventing AIDS. BMJ 1991; 303:1527–9.

10. Toole M. Improving psychosocial survival in complex emergencies. Lancet 2002; 360:869.

11. Food and Agriculture Organization. The state of food insecurity in the world. Rome, Italy: FAO, 2002.

12. Messer E, Cohen MJ, Marchione T. Conflict: a cause and effect of hunger. A draft review by the International Food Policy Research Institute (IFPRI). IFPRI, 2001. Available at www.ifpri.org. Accessed January 13, 2005.

13. Macrae J, Zwi A, eds. War and hunger: rethinking international responses to complex emergencies. London, U.K.: Zed Books, 1994.

14. Toole MJ, Waldman RJ, Zwi A. Complex humanitarian emergencies. In: Merson M, Black R, Mills A, eds. International public health. New York, N.Y.: Aspen Publications, 2000.

15. Toole MJ, Waldman RJ. Refugees and displaced persons: war, hunger, and public health. JAMA 1993;270:600–5.

16. United Nations High Commissioner for Refugees. Convention and Protocol Relating to the Status of Refugees. Geneva, Switzerland: UNHCR. Available at: http://www .alhaq.org/references/laws/law_refugees1. Accessed January 13, 2005.

17. Perrin P. War and public health. Geneva, Switzerland: International Committee of the Red Cross, 1996:381.

18. Medecins Sans Frontieres. MSF 2000. International activity report. Available at: http:// www.msf.org. Accessed February 25, 2005.

19. Coghlan B, Brennan R, Ngoy P, et al. Mortality in the Democratic Republic of Congo: results from a nationwide survey. New York, N.Y.: International Rescue Committee and Burnet Institute, 2004.

20. Cincotta R, Engelman R, Anastasion D. The security demographic. Washington, D.C.: Population Action International, 2003.

21. Duffield M. Introduction: global governance and the new wars. In: Global governance and the new wars. London: Zed Press, 2001.

Part III

How Social Injustice Affects Health

12

MEDICAL CARE

H. Jack Geiger

Introduction

In the United States, medical care—that is, access to personal medical services, both preventive and curative—is ironically a grave area of social injustice. Deep dysfunctions in the organization, financing, and distribution of medical care have profound consequences for individuals in avoidable suffering and preventable death, cumulatively damaging the health status and life prospects of whole populations and incurring staggering costs to the larger society.

These costs and damages in our country are not the inevitable result of fundamental economic laws or the nature of health care itself, as the much better experience of all other modern industrialized democracies attests. They are instead the consequence of a deliberate ideological and political choice: to treat medical care as a market commodity, to be rationed by ability to pay—rather than as (a) a social good to be distributed in response to medical need, (b) a responsibility of government, and (c) a fundamental right embodied in a social contract. As a consequence, the opportunities to maintain a healthy and longer life and to fulfill one's human potential are skewed in the United States by income, education, primary language, race, ethnicity, and area of residence. This injustice is not the consequence of random chance in the distribution of disease. It is injustice by design.

The roots of this injustice lie in American political culture and history. In the United States, neither government nor the shared beliefs of the public have ever fully recognized a human right to health care, as they have done—albeit in a slow political evolution—for other social goods, such as education. While the health status of the U.S. population is now clearly seen as a matter of essential national interest, massive inequalities in the health status of variously disadvantaged or marginalized population groups—by race, ethnicity, social class, and gender—are officially viewed, at best, as problems requiring intervention but not as issues of social justice. Indeed, they have been often viewed as the fault of those populations themselves, on grounds of alleged biological inferiority or deliberate lifestyle choices.

While nominal "fairness" is seen as an important criterion for many policy choices, health care in the United States is not widely considered a part of what John Rawls has defined as "primary social goods" (p. 43): rights and liberties, powers and opportunity, income and wealth, or a social basis of self-respect.[1] Views on health care are thus reflective of the society's willingness to tolerate very large inequalities in income, wealth, and economic and political power. As many recent studies have shown, the more unequal a society is in economic terms, the more unequal it is likely to be in health terms.[2] Yet many ethicists, following Rawls, have argued that health care is special and that, in this domain, inequity is injustice—because poor health care and poor health so profoundly limit opportunities, throughout the life cycle, for the full realization of one's potential for employment, relationships, and social and political participation. In this view, justice in health care is good for the public's health, and the public's good health, in turn, broadens opportunities and facilitates a more just society.[3]

The Impact of Social Injustice in Medical Care

The consequences of this social injustice for public health are complex. Personal medical services make only a modest contribution to the health status of any population—in terms of its morbidity and mortality, life expectancy, or health-related quality of life. Health is not merely a function of access to medical care: to a much greater extent, it is a function of the cumulative experience of social conditions over the course of one's lifetime.[4] The most powerful forces in public health are its social determinants: income levels; rates of employment; the quality and affordability of housing; educational opportunity; workplace safety; the quality of air, water, and food; sanitation; and less tangible, but pervasive, factors such as racism, class bias, and political inequality.

Medical care, however, makes a difference to both personal and public health—one that is most clearly revealed when care is absent or denied. For example, failures to provide immunization have repeatedly led to outbreaks—sometimes lethal—of measles, polio, and other contagious diseases among children of the poor and disadvantaged. Lack of prenatal care is associated with higher rates of infant and maternal mortality among minorities and the uninsured. Studies of poor adults removed from programs that fund access to care, such as Medicaid, have documented the occurrence of uncontrolled illness—and some preventable deaths—within a year of removal. An analysis by the Institute of Medicine concluded that lack of health insurance annually causes approximately 18,000 unnecessary deaths in nonelderly U.S. adults and costs the nation from $65 to $130 billion annually in lost productivity.[5]

On a personal level, the consequence of inaccessible care is the enforced and unjust assumption of risk, as when untreated hypertension leads to a crippling stroke or a lethal heart attack. Poor and uninsured adults consistently assume such risks, even though most of them are full-time workers. So do elderly low-income patients suddenly abandoned when their private-sector, for-profit Medicare health maintenance organizations (HMOs) cancel their coverage and withdraw from the health care marketplace because they find it insufficiently profitable.[6] Whole communities may be affected: neighborhoods with high rates of uninsurance attract few physicians and health care facilities, making access more difficult for everyone—even those who do have coverage. Consequences ripple through the health care system: Hospitals burdened with the huge expenses of unreimbursed emergency department visits and inpatient care by the uninsured shift those costs by increasing their rates for insured patients, thus driving up the cost of health insurance premiums.

There is now overwhelming evidence, from hundreds of careful peer-reviewed studies, that minorities and the poor who do gain access to medical care receive less-comprehensive and lower-quality diagnosis and treatment compared with others—even when insurance status, severity of disease, and other potentially confounding variables are comparable.[7] These minority and poor populations thus bear a triple burden: they live, on average, in the most dangerous biological and physical environments and are exposed to the worst social determinants of health status; they have the least access to care; and, when care is provided, it tends to be of poorer quality. These are long-standing patterns; at no time in the history of the United States has the health status of African-Americans, Hispanic-Americans, Native Americans, and a number of Asian-American subgroups equaled or even approximated that of the white majority. It is largely because of such systemic defects that the United States, while making the world's highest per-capita expenditures for medical care, lags far behind other nations—not just advanced industrial societies but even much poorer countries, such as Cuba and Costa Rica—in such classic indicators as infant mortality and life expectancy.

After prolonged political struggle, and in a time of broader social change, a significant advance toward the assumption of social responsibility for medical care was made in the 1960s with the passage of Medicare to insure the elderly and Medicaid to insure at least some of those with low incomes. However, a fundamental ambivalence in U.S. policy remained. Medical care continued to be treated as a consumer good, subject to the rules of the marketplace and alleged competition, even as these programs represented a partial recognition of the principle that justice is embodied in a shared social responsibility. The strength of that recognition has fluctuated over subsequent decades. With no effective control over total health care costs, including health insurance and prescription drug costs, in a mainstream system that depended on employer provision of health insurance as a workplace benefit, more employers—and more patients—were priced out of the market. Pressures mounted for incremental increases in publicly funded coverage, especially for children, further increasing total health expenditures. By the first decade of the twenty-first century, the medical care system in the United States—the world's only advanced industrial democracy without universal health insurance—was accelerating its long drift into crisis.

The Health Care Crisis and Social Justice

The crisis has three dimensions: access, cost, and quality. Each has implications for social justice.

Access

In a system in which citizens have no legal right to health care (beyond emergency treatment) and no guarantee of access to adequate care unless they have the means to pay for it, some 44 million Americans in 2003 lacked private or public health insurance of any kind. That number has been increasing at a rate of 2 million a year. It includes at least 20 million workers (about 80 percent of uninsured adults) and 8.5 million children.[8] The distribution of the uninsured follows the race- and ethnicity-specific discriminatory patterns that characterize social injustice in the larger society: Among all working adults, 11 percent of whites, 18 percent of African-Americans, and 35 percent of Hispanics are uninsured.[9] (Surveys that count persons who have lacked insurance for just part of the past year find startlingly higher percentages among these same disadvantaged groups.)

The consequences of the lack of health insurance for access are profound. They are best revealed by a comparison of the uninsured with those who have coverage. A study by the Robert Wood Johnson Foundation found that approximately 20 percent of uninsured adults went without urgently needed medical care in the past year, compared with about 5 percent of insured adults. More than half of uninsured adults (56 percent) said they did not have a personal physician or usual source of care compared with 16 percent of the insured. Among uninsured women in at-risk age groups, 46 percent did not receive a mammogram compared with 20 percent of insured women; among uninsured men of appropriate age, 70 percent did not receive a prostate cancer screening test compared with 47 percent of insured men. About 20 percent of uninsured adults rated their own health as only "fair" or "poor"—prognoses associated with earlier mortality—compared with only about 10 percent of insured adults.[9] Thus, lack of insurance—primarily a function of inability to pay for it despite full-time employment—translates directly into inequitable risk and both poorer health and the diminished opportunities that accompany it. These data do not include the millions more who are underinsured, either because of the unaffordable cost of truly adequate coverage or because of insurance policies that limit coverage to those with preexisting disease.[10] And even among those who do have insurance, an estimated 36 million persons (including those eligible for Medicare or Medicaid) are unable to access care because there are too few providers in their communities—or none who will accept public-insurance reimbursement.[11]

These poeple—an estimated 12 percent of the population—are medically underserved.[12] Thus, the health care system arbitrarily but selectively increases inequality in ways that have little to do with individual merit, and (with the exception of the original passage of Medicare) reflects an abandonment of the concept of shared social responsibility—a general obligation to protect the individual against disease, disability, and premature death.[3]

Lack of insurance does not, of course, mean absence of illness, from minor to disabling and life threatening. Some care is delivered to uninsured patients in emergency department visits and in unavoidable, but uncompensated, hospitalizations. The Kaiser Family Foundation's Commission on Medicaid and the Uninsured estimated that the medical costs for all uninsured persons in the United States would reach $125 billion in 2004, adding to the second dimension of crisis: cost.[12]

Cost

In 2003, the most recent year for which complete data are now available, health care spending in the United States totaled $1.7 trillion—more than 15 percent of the total U.S. economy. This amount represented an average expenditure of $5,440 per person—the highest level in the world. Health care spending is projected to grow to 17.7 percent of the economy by 2012 if the system does not change. The premiums that employers paid to provide health insurance coverage to their employees jumped 50 percent from 1996 to 1999, doubled from 1999 to 2002, and are rising by 12 to 16 percent in 2004. In response, many employers reduced benefits, increased deductibles and co-payments, and required their workers to pay a steeply rising share of the premiums; some employees could not afford to pay those costs and joined the ranks of the uninsured, or dropped coverage for other family members. Other employers cut off insurance benefits for retirees or no longer offered health insurance benefits at all. And the coverage that did continue was almost always incomplete. For individuals, out-of-pocket costs not covered by insurance rose $12 billion in 2003 to $212.5 billion. These costs were compounded by fragmentation of care—the consequence of an employer-based system that relies primarily on thousands of private-sector insurers, mostly for-profit concerns with wildly varying benefit packages, frequent limitations on patient choice of physicians and hospitals, and complex regulations. The costs of administering this system—to employers, insurance companies, hospital administrators, and the billing offices of physicians and other providers—is high: Administrative costs add $1,059, on average, to the cost of health care for every insured patient in the United States, compared with only $307 in Canada's government-run, single-payer system.[13]

The cost crisis does not occur only at the federal level. Tax cuts and the slumping national economy produced state fiscal crises in 2003 and 2004, with total state budget shortfalls for 2004 estimated at $78 billion. About 1.6 million people, including about 500,000 children, lost coverage under Medicaid, Supplemental Children's Health Insurance Programs (SCHIP), and other state-funded health insurance programs.[14] (At their peak, these means-tested programs had provided coverage for one-third of all the children in the United States but still had failed to cover all the children of the poor and near-poor.) In Florida, for example, 63,000 children were placed on "waiting lists" for access to care after enrollment was cut off. In Georgia, eligibility rules changes removed almost 20,000 pregnant women from coverage. Mississippi ended coverage for 65,000 low-income patients. Texas ended SCHIP coverage for nearly 160,000 children in working families. In addition, over the past 2 years, 38 states added or raised co-payments for these programs, despite evidence that co-payments are a significant deterrent to the use of essential medical care and prescription drugs among low-income populations and that there are adverse health consequences when such treatment is foregone or delayed. In other states, the scope of covered benefits was reduced and payments to providers were cut dramatically, as were outreach efforts for enrollment. Long and complicated application forms were devised, and extensive documentation and frequent recertification for eligibility was required. Texas, which used all these techniques, added a unique new hole to its safety net: Health insurance coverage did not begin for 90 days after enrollment, even for newborns. In sum, as state governments struggled to balance their budgets, a major stratagem was denial of responsibility for the health care of the poor.

Quality

Vast expenditures, however, do not ensure quality of care. Repeated studies over many decades have documented wide variations in the appropriateness and comprehensiveness of the medical care that patients receive; one government agency has called the gap between what is done and what should be done a quality chasm.[15] A recent study of the quality of care in 12 metropolitan communities across the United States found that patients in all parts of the country are at risk for receiving poor-quality care, receiving only 50 to 60 percent of recommended treatments for any of 30 acute and chronic conditions, such as diabetes, asthma, high blood pressure, and heart disease, as well as reduced preventive care.[16] A congressionally mandated national report card on disparities in care for African-Americans, Hispanics, and other minorities concluded that the problem of lower-quality, less-comprehensive care for these populations is pervasive and systemwide, resulting in serious personal and social costs.[17] Despite its international leadership in biomedical research and technological innovation in health care and repeated claims that its market-based health care system is the best in the world, the United States, despite massive health care expenditures, has neither ensured quality of care nor produced uniform improvements in health status.

Medicare "Reform" and the Triumph of Injustice

In the four decades since the institution of Medicare and Medicaid, incremental expansions of coverage have, at least in principle, given support to the mechanism of government action to assume responsibility for access to health care. However, reliance on employment-based health insurance has, in fact, meant that the proportion of the population covered has waxed and waned with advances or downturns in the national economy. In 2004, this pattern of incremental, but varying, improvement was reversed. An assault was launched on the principle of social cohesion to ensure health care for all. Nothing better illustrates this tilt toward social injustice than the Medicare changes enacted by the U.S. Congress and signed into law by President George W. Bush in 2004.

The new Medicare legislation was characterized by its proponents primarily as a means to help elderly patients pay for the staggering costs of prescription medications—a goal that its drug provisions will accomplish only minimally. (There are gaping holes in its drug coverage and, in any case, its core provisions will not take effect for several years.) However, the legislation's other, less-emphasized, provisions reveal a much broader purpose: the effect, and clearly the intent, will be to abandon Medicare as a social insurance system in which risks and costs are shared across the entire population of the elderly—healthy and ill, rich and poor alike, with free choice of physicians and hospitals, all under a government guarantee to pay for their medical care as an entitlement—a right. Instead, the new law creates multiple strategies to (a) fragment this common-risk pool; (b) move most of the elderly into a spuriously competitive, private-sector, profit-driven marketplace of choice-limited managed-care plans; and (c) transform entitlement into a voucher for the purchase of care as a commodity. The driving principle of this new effort is the use of government funds to subsidize the for-profit and private sector's efforts to establish exclusive dominion over the provision of care.[18]

The first of these stratagems is indeed a subsidy. The government will make huge preferential payments to private-sector health maintenance organizations (HMOs) and managed care organizations, enabling them to lower their monthly premium charges to patients, offer more generous prescription drug coverage, and "compete" on a tilted playing field with traditional fee-for-service Medicare. The field is made still more uneven by provisions allowing these firms to negotiate with pharmaceutical companies for lower drug prices but specifically prohibiting traditional Medicare—with its massive bulk purchasing power—from doing the same. (This is a startling deviation by advocates of a free market.) But there is still more. The law allows elderly beneficiaries—if they are wealthy enough to make this choice—to withdraw from Medicare almost entirely, by establishing large, tax-free "health savings accounts" or tax shelters, using their own money to pay for medical expenses rather than paying monthly premiums for Medicare coverage and remaining in the common-risk pool of all the elderly. The predictable effect of these provisions is that the healthiest and wealthiest of the elderly—those with the greatest means and the lowest risk of needing prolonged and expensive care—will join private-sector plans and effectively withdraw from Medicare, while the poorest and sickest will remain. The increased medical needs and costs of the poorest and sickest will inevitably drive up traditional Medicare's expenses, requiring its premiums to rise sharply, and escalate Medicare's drain on general government revenues. (Since the tax-sheltered "health savings" provisions apply to everyone, not just the elderly, the selective flight of the healthy and wealthy will similarly also drive up the cost of employment-based health insurance.) To ensure that these outcomes appear to be a triumph of the private marketplace and to ensure that the principle of social insurance is demeaned, the law arbitrarily asserts that when more than 45 percent of traditional Medicare's costs come from general revenues, Medicare will be declared to be in crisis—by fiat, rather than fact, an unaffordable failure.

At the first level of analysis, what is striking is the extent to which these stratagems fly in the face of well-established evidence. Careful studies of

Medicare managed-care plans (euphemistically named Medicare + Choice) have shown that they cost more than fee-for-service Medicare, incur higher out-of-pocket costs for subscribers, frequently deny services (sometimes with disastrous medical results), and often require limitation or elimination of patients' free choice of health care providers. Some plans abandoned their subscribers entirely when profits turned into losses. For example, between 1999 and 2003, Medicare HMOs dropped 2.2 million elderly patients from their rolls.[19] The administrative costs of commercial health insurers and private-sector, managed-care plans are approximately seven times higher than the 2 percent rate of administrative costs in traditional Medicare. Finally, health economists have long demonstrated that health care, unlike real commodities, cannot be efficiently managed by the marketplace.[20]

To stop at this level of analysis, however, is to miss the real goal of these efforts, which is to abandon the principle of shared social responsibility—government action to embody a right—in favor of an intrinsically unjust allocation of resources, favoring the most affluent and those least in need. In effect, the new law creates an Orwellian choice: We can all equally be involved in this task of providing health care, or some people can be more equal than others. That choice becomes clearer if we examine it in relation to another primary social good, a system that is widely understood to be a government responsibility designed to serve the whole population: police protection for the security of individuals and property. Of course, in addition to the police, there are private guards and security firms already in existence. But suppose the government now began to use public funds to subsidize these private firms to lower their rates and expand their services. Imagine, further, that legislation created tax-sheltered "security savings accounts," so that citizens with the means could use their own money to hire bodyguards and private patrols, while reducing their local property taxes by one-third on the grounds that they no longer depended primarily on the public police system. Inevitably, those with the highest incomes, the most property to protect, and the most to gain from tax shelters would be those most likely to enter this subsidized marketplace for commercial security services. Just as inevitably, local governments' revenues from property taxes would fall, forcing them to either raise taxes on everyone else or close police stations and fire police officers, making life more dangerous for the middle class and the poor. Either way, the principle of collective security would be abandoned. That is precisely what is now threatened by the planned de-socialization and de-universalization of health insurance. In both cases, what is denied is a general social obligation to provide systems of protection for individuals and families. In the case of health care, this involves the willingness of more affluent and healthy people to share in the cost of care for people who are sicker and less well off—a matter of distributive justice.

Root Causes of Paradox and Failure

There is a political paradox in these new plans. Public opinion polls consistently show that Americans, dissatisfied with incremental expansions, favor universal health coverage—as do substantial numbers of physicians and other health care providers.[18] The same polls reflect deep public concern about exploding costs and shrinking and uncertain coverage, access, and quality. Even among Medicare beneficiaries seeking help for the unmanageable costs of prescription drugs, a large majority wish to remain in the traditional fee-for-service program— rather than to receive such assistance by relying on the marketplace and its promises of "competition" and "efficiency," while limiting choices. Yet all attempts to establish universal coverage and access have failed.

Political analysts attribute this failure to the power of two basic American cultural beliefs: (a) a persistent mistrust of government and (b) an ideological commitment to individual autonomy and entrepreneurship. Other factors are structural, such as the long-term political absence in the United States of a labor party—a key supporter of universal health coverage in other advanced democracies. More important than these factors, however, is a federalist political system designed to resist populist pressures and constrain large-scale changes, even when they have widespread public support. In this view, the passage of Medicare itself was an aberrant event, the product of a rare period of control by one party of the White House and both branches of Congress by lopsided margins.[18] The most important factor of all, however, is the organized power and money of corporate interests to influence the political process, at both the state and federal levels, through campaign contributions, lobbying, and advertising. A recent "Op-Chart" in the *New York Times* succinctly outlined this process in the passage of Medicare's "reform" legislation by simply presenting a series of numbers. It identified the multi-billion dollar profits expected to accrue to the drug and insurance industries, the multi-million dollar total of contributions made by those industries to political parties, the number of industry lobbyists involved in the effort to shape legislation, the rapid benefits that will accrue to marketplace entities, and the limited and delayed benefits for patients.[21] Against this power, progressive change is difficult. The uninsured have no organized constituency or voting block.

What Needs to Be Done

Forty years of incremental remedies have ameliorated, but not fundamentally changed, the inequities and inefficiencies in the U.S. health care system. And, as data from state Medicaid programs demonstrate, these "remedies" have been profoundly regressive. The effort to establish access to health care as a right in the United States has been an unsteady march—and will likely continue to be so unless changes occur both within and outside the health care system.

At the root of these difficulties is an unresolved ideological conflict in the political and social thinking of the American public, a conflict between (a) those who see government as an instrument of shared social responsibility, and (b) those who view government action as a threat to individual freedom and autonomy and argue—in the face of the evidence—that, in health care as in other areas, the marketplace and entrepreneurship are the most effective mediators. This conflict, however, is susceptible to resolution on pragmatic grounds: if the crisis of exploding costs, deteriorating access, and uncertain quality becomes an implosion, the American public—already in favor of universal coverage, in principle, but divided as to the best means to achieve it—may then be ready to embrace fundamental change.

To be effective, fulfillment of that wish will require change outside the health care arena, most conspicuously in the achievement of real campaign finance reform, so that corporate money cannot have its present power to block legislation or to shape it to its own interests, rather than the public interest. Such reform, important to many issues in addition to health care, is also essential to the restoration of a public belief in the integrity of the political process, the absence of which is reflected in nearly half of all registered voters not voting in major elections.

Federalist sentiments and traditions may provide an intermediate step. Legislatures in Maryland, Maine, and other states are now considering state-level plans to provide universal coverage to their residents, albeit with a mix of private and public funding and mechanisms. While a patchwork of widely varying state programs is no substitute for a uniform and efficient national program, any success at the state level may spur support for federal initiatives.

Effective change will also require new alignments within the health care sector—most notably, a recognition of the common interests of health care providers and patients, the twin victims of the present system of corporate and marketplace control. The two groups share profound concerns about the loss of autonomy, the uncontrollable costs, the exhausting burdens of administration and paperwork, and the difficulties of providing or receiving appropriate and high-quality care. The egalitarian and ethical commitments of health care providers and the self-interest of patients are in alignment. What may be necessary for both groups is to recognize that the present system is not merely unsatisfying but rather profoundly unjust.

Conclusion

Social injustice is built into the very fabric of the American health care system. The United States is the only advanced industrial nation that does not define health care as a right of its citizens and a social responsibility of government, and therefore does not provide universal health care coverage. Instead, access to health care is treated as a commodity to be purchased by those with the means to pay, or as a partially subsidized benefit of employment, in a system that is increasingly dominated by for-profit insurance companies, pharmaceutical manufacturers, and corporate medical providers. As a consequence, 44 million people, including members of many working families, lack any ensured access to health care; millions more are inadequately insured; and the overall financial costs of the system—the highest per-capita expenditures in the world—have escalated to the point of crisis. The other costs—unattended illness, disability, and preventable mortality, limiting the opportunities for social, political and economic participation—violate fundamental principles of distributive justice.

These burdens fall most heavily on the poor and racial and ethnic minorities— the very populations at greatest risk and in greatest need—and contribute significantly to the poorer health status of these groups, already impaired by their exposure to more dangerous physical, biological, and social environments and other social determinants of health. During the last third of the twentieth century, one true form of social health insurance—the Medicare program for all the elderly—was established, and a variety of means-tested programs and safety-net systems provided some access to medical care for the poor. In the first years of the twenty-first century, however, even these programs have come under attack, most ominously in legislation encouraging the wealthiest and healthiest to withdraw from systems of shared risk and cost in favor of the tax-sheltered purchase of private protection.

At the root of these injustices are ideological and political choices: (a) to rely on the mechanisms of the marketplace—ill suited to such a basic human need as health care; (b) to invoke a suspicion of government action; and (c) to permit enormous expenditures by corporate health-sector interests to influence legislation and governmental regulation. The present system, which leaves the United States far behind other advanced nations in population health status, is drifting toward financial and social chaos. In contrast, universal health access through public-sector social insurance must become part of the American social contract, restoring the primacy of the interests of patients and providers in a just and equitable system.

References

1. Rawls J. A theory of justice. Cambridge, Mass.: Harvard University Press, 1971.
2. Kawachi I, Kennedy BP, Wilkinson RG, eds. Income inequality and health. New York, N.Y.: W.W. Norton and Company, 1999, p. xvi.

3. Daniels N. Justice, health and health care. In: Rhodes R, Battin MP, Silvers A, eds. Medicine and social justice. New York, N.Y.: Oxford University Press, 2002.

4. Berkman LF, Kawachi I, eds. Social epidemiology. New York, N.Y.: Oxford University Press, 2000.

5. Institute of Medicine Committee on the Consequences of Uninsurance. Insuring health: hidden costs, value lost. Washington, D.C.: National Academies Press, 2003.

6. Bodenheimer T. The human faces of Medicare privatization. San Francisco, Calif.: Senior Action Network, 2003. Available at: http://www.SeniorActionNetwork.org. Accessed January 14, 2005.

7. Institute of Medicine Committee on Understanding and Eliminating Racial and Ethnic Disparities in Health Care. Unequal treatment: confronting racial and ethnic disparities in healthcare. Washington, D.C.: National Academies Press, 2001.

8. News summary on health care access and quality. Available at: http://www.community-voices.org. Accessed January 14, 2005.

9. Robert Wood Johnson Foundation. Available at: http://www.rwjf.org. Accessed January 14, 2005.

10. Institute of Medicine Committee on the Consequences of Uninsurance. Insuring America's health: principles and recommendations. Washington, D.C.: National Academies Press, 2004.

11. National Association of Community Health Centers. Available at: http://www.nachc.org. Accessed January 14, 2005.

12. Kaiser Family Foundation Commission on Medicaid and the Uninsured. Available at: http://www.kff.org, at "Health Coverage and the Uninsured." Accessed January 14, 2005.

13. Woolhandler S, Campbell T, Himmelstein DU. Costs of health care administration in the United States and Canada: micromanagement, macrocosts. Int J Health Serv 2004;34:65–78.

14. Center for Budget and Policy Priorities. Available at: http://www.cbpp.org. Accessed January 14, 2005.

15. Institute of Medicine Committee on the Quality of Health Care in America. Crossing the quality chasm: a new health system for the 21st century. Washington, D.C.: National Academies Press, 2001.

16. Kerr EA, McGlynn EA, Adams J, et al. Profiling the quality of care in 12 communities: results from the CQI Study. Health Affairs 2004;23:247–56.

17. Agency for Healthcare Research and Quality. National report card on disparities in health care. Available at: http://www.ahrq.gov. Accessed January 14, 2005.

18. Vladek B, Fishman E. Unequal by design: health care, distributive justice, and the American political process. In: Rhodes R, Battin MP, Silvers A, eds. Medicine and social justice. New York, N.Y.: Oxford University Press, 2002.

19. Davis K, Schoen C, Doty M, et al. Medicare versus private insurance: rhetoric and reality. Health Aff (Millwood). 2002;Jul–Dec(Suppl Web Exclusives):W311–24.

20. Savedoff, WD. Kenneth Arrow and the birth of health economics. Available at: http://www.who.int/bulletin/volumes/82/2/en/PHCC.pdf. Accessed January 14, 2005.

21. Brown S, Doyle S. Op-Chart: the Medicare index. *The New York Times*, January 28, 2004, p A25.

13

INFECTIOUS DISEASES

Joia S. Mukherjee and Paul E. Farmer

Introduction

Bubonic plague—the "Black Death"—is the epitome of a devastating infectious disease epidemic. In 1348, Europe was ravaged by the first attack of *Yersinia pestis*. Over the next 300 years, as many as 40 million people perished.[1] Plague-stricken communities lacked strategies to deal with the rapidly spreading disease and resorted to extreme measures, such as burning masses of people alive—a method considered to be a rational public health strategy at the time. Other defensive measures included banishing members of society who followed lifestyles seen as offensive to God, partaking in public processions to appease angry deities, and simply awaiting a realignment of the planets.

The plague claimed the lives of up to half of many urban populations, but it did not affect Europe's entire population equally. The wealthy could avoid the plague by physically running away from it: "by fleeing early, fleeing far, and returning late."[2] Indeed, many physicians, being of greater means themselves, moved to safer, less plague-ridden areas.[3] To exercise this option required money, employment, housing, land ownership, and access to transportation. Only if these resources were available could one escape the transmission of the plague.

Today, despite many advances in prevention and treatment, infectious diseases continue to plague humanity (fig. 13-1). Tuberculosis (TB) accounts

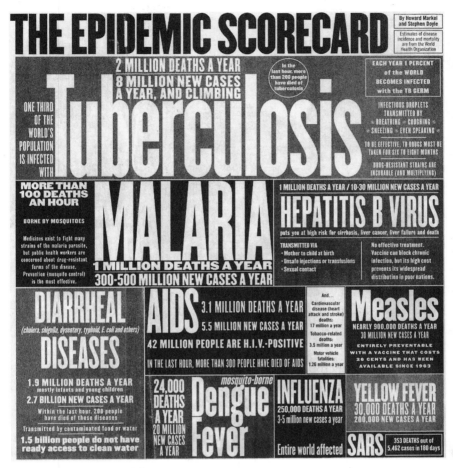

Figure 13-1 The Epidemic Scorecard: The sudden appearance of an epidemic typically inspires rapt attention, panic, and action. Once the crisis subsides, public attention wanes although the threat of contagion continues, especially among the world's poor. Compare our response to severe acute respiratory syndrome (SARS) with the more familiar germs that plague us daily. Compare it with the dangers of smoking or getting into a car and heading out on the road. Every life is precious, but when you look at the numbers, SARS just is not as formidable a threat as we have made it out to be. When the facts are few, it is easy for fear to fill the vacuum. (From Markel H, Doyle S. The epidemic scorecard. *New York Times*, April 30, 2003, p. A31.)

for 8 million new cases and 2 million deaths a year; one-third of the world's population is infected with the tubercle bacillus. Malaria accounts for 300 to 500 million new cases and 1 million deaths a year. Approximately 40 million people are infected with HIV—mainly in less developed parts of the world (fig. 13-2)—and approximately 3 million die of AIDS each year. Millions of

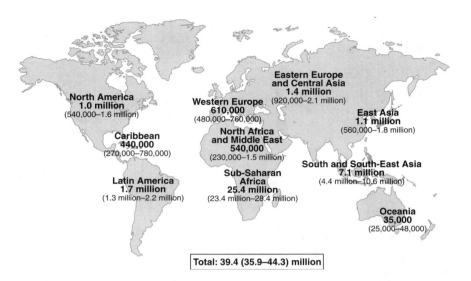

Figure 13-2 Number of adults and children estimated to be living with HIV in various regions as of the end of 2004. (From UNAIDS. AIDS Epidemic Update 2004. Geneva, Switzerland: Joint United Nations Program on HIV/AIDS [UNAIDS] and World Health Organization [WHO], 2004, 77.)

other people suffer from and die of diarrheal, respiratory, hepatic, and other infectious diseases annually.

Long before the development of the germ theory of disease, it was recognized that overcrowding, lack of sanitation, and poverty exacerbate the spread of epidemic diseases. For centuries, individuals with agency over the basic aspects of their lives—such as where to live and work and what to eat and drink—have experienced a significantly lower risk of contracting infectious diseases than those who have not enjoyed such choices. Structural risks and lack of agency, largely borne by the poor, have proved to be central factors in most infectious disease epidemics.[4] Thus, disease prevention programs that do not address issues of structural violence are inevitably limited in their effectiveness.

Communities most heavily affected by infectious diseases also tend to have the least access to treatment. One of the most vivid and dramatic examples occurred when envelopes containing *Bacillus anthracis* were mailed to U.S. senators and news media leaders in October 2001. Countless Americans were thought to be at risk. Yet, nationally, only five fatalities occurred as a result of this sinisterly engineered outbreak. One of the few consolations during this national scare was that anthrax can be treated with ciprofloxacin or even cheaper alternatives, such as penicillin or doxycycline. The U.S. government, concerned for the welfare of its people and perceiving a national emergency, exerted its substantial influence and persuaded the Bayer Corporation to lower the price of ciprofloxacin from about $1.80 per tablet to $1.00 per tablet, reducing the cost of a 6-week course of therapy from about $150 to about $80.

Meanwhile, numerous anthrax cases have been reported from Haiti since the mid-1970s. Less than 10 percent of Haiti's population has access to basic health care—let alone drugs such as penicillin or doxycycline. Clearly, treatment access is not proportional to need. Even in the context of a disease as deadly as anthrax, drugs are neither developed nor made accessible if the target population does not represent a lucrative market for the pharmaceutical industry. While the U.S. annual health expenditures exceed $4,800 per person, that of Haiti is the equivalent of US$12 per person. Haiti is only one example of an extremely poor and heavily disease-burdened country that lacks the economic bargaining power to effectively pressure pharmaceutical companies who boast corporate profits that are often of greater magnitude than the gross national product (GNP) of poor nations.

Another important issue of social injustice related to infectious disease concerns the cost of treatment. Efforts to prevent an infectious disease epidemic are often significantly cheaper than providing treatment afterward. Therefore, cost constraints often lead to public health policies focusing on prevention in lieu of treatment. In schools of public health and global public health institutions, the underlying assumption that resources are limited drives an ethic that favors programs with the lowest cost and the broadest reach—without regard to equity, justice, or disease burden. Such utilitarian decision-making not only neglects the lives of the sick but also promotes the spread of untreated infections through poor neighborhoods. The global community has not fully appreciated the long-term costs wrought by public health and economic policies by which entire communities live and die without access to modern medicine.

This chapter focuses on the causative relationship between social injustice and infectious diseases and the processes by which the disproportionate burden of infectious diseases on the poor further a vicious cycle of poverty and injustice. The remediation of social injustice must be at the root of global efforts to successfully prevent, treat, and control infectious diseases. Thus, current public health paradigms for the prevention and treatment of infectious diseases must be altered to incorporate an ethos of social justice and human rights.

The Impact of Social Injustice on Infectious Diseases

The burden of infectious disease cases and deaths falls most heavily on developing countries, as illustrated in table 13-1 for malaria and respiratory infections. These marked disparities are also reflected in table 13-2, which demonstrates a much higher prevalence of HIV infection and a much higher incidence of tuberculosis among people living in developing countries.

TABLE 13-1   Estimated Burden of Disease and Deaths, for Selected Diseases, by Areas of the World, 2002

WHO Region and Mortality Stratum	Burden of Disease (in thousands of DALYs*), by Cause		Deaths (in thousands), by Cause	
	Malaria	Respiratory Infections	Malaria	Respiratory Infections
Africa				
High child and adult mortality	19,429	16,569	538	533
High child, very high adult mortality	19,736	16,134	549	538
The Americas				
Very low child and adult mortality	0	390	0	72
Low child and adult mortality	86	1,872	1	107
High child and adult mortality	24	1,120	0	49
Eastern Mediterranean				
Low child and adult mortality	92	559	2	20
High child and adult mortality	2,112	10,458	55	345
Europe				
Very low child and adult mortality	1	690	0	174
Low child and adult mortality	18	1,437	0	60
Low child, high adult mortality	0	625	0	39
Southeast Asia				
Low child and adult mortality	502	1,499	12	108
High child and adult mortality	2,253	30,286	53	1,285
Western Pacific				
Very low child and adult mortality	0	372	0	108
Low child and adult mortality	433	8,165	11	403

*DALYs are disability-adjusted life years.

Adapted from World Health Organization. The world health report 2003. Geneva, Switzerland: World Health Organization, 2003, pp. 154–55, 160–61.

Structural Inequities and the Disproportionate Burden of Infectious Diseases on the Poor

It is often said that infectious diseases know no boundaries. While it is true that transmissible diseases can freely cross national borders, it is also the

TABLE 13-2   Prevalence of HIV Infection (2001) and Incidence of Tuberculosis (2002) in Selected Developing Countries and the United States

Country	Prevalence of HIV (in percent)		Incidence of Tuberculosis (per 100,000 people)
	Males Aged 15–24	Females Aged 15–24	
Afghanistan	NA	NA	333
Guatemala	0.90	0.85	77
Haiti	4.06	4.96	319
Iraq	NA	NA	167
Kenya	6.01	15.56	540
Pakistan	0.06	0.05	181
Peru	0.41	0.18	202
Sierra Leone	2.48	7.53	405
South Africa	10.66	25.64	558
Vietnam	0.31	0.17	192
United States	0.5	0.2	5

From The World Bank. 2004 World development indicators. Washington, D.C.: The World Bank, 2004.

case that socioeconomic boundaries are not nearly as porous as national frontiers. For example, a man living in South Africa may travel to Botswana to work in a diamond mine. While isolated and away from home for many months, he may acquire HIV from a commercial sex worker who was herself infected at age 15, when she was raped by an older man in her village in Namibia for whom she had worked as a domestic servant. Both the South African man and the Namibian woman may then spread the virus in their home villages and countries.

Yet it is unlikely that this infected couple will spread HIV to a wealthy banker in Durban or a research scientist in the United States. Why? The same structures that create a disproportionate burden of infectious diseases among the poor— lack of housing, employment, land ownership, and education—also serve to physically and socially separate the poor from the wealthy. Such structural divisions effectively concentrate and magnify the impact of infectious diseases to epidemic proportions in the world's most impoverished and vulnerable communities. Because these forces are embedded in ubiquitous social structures and occur wherever people are disadvantaged by political, legal, economic, or cultural traditions, prevention programs must address these fundamental and widespread inequities in order to significantly decrease the transmission of infectious disease to and within the most vulnerable populations.

Thanks to the fruits of modern medicine, life expectancy for women in developed countries has now reached a high of 78 years. Yet over the past two decades, life expectancy for men in sub-Saharan Africa has plummeted to 46 years.[5] The vast difference in life expectancy trends in rich and poor nations can largely be explained by disparities in infectious disease prevalence and mortality. For example, 60 percent of all adult deaths in Africa are caused by infectious diseases, compared with only 10 percent of all adult deaths in developed countries.

The statistics for children are equally grim. Both child and infant mortality rates were greatly reduced in the 1970s and 1980s, largely due to the widespread implementation of oral rehydration therapy and infant vaccination. But these gains have been virtually reversed over the past decade in the world's poorest countries. Diarrheal diseases, pneumonia, and malaria are now the leading causes of child and infant mortality. In 2001, the average under-5 mortality rate in low-income countries was 121 deaths per 1000 live births; in lower-middle-income countries, 41; in upper-middle-income countries, 27; and in wealthy countries, fewer than 7. The 17-fold difference in under-5 mortality rates between low-income and wealthy countries can largely be explained by the high rate of gastrointestinal disease in poor countries.[6–8] Yet even in developed countries, poor children suffer disproportionate morbidity from diarrheal disease related to structural factors, including inadequate maternal education and substandard, transient housing.[9] Lack of access to sanitation and clean water have also been determined to be major risk factors for gastrointestinal disease.[10] In a comprehensive study using aggregated World Bank and UNICEF data from 22 countries in Latin America and the Caribbean, the following five structural factors were found to be inversely related to under-5 mortality rates: the use of oral rehydration therapy, access to safe water, vaccination levels, female literacy, and per-capita GNP.[11]

Roots and Underlying Factors

Preventive interventions, such as the use of DDT to control malaria north of the Panama Canal[12] and the decline of child mortality as a result of vaccination,[13] have been great victories in public health. Social injustice, however, underpins the enormous differences in the distribution of diseases. Prevention can be defined as the mitigation of risk, but when unequal access to food, water, housing, and employment promote the transmission of infectious diseases, the world's most impoverished and vulnerable communities have neither the resources nor the agency at the governmental, community, and personal levels to mitigate disease risk.

Inadequate Support for Public Works and Infrastructure

Risk factors for the spread of infectious diseases are often directly related to public works and infrastructure, or the lack thereof. This relationship was first recognized in 1854 when John Snow traced a London cholera epidemic to unclean water originating from one isolated pump.[14] Snow removed the handle of the pump and effectively stopped a cholera epidemic with one simple intervention. However, the structural inequalities affecting access to clean water are usually far more widespread and complex. In 2003, the United Nations Development Program estimated that over 1.2 billion people lack access to clean drinking water and over 2.4 billion lack access to proper sanitary facilities.[15] The ability to construct basic public works, such as wells and sanitation systems, lies far beyond the economic means of many of the world's poorest governments. Furthermore, under the guise of development programs and loans, international financial institutions often impose structural adjustment policies that further constrain the ability of poor countries to provide basic services to their citizens.[16] (See chapter 21.)

For example, South Africa, although not as poor as many of its neighbors, still struggles to overcome the well-documented inequalities stemming from decades of oppression and injustice under apartheid. Only after the transition to democracy in 1994 did South Africa begin to provide sanitary water to residents of the former homelands. However, bowing under pressure from international financial institutions, these water programs were subsequently privatized, and user fees were imposed. Not surprisingly, a cholera epidemic in KwaZulu Natal in 2000 was directly linked to the cessation of sanitary water provision to an informal settlement whose residents were unable to pay the new user fees.[17]

All too often, prevention strategies fail to address the structural inequities that perpetuate disease at the most basic level. For example, decentralizing and privatizing health care—another tenet of structural adjustment and neoliberal economic reform—has severely weakened the public health infrastructure in many poor countries.[18,19]

The public sector in all countries serves the poor. This is true for both health and education, two strong determinants of public health. Privatization of the health sector and the imposition of user fees in the public sector reduces the utilization of services, especially by the poor.[20–22] Such cost recovery measures, although widely considered as regressive, are still being implemented to force poor countries to spend less in the public sector and move toward market economies. As countries face the mounting HIV/AIDS crisis, such policies have been called into question. In 2003, Uganda was awarded a grant from the Global Fund to Fight AIDS, Tuberculosis, and Malaria to implement an HIV treatment program. Pursuant to preexisting stipulations handed down by the international financial institutions, however, the grant would have exceeded health care spending limits. It was thus suggested by the Ugandan government, afraid of repercussions from the international financial institutions, that the money be put into the financial sector.[23] Even a physician without formal economic training soon starts to wonder if the neoliberal agenda of the international financial institutions might be increasing the risk of infectious diseases, as these institutions "slap the hands" of those who dare to treat the destitute sick.

Social and Economic Rights

The spread of infectious diseases is strongly linked not only to the services to which people have access but also to the conditions in which people live. However, fulfilling basic social and economic rights, such as the right to adequate housing, education, and food, is not often linked to strategies that are developed to prevent infectious diseases. Disparities in housing, level of education, and nutritional status are causally linked to the disproportionate burden of infectious disease in impoverished communities. This relationship is clear in the spread of airborne diseases, most notably TB, among the poor. Conditions of urban poverty—overcrowding, poor housing, and poor nutrition—continue to drive the spread of TB worldwide. While TB treatment is highly effective, it was not treatment but the improvement of living conditions that first reduced TB occurrence in developed countries.

In the 1940s, before the advent of effective treatment, the rate of active TB plummeted in New York City, mainly due to the post–World War II economic boom and the migration of people from tenements in cities to single-family homes in the suburbs. TB then made a striking reappearance in the United States in the 1990s,[24] fueled by HIV and structurally associated with overcrowding in prisons, increased rates of homelessness, and funding cuts that led to deterioration of the public health infrastructure.[25] Similarly, the incidence of childhood acute respiratory infection in developing countries has been directly linked to conditions in the home environment, including inadequate food, concomitant diarrheal illness, little maternal education, and indoor cooking fires.[26,27] Yet current strategies to eradicate respiratory diseases are primarily focused on secondary prevention, such as raising awareness and prompting the affected to seek treatment.[8] As is true with all infectious diseases, true eradication of respiratory diseases will require remediating the conditions of poverty that initially place people at risk and subsequently impede effective treatment.

Economic Freedom and Agency

The spread of sexually transmitted infections brings the concept of structural violence to an individual level. HIV/AIDS is the worst epidemic disease of our time. It spreads with a strikingly unequal distribution among populations, both locally and globally. Methods promoted by global health experts to prevent the sexual transmission of HIV/AIDS include delaying the onset of sexual intercourse, decreasing one's number of sexual partners, and using condoms. "Knowledge, attitudes, and practices" surveys and prevention strategies based on their results have been used for almost two decades to try to limit the spread of HIV/AIDS. The risk of acquiring HIV depends less on knowledge of how the virus is transmitted, however, and more on freedom to apply this knowledge. Poverty is a major factor limiting such freedom. Many who acquire HIV infection do so despite having enough information to protect themselves. Studies indicate that migration for work, domestic servitude, and sex for food, money, and survival are among the main risk factors fueling the epidemic.[1,28,29] While sub-Saharan Africa is wracked by violence, little has been written about the increase in HIV infection after political conflict, war, or genocide.[30,31] Yet rape as a war crime is front-page news when it occurs on the European continent.[32] Risk groups in the modern HIV era consist of those who live lives of constrained choices: from child servants who are raped by their masters, to men who work in mines far from their home villages, to married women remaining faithful to one man who has multiple partners. Often, their very survival may be contingent on maintaining or enduring the situations that put them at risk.

Access to Treatment

The improved treatment of infectious diseases has been a hallmark of modern medicine. The discovery of penicillin in the 1940s was quickly followed by the discovery of other antimicrobials, most notably streptomycin for TB treatment. In the 1950s, cures for previously fatal bacterial diseases such as pneumonia, endocarditis, and tuberculosis became normative in Western medicine. HIV/AIDS, when it came along, presented one of the first widespread incurable infections. As a retrovirus, it is a unique pathogen against which to target pharmaceuticals. Highly active antiretroviral therapy (HAART), which was developed 15 years after the first reported cases, has dramatically prolonged and enhanced the lives of those affected by HIV.[33]

Drug Development and Market Forces

The treatment of TB is one of the most illustrative examples of how market forces—rather than disease burden—drive the development of drugs. Worldwide, 1.8 billion people are infected with the TB bacillus; resistance to anti-TB drugs is growing; and more than 5,000 deaths each day are attributable to TB. Yet there has not been a new drug developed for TB since the 1970s. Drugs are not developed if there is no market able to pay for treatment—even for the most devastating diseases in the world. Although manufacturers claim that it takes years to recoup the cost of research and development of a new drug, they in fact spend twice as much on marketing than on research and development.[34]

In wealthy countries, determined constituents are sometimes able to circumvent market-driven research and development agendas, even when no obvious market exists. In 1983, the U.S. Congress passed the Orphan Drug Act. The purpose of this law was to encourage the development of drugs for "orphan diseases"—6,000 known rare diseases and conditions that each affect, on average, about 40,000 Americans. Brought about through lobbying by those afflicted by these rare diseases, the act enabled the government to safeguard pharmaceutical companies—through tax incentives—against financial losses that they might incur in the research and development of therapies expected to generate relatively small sales.[35,36] The hundreds of millions of people worldwide who are suffering from TB, whose ability to pay for life-saving drugs is limited, have no such lobbying power.

The Use of Substandard Therapies

Utilitarian public health strategies have promoted a nihilistic approach toward treatment regimens. For example, the standard treatment for diarrheal disease is oral rehydration therapy (ORT). While ORT is a life-saving intervention, invasive bacterial gastrointestinal infections, such as typhoid, often require antibiotics and occasionally surgical management. Case-fatality rates of untreated typhoid range from 10 to 50 percent, and children 1 to 5 years of age are at the highest risk of death. However, antibiotics are not the standard of care for diarrheal diseases, even when dysentery is present. Constrained choices are cited as the reason for focusing solely on ORT.[37–39]

A similar choice has been made historically in the treatment of drug-resistant TB. While multidrug-resistant tuberculosis (MDR TB) is treatable, duration of treatment is 18 months or more with second-line anti-TB drugs, which are expensive.[40] Because of the cost of second-line treatment and constrained choices, however, the international public health community has continued to promote the use of standard anti-TB drugs to treat patients known to have MDR TB. This misguided policy has resulted in disability and death for those infected, and ongoing transmission of resistant TB strains.

Neglecting the Sick: The False Dichotomy of Prevention Versus Treatment

Much of the ongoing debate over how best to address the AIDS pandemic centers on the relative merits of prevention versus treatment efforts, as if the two are mutually exclusive. While AIDS claims 8,500 lives daily in poor countries, it is in fact a treatable disease. Where available, highly active antiretroviral therapy has resulted in a 90 percent reduction in mortality and marked improvement in quality of life for people in treatment.[41] As of July 2002, however, less than 5 percent of people worldwide who required therapy had access to HAART. Fewer than 50,000 Africans with AIDS are currently receiving HAART—less than 2 percent of those who need it.[42]

Even in the face of the mounting death toll, some experts argue that, based on cost-effectiveness considerations, prevention efforts should take priority over AIDS treatment in Africa.[43,44] Cost-effectiveness analyses fail in their accounting of the most important reason for implementing widespread HIV treatment: treating the sick. Prevention strategies do nothing to improve the quality or length of life of the millions of people currently living with HIV. Failure to treat this population leads to a range of huge indirect costs, including orphanhood, economic decline, famine, stigma, and burnout of health professionals. Moreover, the very programs considered to be "cost-effective" are even more effective when linked with the provision of treatment.

One of the most critical components of a comprehensive strategy against HIV/AIDS is widespread access to voluntary counseling and testing (VCT). Data from VCT programs indicate that the most effective way to catalyze behavior change is by enabling people to know their HIV serological status.[45] However, 95 percent of people in Africa have no access to testing and therefore remain unaware of their HIV status. The linkage between this prevention modality and treatment is critically important, as the availability of treatment increases the demand for VCT. For example, voluntary counseling and testing at the Partners In Health hospital in rural Haiti increased four-fold after the introduction of HAART.[41] Similar results have been reported from anti-retroviral treatment programs in African countries.[46]

Access to VCT has been implemented most successfully in Brazil, one of the few resource-poor countries to offer its residents comprehensive access to HAART. Under a national control strategy, annual incidence of HIV infection in Brazil declined from 24,816 in 1998 to 7,361 in 2001.[47]

Treatment provides an obvious avenue of contact with health care providers who can reinforce prevention messages. New prevention strategies proposed by the U.S. Centers for Disease Control and Prevention emphasize this "secondary prevention" approach, targeting HIV prevention messages to those who are known to be sero-positive.[48] From cholera to syphilis, from tuberculosis to AIDS, infectious-disease epidemics have taught the public health community that successful disease control involves a combination of prevention, education, and treatment rather than a dichotomization of these complementary components.

What Needs to Be Done

The World Health Organization (WHO) declaration at Alma-Ata in 1978 for "health care for all by the year 2000"[49] was the last time we heard such an ambitious and rights-based call for access to health care. The rights-based goals of Alma-Ata were straightforward: (a) 90 percent of children should have a weight-for-age that corresponds to reference values; (b) every family should be within a 15-minute walk of potable water; and (c) women should have access to medically trained attendants for childbirth. In addition, it was widely agreed that these goals could not be achieved without increased international aid. However, the right to universal basic health care proposed in the Alma-Ata declaration was attacked by international experts as naïve and too expensive. Since 1978, distribution of limited resources for health has been determined more by markets than by rights.[50] With foreign debt mounting, poor countries were called upon by the international financial institutions to decrease the proportion of their gross national product spent on health as they moved toward market economies. Reforms in the health sector emphasized user fees, privatization, and other cost-recovery measures. The effects of these so-called reforms have been devastating in most of the countries in which they were implemented.

Revitalizing the public health infrastructure and improving the delivery of essential services, such as immunization, sanitation, and the provision of clean water, are critical if we are to address the social injustices that underlie and perpetuate infectious disease. Governments need to assume responsibility for the health of their people by setting rational, stable, and rights-based policies that guarantee health care for even the poorest and most vulnerable citizens. Poorly planned, sweeping reforms of the health sector in developing countries have often resulted in (a) chaotic implementation of services; (b) unclear lines of authority for specific tasks, such as drug purchasing; and (c) a lack of institutional memory. For example, poor planning and health system changes have adversely affected TB control efforts in many countries.[51,52]

While many say this responsibility rests with the governments of the poorest countries, these governments cannot realistically begin to address the right to health without substantial financial assistance. Advocacy efforts to address social injustice and the health of the poor must recognize that international financial institutions, in calling for restrictions on health spending, promote inequity in health care and perpetuate social injustice. Recent calls for debt relief are rooted in the argument that governments that spend less of their budget paying off debt can invest more money in health and education. In addition, novel strategies to dedicate more money to the health sector have been initiated over the past several years, including the Global Fund to Fight AIDS, Tuberculosis, and Malaria (the largest multilateral public health fund) and calls for debt relief. In 2003, the Global Fund disbursed $1.5 billion to 160 programs in 85 countries—a remarkable achievement for a program just 2 years old. Yet the Global Fund continues to face budgetary shortfalls due to the desire of donor countries to maintain political control over their aid monies.

Another important principle in remediating inequalities of access to health care is to ensure that treatment gets to the people who need it the most. WHO's list of essential drugs serves as a guide to the medications that have the greatest impact on health, but access to even essential drugs is severely limited in poor settings. The Millennium Development Goals (table 21-7 on p. 394) were established to improve factors that most affect health and development, one of which is access to essential medicines. These goals, however, are not within the reach of poor countries without external help.[53] The newly created Global Drug Facility was initiated to coordinate the bulk procurement of low-priced, quality-assured anti-TB drugs. Governments of poor, heavily indebted countries can apply to the Facility to obtain these drugs free of charge. Price reductions and tiered pricing systems are additional methods of decreasing inequities in treatment.[54] Advocacy efforts led by Médicins Sans Frontières, the Clinton Foundation HIV/AIDS Initiative, and other organizations has helped to lower the annual cost of anti-AIDS medication from $10,000 in 2001 to about $140 in 2003. Advocating for the progressive interpretation of trade laws would allow poor countries to access less-expensive generic medications.[55] Recently, the Global Alliance for Tuberculosis Drug Development, a nonprofit organization, was created to encourage pharmaceutical companies to undertake research on new anti-TB drugs.[56]

The magnitude of human suffering due to infectious diseases can be alleviated only if social injustice is comprehensively addressed by governments of both developed and developing countries, as well as by the international business and financial communities. All governments have the responsibility to ensure basic social and economic rights, including the right to health care, education, and access to food, water, and shelter. However, the governments of deeply impoverished countries suffer profound economic stress because of large debt burdens. The responsibility of the donor community is to abolish punitive structural-adjustment policies and grant debt relief, which would allow poor countries to spend more money ensuring the right to health and addressing the social injustices that underlie ill health. Additionally, novel approaches to drug development and intellectual property law are needed to ensure that the advances of science are shared equitably worldwide.

Conclusion

Risk mitigation, prevention, and care for those suffering from infectious diseases must be seen as a public good. The justifications for such ambitious initiatives are many: the needs of those already sick, the prevention of ongoing transmission, and the rectification of previous clinical and policy errors. Perhaps the most compelling justification is the ethical unacceptability of tolerating a lower standard of care for the poor. If we are to truly improve global health, social justice must become a central component of public health.

Focusing solely on prevention fails to address the needs of those already infected or sick. Prevention is considered cheap when compared to treatment, and yet real preventive measures—the provision of safe water sources, adequate housing, and gainful employment—have not yet been promoted as integral components of public health strategies. Rather, these factors are relegated to the "development" sphere and most often linked with reform of markets that exclude the poorest and most vulnerable populations.

We can undermine faith in medicine and public health by making unreasonable, excessive, or propagandistic claims. Arguing, for example, that "education is the only vaccine" is neither accurate nor appropriate. We cannot show that cognitive interventions have been highly effective in preventing HIV infection among the poor, and it would thus seem unwise to rely exclusively on such methods. We keep hearing that we live in "a time of limited resources." Yet the wealth of the world has not dried up—it has simply become unavailable to those who need it most.

Improving the lives of the destitute sick requires large-scale, novel, multilateral, and innovative funding strategies (such as the Global Fund) and coordinated political activities (such as debt relief and reinterpretation of intellectual property rights laws and trade agreements). The global community has been slow and less than generous in addressing the inequalities that promote the occurrence of infectious diseases. Social justice in global public health requires a commitment to eliminating the structural violence that puts communities at risk and to treating the populations most heavily affected by infectious diseases. Without a social justice approach, public health will be relegated to the historical ledger as having offered cheap and inadequate palliation, rather than sustainable remediation, in the face of global cataclysm.

References

1. Quinn TC. Population migration and the spread of HIV types 1 and 2 human immunodeficiency viruses. Proc Natl Acad Sci USA 1994;91:2407–14.
2. Watts S, ed. Epidemics and history. New Haven, Conn.: Yale University Press, 1997.
3. Kiple K, ed. The Cambridge world history of human disease. Cambridge, U.K.: Cambridge University Press, 1993.
4. Burris S. Law as a structural factor in the spread of communicable disease. Houston Law Rev 1999;36:1755–86.
5. World Bank. World development indicators 2004. Available at: http://www.developmentgoals.org/sub-Saharan_Africa.htm. Accessed February 22, 2005.

6. Porignon D, Noterman JP, Hennart P, et al. The role of the Zaïrian Health Services in the Rwandan refugee crisis. Disasters 1995;19:356–60.
7. Bern C, Ortega Y, Checkley W, et al. Epidemiologic differences between cyclosporiasis and cryptosporidiosis in Peruvian children. Emerg Infect Dis 2002;8:581–5.
8. Akram DS, Agboatwalla M. A model for health intervention. J Trop Pediatr 1992; 38:85–7.
9. Baker D, Taylor H, Henderson J. Inequality in infant morbidity: causes and consequences in England in the 1990s. ALSPAC Study Team. Avon Longitudinal Study of Pregnancy and Childhood. J Epidemiol Commun Health 1998;52:451–8.
10. Abate G, Kogi-Makau W, Muroki NM. Health seeking and hygiene behaviours predict nutritional status of pre-school children in a slum area of Addis Ababa, Ethiopia. Ethiopia Med J 2000;38:253–65.
11. Moore D, Castillo E, Richardson C, et al. Determinants of health status and the influence of primary health care services in Latin America, 1990–98. Int J Health Plann Manage 2003;18:279–92.
12. Najera JA. Malaria control: achievements, problems and strategies. Parassitologia 2001;43:1–89.
13. Morley D. Saving children's lives by vaccination. BMJ 1989;299:1544–5.
14. Vinten-Johansen P, Brody H, Paneth N, et al, eds. Cholera, chloroform, and the science of medicine: a life of John Snow. New York, N.Y.: Oxford University Press, 2003:115–6.
15. United Nations Development Program. Clean water and sanitation for the poor. New York, N.Y.: United Nations Development Program, 2003.
16. Kim JY, Millen J, Irwin A, eds. Dying for growth: global inequality and the health of the poor. Monroe, Me.: Common Courage Press, 1999.
17. Pauw J. The politics of underdevelopment: metered to death—how a water experiment caused riots and a cholera epidemic. Int J Health Serv 2003;33:819–30.
18. Hanson S. Health sector reform and STD/AIDS control in resource poor settings—the case of Tanzania. Int J Health Plann Manage 2000;15:341–60.
19. Yoder RA. Are people willing and able to pay for health services? Soc Sci Med 1989;29:35–42.
20. Benson JS. The impact of privatization on access in Tanzania. Soc Sci Med 2001; 52:1903–15.
21. Ching P. User fees, demand for children's health care and access across income groups: the Philippine case. Soc Sci Med 1995;41:37–46.
22. Mbugua JK, Bloom GH, Segall MM. Impact of user charges on vulnerable groups: the case of Kibwezi in rural Kenya. Soc Sci Med 1995;41:829–35.
23. Wendo C. Uganda and the Global Fund sign grant agreement. Lancet 2003;361:942.
24. Frieden TR, Sherman LF, Maw KL, et al. A multi-institutional outbreak of highly drug-resistant tuberculosis: epidemiology and clinical outcomes. JAMA 1996;276: 1229–35.
25. Brudney K, Dobkin J. Resurgent tuberculosis in New York City: human immunodeficiency virus, homelessness and the decline of tuberculosis control programs. Am Rev Respir Dis 1991;144:745–9.
26. Hortal M, Contera M, Mogdasy C, et al. Acute respiratory infections in children from a deprived urban population from Uruguay. Rev Inst Med Trop Sao Paulo 1994;36: 51–7.
27. Denny FW, Loda FA. Acute respiratory infections are the leading cause of death in children in developing countries. Am J Trop Med Hygiene 1986;35:1–2.

28. Jochelson K, Mothibeli M, Leger JP. HIV and migrant labor in South Africa. Int J Health Serv 1991;21:157–73.

29. Kelly RJ, Gray RH, Sewankambo NK, et al. Age differences in sexual partners and risk of HIV-1 infection in rural Uganda. J Acquir Immune Defic Syndr 2003;32:446–51.

30. Donovan P. Rape and HIV/AIDS in Rwanda. Lancet 2002;360(suppl):S17–8.

31. Smallman-Raynor MR, Cliff AD. Civil war and the spread of AIDS in Central Africa. Epidemiol Infect 1991;107:69–80.

32. Acheson D. Health, humanitarian relief, and survival in former Yugoslavia. BMJ 1993;307:44–48.

33. Hammer SM, Squires KE, Hughes MD, et al. A controlled trial of two nucleoside analogues plus indinavir in persons with human immunodeficiency virus infection and CD4 cell counts of 200 per cubic millimeter or less. AIDS Clinical Trials Group 320 Study Team. N Engl J Med 1997;337:725–33.

34. Families USA. Off the charts: Pay, profits and spending by drug companies. Washington, D.C.: Families USA Foundation, 2001:3.

35. van Woert MH. Orphan drugs: proposed legislative help. N Engl J Med 1981; 304:235.

36. Asbury CH, Stolley PD. Orphan drugs: creating a policy. Ann Intern Med 1981;95: 221–4.

37. Bhandari N, Bahl R, Taneja S, et al. Pathways to infant mortality in urban slums of Delhi, India: implications for improving the quality of community- and hospital-based programmes. J Health Popul Nutr 2002;20:148–55.

38. Goldman N, Pebley AR, Beckett M. Diffusion of ideas about personal hygiene and contamination in poor countries: evidence from Guatemala. Soc Sci Med 2001;52: 53–69.

39. Goldman N, Pebley AR, Gragnolati M. Choices about treatment for ARI and diarrhea in rural Guatemala. Soc Sci Med 2002;55:1693–712.

40. Mukherjee J, Rich M, Socci A, et al. Programmes and principles in treatment of multidrug-resistant tuberculosis. Lancet 2004;363:474–81.

41. Farmer P, Léandre F, Mukherjee J, et al. Community-based treatment of advanced HIV disease: introducing DOT-HAART (directly observed therapy with highly active antiretroviral therapy). Bull WHO 2001;79:1145–51.

42. Mukherjee JS, Farmer PE, Niyizonkiza D, et al. Tackling HIV in resource poor countries. BMJ 2003;327:1104–6.

43. Marseille E, Hofmann PB, Kahn JG. HIV prevention before HAART in sub-Saharan Africa. Lancet 2002;359:1851–6.

44. Creese A, Floyd K, Alban A, et al. Cost-effectiveness of HIV/AIDS interventions in Africa: a systematic review of the evidence. Lancet 2002;359:1635–43.

45. Roth DL, Stewart KE, Clay OJ, et al. Sexual practices of HIV discordant and concordant couples in Rwanda: effects of a testing and counselling programme for men. Int J STD AIDS 2001;12:181–8.

46. Anonymous. Efficacy of voluntary HIV-1 counselling and testing in individuals and couples in Kenya, Tanzania, and Trinidad: a randomised trial. The Voluntary HIV-1 Counseling and Testing Efficacy Study Group. Lancet 2000;356:103–12.

47. Dados epidemiológicos de Brasil. Boletin Epidemiológico—AIDS, 27ª a 40ª Semanas Epidemiológicas Julho a Setembro de 2001, 2002;15(1): n.p.

48. Centers for Disease Control and Prevention. Adoption of protective behaviors among persons with recent HIV infection and diagnosis—Alabama, New Jersey, and Tennessee, 1997–1998. MMWR Morb Mortal Wkly Rep 2000;49:512–5.

49. Declaration of Alma-Ata. International Conference on Primary Health Care, Alma-Ata, USSR, 6–12 September 1978. Geneva, Switzerland: World Health Organization, n.p. Available at: http://www.who.int/hpr/NPH/docs/declaration_almaata.pdf. Accessed February 22, 2005.

50. Hall JJ, Taylor R. Health for all beyond 2000: the demise of the Alma-Ata Declaration and primary health care in developing countries. Med J Aust 2003;178:17–20.

51. Kritski AL, Ruffino-Netto A. Health sector reform in Brazil: impact on tuberculosis control. Int J Tuberc Lung Dis 2000;4:622–6.

52. Bosman MC. Health sector reform and tuberculosis control: the case of Zambia. Int J Tuberc Lung Dis 2000;4:606–14.

53. Anonymous. Health-related Millennium Development Goals out of reach for many countries. Bull WHO 2004;82:156–7.

54. Berman D. AIDS, essential medicines, and compulsory licensing. J Int Assoc Physicians AIDS Care 1999;5:24–5.

55. Elliott R. TRIPS from Doha to Cancun . . . to Ottawa: global developments in access to treatment and Canada's Bill C-56. Can HIV AIDS Policy Law Rev 2003;8:1,7–18.

56. Walgate R. New non-profit organization will support research to combat neglected diseases. Bull WHO 2002;80:842–3.

14

NUTRITION

J. Larry Brown

Introduction

Poor nutritional status leads to adverse health outcomes. In both developing and developed countries, there is a strong association between poor nutrition in vulnerable populations and poverty, inequality, and other manifestations of social injustice (fig. 14-1). (See box 21-2 on p. 388 concerning inadequate nutrition in developing countries.)

Inadequate Nutrition: The U.S. Context

In 1966, a team of physicians commissioned by the Field Foundation studied areas of endemic poverty in the United States: migrant labor camps, Indian reservations, urban slums, and small towns in the Mississippi Delta. In their report to the U.S. Congress the following year, they underscored the desperate circumstances they had found: "If you go look, you will find America a shocking place. No other Western country permits such a large population of its people to endure the lives we press on our poor. To make four-fifths of a nation more affluent than any other people in history, we have degraded one-fifth merci-lessly."[1,2] It was common, the team reported, for poor infants and young children to have no milk to drink because their parents did not have the money to purchase

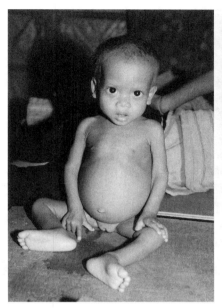 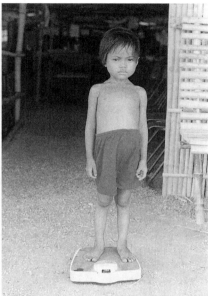

Figure 14-1 Malnutrition among children in a Cambodian refugee camp. Left: young child with kwashiorkor, a severe form of malnutrition. Right: Seven-year-old girl with severe malnutrition, who weighed only 27 pounds. Much hunger and malnutrition occurred among Cambodians during the genocidal regime of Pol Pot in the late 1970s. (Photographs by Barry S. Levy.)

it. Hunger was widespread. Many households had little, or sometimes nothing, to eat for several days each month. Kwashiorkor, a form of severe malnutrition usually associated with Third World conditions of starvation, was not uncommon. It was seen in African-American children whose black hair had turned yellow, in Native American children with sunken eyes and rotted teeth, and in the protruding abdomens and thin limbs of children in migrant camps and city slums. (See box 14-1 for definitions of hunger, malnutrition, and related terms.)

These shocking findings provoked enough public outrage to galvanize a Republican President, Richard Nixon, and a Democratic Congress into action.[3] The Food Stamp Program was expanded from a pilot effort reaching only 2 million poor households to a national program covering 10 times that number.[4] The federal School Lunch Program was augmented with a parallel School Breakfast Program, elderly feeding programs were begun, and the Special Supplemental Food Program for Women, Infants, and Children (WIC) was established.[5] This collective policy response, viewed by political leaders as a wise investment in the nation's future,[6] produced remarkable results. A decade later, the team of physicians returned to the same areas of the nation and reported to Congress that, while poverty remained a significant problem,

---

BOX 14-1   Definition of Key Terms

Food deprivation

Involuntary lack of access to an adequate diet typically associated with poverty and low income status.

Food insecurity

The condition of not knowing where one's next meal will come from, going without enough to eat, cutting back on adequate nutritional intake, and/or reliance on charitable hand-outs.

Hunger

Defined by the federal government as a "painful sensation" associated with inadequate food intake. The scholarly community considers hunger to be the chronic underconsumption of adequate food and nutrients associated with inadequate income.

Malnutrition

A general term referring to severe impairment of health and/or mental function that results from chronic failure to receive adequate nutrients in the diet.

---

hunger was no longer widespread.[5] This conclusion was later borne out by university-based scholars and national nutrition surveys.[7,8]

The success, however, would be short-lived. The first official recognition that hunger had reappeared came in 1982, from the U.S. Conference of Mayors.[9] Since the beginning of the 1980s, the news media had been reporting locally and regionally on what would become a national phenomenon: increasing bread lines and soup kitchens in the United States.[10] The mayors termed hunger "a most serious emergency," and some, like the mayors of Detroit and Salt Lake City, called the situation "a national tragedy and a national disgrace."[11] In 1983, a study commissioned by the U.S. Department of Agriculture (USDA) found that hunger was growing across the nation "at a frenetic pace,"[12] but the White House ordered that these findings not be released. They became known only because lower-level civil servants, angered by the suppression of the study, gave copies to the media.[13]

The first authoritative calculation of the extent of hunger in the United States was published in the 1985 report of the Harvard-based Physician Task Force on Hunger in America entitled *Hunger in America: The Growing Epidemic.* This group estimated the number of people affected by hunger to be

20 million,[11] or 9 percent of the U.S. population—a number challenged by the Reagan Administration, for which the problem had political overtones.[14]

At the time there was no universal definition of hunger. The Harvard-based physician group defined hunger as "chronically inadequate nutritional intake due to low income status."[11] Whether chronic or episodic in nature, hunger was the lack of sufficient calories and nutrients for physical growth or the maintenance of good health. Frequently extending over longer periods, hunger can lead to serious chronic health conditions in both children and adults.

Since 1995, the federal government has used its own measure of nutritional deprivation based on an annual survey conducted by the U.S. Census Bureau as part of its Current Population Survey. Known as the "Federal Hunger and Food Security Module"[15] and annually released by the USDA, this survey consistently supported estimates that the number of Americans living in households with serious food problems is more than 30 million. The latest report (for 2002) put the number above 35 million.[16] Representing more than 12 percent of the population, this proportion is significantly higher than the somewhat more conservative Harvard estimate, although the federal data are based on a slightly different definition of hunger.

The federal standard labels anyone having food-access problems as "food insecure," including (a) people experiencing the pangs of hunger, (b) families who do not eat what they know they need because they cannot buy it, and (c) those who have no idea from where their next meal will come. However, the federal standard also has a subcomponent: households that it terms "hungry." Oddly, its official definition of hunger is far more conservative than its own survey justifies. Hunger is defined as a "painful sensation," meaning that its victims must hurt in their stomachs before they are considered hungry.[15] Not only is this definition not reflective of their survey questions, but it also has little basis in science. Pain is neither the first nor the only consequence of being hungry. Moreover, many people who experience hunger report no pain at all; others who experience pain report that it passes with time.[17,18] In other words, "pain" is neither a necessary nor sufficient definition of hunger. Whether or not people experience pain, their nutrient intake may be inadequate for optimal health and productivity.

It is with this backdrop—a nation carrying the burden of more than 30 million people consistently without adequate nutrition—that we can examine what hunger does to its victims and why it occurs amid extravagant wealth.

The Impact of Social Injustice on Nutrition

While debate about the causes and remedies of hunger is conducted in the political arena, hunger itself is a public health issue. The adverse consequences of chronic undernutrition, as well as the social sequelae, make hunger a critical problem for the nation. Moreover, an increasing body of knowledge points to the problem of obesity as a health consequence frequently associated with inadequate income and even hunger[19] (box 14-2).

In the United States, hunger presents quite differently than it does in developing nations. (See box 21-2 on p. 388.) Protein-calorie malnutrition, or marasmas, and kwashiorkor, characterized by adequate calories but extreme protein deficiency, now occur in the United States only rarely.[20] Rather, hunger in this country typically takes the form of what the World Health Organization calls "silent undernutrition."[21] It is reflected in young children who are several pounds beneath the low end of the pediatric growth chart. They may look simply like thin children, but a trained health professional will recognize that they are experiencing growth failure. Although their symptoms are different from those of malnourished children in developing countries, they are, from a health perspective, in difficulty. (See box 5-1 on p. 92 for a comparison between the United States and other developed countries.)

Because children grow and their height and weight gains are plotted on internationally used pediatric growth charts, they are perhaps the easiest population group in which to detect the consequences of inadequate nutrition. Typically, youngsters who fall below the fifth percentile in weight or height for age on growth charts are candidates for further investigation. To be certain, it is expected that normally 5 percent of any population would fall in this low end of the range; but in studies of low-income children, 10 to 15 percent do so. This indicates that what is being observed is not normal genetic variation but rather a "human-made" outcome. Moreover, this analysis is confirmed in the work of child development clinics in urban teaching hospitals across the United States, where children experiencing growth failure due to poverty are nursed back to health with appropriate nutrition.

While the relationship between inadequate nutritional intake and health status reflected in the height and weight of children is well established, scientific research in recent years has broadened our understanding of other insidious effects. Direct links exist between inadequate food intake and a variety of poor developmental outcomes in children. The health status of children from impoverished homes experiencing hunger and food insecurity is much worse than that of other children. They get sick more often, have much higher rates of both iron-deficiency anemia and serious ear infections, and are hospitalized more frequently.[22]

As a result, low-income children miss more days of school and are less prepared to learn when they do attend, making the relationship among food intake, health status, and learning far more poignant than previously understood. Further exacerbating this interactive impairment of young bodies and minds are behavioral and emotional outcomes that accompany food deprivation. Poorly

BOX 14-2 Obesity

Recent research is beginning to shed light on the paradox of obesity among low-income households that experience food insecurity and hunger. Obesity itself is now at epidemic proportions in the United States, as more and more people are affected by the social causes of high energy consumption and/or too little expenditure through exercise. Ironically, this problem also affects poor people. It is reasonable to wonder how households that do not get enough to eat can produce people with obesity.

Hunger exists when people lack access to an adequate diet because they do not have enough money to purchase what they need to eat. Their dietary purchases are limited to cheaper, more-filling foods that produce the sensation of being full. Healthier foods, such as vegetables and fruit, especially those with necessary micronutrients, cannot be purchased.[1] Instead, many poor families rely on diets of macaroni and cheese, biscuits and gravy, and hamburgers and French fries at fast-food restaurants—a "good buy" from a caloric perspective, filling the body with cheap calories to stave off hunger. In the short term, the stomach is not an intelligent organ; it knows when it is full, not whether it has had an adequate meal.

The research community is now looking into several aspects of the hunger–obesity relationship.[2,3] One consists of the needs mentioned in the text of this chapter to maximize caloric intake on limited food dollars to stave off hunger. The greater the economic constraints, the harder it is for families to achieve the nutritional quality they need in their diets.[2,4] This "economic roulette," in turn, produces a tradeoff between quantity and quality of food. Households go through a succession of coping strategies to try to get by. They first reduce overall food expenditures, they then change the quality and variety of their intake, and ultimately, if forced, they reduce the quantity of their intake as well. Parents consistently reduce their own intake first to protect that of their children, but often both children and parents suffer this circumstance. Overall, the primary goal of households faced with not enough money to eat right is to consume enough to not feel hungry. Theirs is a tradeoff of quantity over quality. The price paid for the circumstance in which they are put is the resulting obesity it produces.

Obesity also can be an adaptive response when food availability is unreliable. Chronic food shortages related to low income leads people to overeat when food is available. This cycle often results in weight gain. The body then experiences physiological changes designed to help conserve energy when it is available. It compensates for periodic shortages by becoming more efficient at storing more calories as fat.

In the future, researchers will learn still more about how the social injustice that produces hunger in America also produces obesity among many of its victims.

(continued)

BOX 14-2 *(continued)*

References

1. Basiotis PP. Validity of the self-reported food sufficiency status item in the U.S. Department of Agriculture's food consumption surveys. In: Haldeman VA, ed. American Council on Consumer Interests 38th Annual Conference: the proceedings. Columbia, Mo.: American Council on Consumer Interests 38th Annual Conference, 1992.
2. Darmon N, Ferguson EL, Briend A. A cost constraint alone has adverse effects on food selection and nutrient density: an analysis of human diets by linear programming. J Nutr 2002;132:3764–71.
3. Radimer KL, Olson CM, Greene JC, et al. Understanding hunger and developing indicators to assess it in women and children. J Nutr Educ 1992;24:36S–45S.
4. Townsend MS, Peerson J, Love B, et al. Food insecurity is positively related to overweight in women. J Nutr 2001;131:1738–45.

nourished children have significantly higher rates of emotional problems, mental disorders, and withdrawn or disruptive behavior.

Household food insufficiency is associated with overall declines in general health.[23,24] In one national study, food-insufficient preschool and school-aged children had elevated rates of stomach aches, headaches, and colds.[23,24]

Other studies have corroborated these results and reported additional ones. In a multistate study of low-income families, hungry children under age 12 had twice the rate of anemia of nonhungry children in low-income households.[25] Hungry children also have higher rates of emergency department and physician visits.[25]

Food deprivation is associated with considerable psychological and emotional distress in children. In controlled studies, low-income children from households with inadequate food were more likely to exhibit impaired psychosocial functioning, including higher levels of anxiety, irritability, hyperactivity, and aggression.[26,27] In a national sample, children from food-deprived households manifested significantly higher levels of aggressive and destructive and withdrawn behavior.[28] Related outcomes apparently extend into the teenage years as well. Two studies have shown that food-insufficient teenagers are more likely to have no friends and to exhibit both depressive disorders and suicidal behaviors.[29] Such efforts, not surprisingly, seem to be expressed in the educational environment as well. Hungry children are much more likely to have had mental health counseling and to require special education services.[27,28]

Nutritional status and cognitive function in children are strongly linked. Children from food-insufficient households do not perform as well on academic achievement tests as do food-sufficient children. In some studies, hungry children not only have higher rates of lateness and absence but also are more likely to have to repeat a grade in school. For example, in two national studies of elementary school children, household food hardships were negatively correlated with school test results and achievement test results.[28–30] In another national study of kindergartners, children from food-deprived households not only entered school less prepared to learn mathematics but also learned less over the course of the year.[31]

Food deprivation impairs cognitive function.[32] In a nutrient-deprived state, the body allocates energy (a) first to critical organ function, (b) then to height and weight gain, and (c) then to the role of the nervous system in one's interaction with the environment, including listening to parents, dealing with peers, and learning. If there is insufficient energy to enable a child to carry out the latter activities, cognitive dysfunction results. Children from hungry and food-insecure homes are more likely to repeat grades,[26,27,29,30] be absent or late,[25,33] and be suspended from school.[29,30] The public health and economic implications of all this evidence are significant.

In general, low-income families know what constitutes a nutritious diet as well as the rest of the population.[34] Because limited income constrains their purchasing choices—for example, fresh fruits and vegetables typically are too expensive for them—their intake of required nutrients is significantly lower than both the Recommended Dietary Allowances (RDAs) and that of the general population.[35]

Pregnancy is a period of significant risk from dietary inadequacy because a woman needs nutrient energy not only for herself but also for the growing fetus. Stores of maternal nutrients may be depleted, and maternal anemia can be one consequence. The primary risk is borne by the fetus, including prematurity (birth at less than 37 weeks' gestation) and low birth weight (less than 2500 grams, or approximately 5.5 pounds). Infants born too early or too small, or both, are not well equipped for extrauterine life. Sequelae include respiratory distress syndrome, weakening of the immune system, and long-term developmental problems. The most paramount threat, however, is death, because low birth weight infants account for 75 percent of deaths to infants in the first month of life (neonatal deaths).[36]

Older people represent another highly vulnerable population for food deprivation. In old age, the risk factors associated with not having enough to eat are heightened by the circumstances associated with aging. Chief among these are chronic conditions, such as hypertension, coronary heart disease, and diabetes, at least one of which affects 85 percent of people over age 65.[13] Other factors impairing health status in the elderly that are associated with food intake are deficiency diseases, such as osteoporosis, and conditions that impair digestion.[37] In addition, the elderly have a heightened vulnerability to infection, and their risk of infection is increased significantly when their diet is constrained by limited income for purchase of appropriate foods.

Roots and Underlying Factors

Why do so many people have an inadequate food supply in the wealthiest nation the world has ever seen? Several factors are commonly cited. I will critique the first two, which are myths, and then address the actual cause:

There Is Not Enough Food to Go Around (Myth 1)

In fact, not only does the United States produce enough food for all its people, but some experts estimate that it has the capacity to feed most of the world's hungry as well.

The Poor Make Bad Purchasing Choices (Myth 2)

Former President Ronald Reagan once suggested that the poor simply are "too ignorant."[38] Scholarly analysis sheds a different light on the situation. All population groups could learn more about getting better nutritional value for their food dollar. Too many non-nutritious purchases are made, and too few healthy diets are the norm. But no evidence suggests that low-income households make poorer purchasing choices than do the rest of the population. Indeed, the Continuing Survey of Food Consumption suggests that poor households do as well as non-poor households in knowing what they should purchase. They simply do not have the money to do it. Moreover, we might come at this notion of ignorance from a somewhat different standpoint, that of common sense. It is well established that hunger in this nation was reduced and then returned and that the rate now varies up and down from year to year. Were we seeing an outcome resulting from ignorance, it is not likely that the impact would vary as it has over time. In other words, when the prevalence of hunger suddenly spikes, it makes little sense to think that this reflects a sudden upturn in nutritional ignorance. Conversely, when the rate of hunger goes down, this cannot be sensibly attributed to a sudden increase in knowledge.

The Underlying Cause

How, then, are we to understand the existence of 35 million people in this country without enough to eat? For this, we must consider some of the components of social injustice: the economy, wages, poverty, and related public policies. Virtually all food deprivation and its adverse health consequences are the direct or indirect outcome of social injustice or, to put it another way, of human actions that include policy decisions.

To see how the human hand can create food deprivation in our nation, let us go back to the 1970s, when domestic hunger seemed largely under control, and the early 1980s, when it returned with a vengeance. Within a few years, bread lines and soup kitchens went from a handful to 300, 400, and even 500 in each of our major cities.[11] Clearly, something quite abrupt had changed the situation. Toward the end of the 1970s and into the early 1980s, a national recession led to high unemployment and unusually high interest rates. Millions of people lost their jobs, thousands and thousands of farmers lost their livelihood, and many people once secure in their middle class existence went through unemployment due to downsizing, only to reenter the labor market with a much lower income. While the recession was significant, it was not unprecedented; the nation had experienced some tough economic circumstances not too many years earlier, but these times had not led to the proliferation of bread lines and soup kitchens. The phenomenon in the 1980s had not been seen since the Great Depression of the 1930s. Something else was at work.

The return of hunger to the nation was ushered in not by the economy per se but rather by new public policy that was adopted as more households were becoming vulnerable. Starting in 1982, the Reagan Administration submitted its first 4-year budget (for the 1982–1985 period)—the Omnibus Budget and Reconciliation Act. It was passed by a Democratic Congress largely as submitted. This budget cut more than $12 billion from the federal food program safety net that had been created during the late 1960s and early 1970s. Nearly $8 billion was cut from the Food Stamp Program, largely through reducing the allotment or value of the stamps to an average of $0.72 per person per meal. An additional $4 billion was cut from child nutrition programs, such as the school breakfast program.

In sum, more people jobless during a recession together with the intentional weakening of federal programs to feed people during tough times led to more bread lines and soup kitchens. Hunger was the inevitable product of political choices made at the time. Although we cannot always predict or control the national economy or the well-being of individual households, we can protect families from the occasional vicissitudes of the economy.

Food deprivation in the United States remained relatively stable, at more than 30 million each year, even during the economic boom from 1992 to 1999. However, the tremendous accumulation of income and wealth by some segments of the population then masked two other factors: (a) the dramatic shift of resources up the income scale and away from working and low-income households, and (b) the shift to a job market based on increasingly lower wages.

At the end of 1999—the peak of the boom—the average hourly wage was $11.87, lower than it had been in 1979: $12.05 (adjusted for inflation). For salaried workers, the median weekly income was $567 in 1999, about the same when it was $558 in the 1970s. In 1999, the per-capita annual income of the poorest quintile of the labor market earned $13,320, compared with $13,540 in 1979 (in constant dollars). In contrast, in this 20-year period, the richest quintile increased its per-capita annual income to $45,000.

In terms of wealth, inequality is even more striking. The bottom four quintiles own 4 percent of the nation's wealth, compared with the richest 1 percent that owns 48 percent.

Hunger and food deprivation exist in the United States because we are tolerating such great inequality. When our nation's nutrition-policy safety net is so threadbare, such economic disparities are destined to have a profound impact.

What Needs to Be Done

Two avenues exist to remedy hunger and other forms of nutritional deprivation in the United States: to treat the symptom and to address the root cause of the problem—the growing inequality in both income and wealth that increasingly affects more people.

It is possible to end hunger without addressing poverty and inequality—the quicker, easier, and less costly approach for now. Hunger in the United States could be ended by the president and Congress within 6 months by fully funding and utilizing existing programs for people in need. For an estimated $8 to $9 billion a year,[39] we could:

- Better fund the Food Stamp Program and extend it to the 45 percent of eligible people that it now fails to reach
- Mandate that all schools offer the federal school breakfast program and that all communities with low-income children participate in the federally funded summer food program
- Expand the provision of after-school snacks
- Increase the coverage of elderly feeding programs.

Implementation of these measures and some fine-tuning of a handful of other federal programs, such as WIC and Head Start, would mean that no one in the United States would go hungry or need to demean themselves by taking their children to eat in a soup kitchen.

We can also work to address the structural injustices that cause hunger. This will require a reconstruction of the social contract—the nature of the relationship between government and households. The social contract that had been the hallmark of social policy since the New Deal has eroded dramatically over the past quarter-century due to regressive social policies that have removed much protection for those most vulnerable.

The most likely policy construct through which a new social contract might be built is referred to as asset development policy.[40] To reach middle-class living standards, households need (a) income; (b) financial wealth, in the form of a home, a savings account, investments, and a retirement plan; and (c) human capital assets, such as a good education and skill-based training. This new policy construct is based on long-standing U.S. government policies. The Homestead Act of another era or, more recently, the GI Bill was a federal policy that invested in asset building through the promotion of property ownership, home ownership, and higher education. Millions of military personnel, for example, entered the middle class through this form of governmental largesse. Currently, many people benefit through other governmental investments, such as pretax retirement accounts, home mortgage deductions, and college loan funds—all of which help household members accrue the assets they need for economic security and well-being.

What has been good government policy for the many, however, has not been extended to the downtrodden. Social policy has seen most Americans as targets of governmental investments but the poor as a drain on the economy. The new vision of asset-based social policy, however, is to treat all households as targets of government investment so that people in low-income households, like other Americans, can acquire the assets they need for greater independence and security.

This transformation can be achieved in numerous ways,[41] as the following examples illustrate:

- By indexing the minimum wage to inflation, and restoring it to at least its purchasing power of, say, the 1970s, we can ensure that no working people bring home paychecks insufficient to feed the family.
- Similarly, the earned income tax credit (EITC) can be expanded, along with its state tax corollary, to ensure adequate household incomes.
- Individual development savings accounts (IDAs) can be provided to help low-income people to accrue wealth.
- Home ownership can be expanded through set-aside savings plans, whereby part of rents paid by public housing tenants are placed into dedicated accounts so they can save for down payments on homes.
- Children's savings accounts (CSAs) can be created whereby, for example, each child born in the United States would receive a $10,000 investment in a dedicated account. The investment could be matched in subsequent years by other federal investments and/or be augmented by family contributions. The original investment could grow to $50,000 or more by the time a child reached college age, and $500,000, if left to accrue until retirement. Moreover, CSAs could be earmarked for specific

purposes, such as a college education, a first home, the establishment of a business, or retirement income.

The beauty of asset development policy is that it is universal in nature, treating rich and poor alike. It is built on the widely shared values of work, responsibility, meaningful opportunity, and reward.

Conclusion

Social injustice in the United States has many adverse effects. Few are as troubling as hunger. Seven thousand years after the first cities were established to ensure food security, the wealthiest civilization in the history of the world somehow finds itself incapable of doing the same. But hunger, as we have seen, stems not from a shortage in the food supply or from lack of capacity and know-how but rather from structural inequalities built into our economy and social system.

While it is possible to end hunger in the United States within a year by better using the federal programs designed to feed those at risk, it is also possible to address the root cause of food insecurity by reframing the nation's social contract. Government policy that invests in all households—rather than some—and narrows disparities in income and wealth—rather than widening them—will end not only hunger but also the many other adverse health outcomes that result from social injustice.

References

1. Citizens' Board of Inquiry into Hunger and Malnutrition in America, Hunger USA. Boston, Mass.: Beacon Press, 1968:4.
2. Subcommittee on Employment, Manpower and Poverty, Committee on Labor and Public Welfare, U.S. Senate. Poverty: hunger and federal food programs background information. Washington, D.C.: U.S. Government Printing Office, 1967.
3. Brown JL. Hunger USA: the public pushes Congress. J Health Soc Behav 1970;11.
4. Select Committee on Nutrition and Human Needs, U.S. Senate. Hunger 1973 and press reaction. Washington, D.C.: Government Printing Office, 1973:1–74.
5. Citizens' Board of Inquiry into Hunger and Malnutrition in America. Hunger USA revisited. New York, N.Y.: Field Foundation, 1977.
6. McGovern G. Testimony before the U.S. House of Representatives, Select Committee on Hunger. Washington, D.C.: USGPO, 1984.
7. Allen JE, Gadson KE. Nutritional consumption patterns of low-income households. In: Elimination of the purchase requirement in the Food Stamp Program. Washington, D.C.: USDA Economic Research Service, 1979.

8. Radzikowski J. National evaluation of school nutrition programs, final report executive summary. Washington, D.C.: USDA Office of Analysis and Evaluation, 1983.

9. U.S. Conference of Mayors. Human services in FY82. Washington, D.C.: 1982.

10. Brown JL, Pizer H. Living hungry in America. New York, N.Y.: Mentor, 1987.

11. Physician Task Force on Hunger in America. Hunger in America: the growing epidemic. Middletown, Conn.: Wesleyan University Press, 1985:12–14.

12. Social and Scientific Systems. Report on nine case studies of emergency food assistance programs. Washington, D.C.: USDA, 1983.

13. Brown JL, Allen D. Hunger in America. Annu Rev Public Health 1988;9:503–26.

14. Bode JW, Bauer GL, Brown JL. Letters. Scientific American 1987;255.

15. Abt Associates, Center on Hunger and Poverty, Cornell University Division of Nutritional Sciences, CAW Associates. Household food security in the United States in 1995. Alexandria, Va.: USDA Food and Nutrition Service, 1996.

16. Food Security Institute Bulletin. Increase in U.S. hunger and food insecurity continues. Waltham, Mass.: Center on Hunger and Poverty, Brandeis University, November 2003.

17. DeCastro J, Elmore DK. Subjective hunger relationships with meal patterns in the spontaneous feeding behaviors of humans. Physiol Behav 1987;43:159–65.

18. Ogden J, Wardle J. Cognitive restraint and sensitivity to cues for hunger and satiety. J Physiol Behav 1990;47:477–81.

19. Center on Hunger and Poverty, Food Research and Action Center. The paradox of hunger and obesity in America. Boston and Washington, D.C.: CHPFRAC, September, 2003.

20. Listernack R, Christoffel K, Pace J, et al. Severe primary undernutrition in U.S. children. Am J Dis Child 1985;139:1157–60.

21. World Health Organization. Toward a better future: maternal and child health. Geneva, Switzerland: WHO, 1980.

22. Center on Hunger and Poverty. The consequences of hunger and food insecurity for children: evidence from recent scientific studies. Manuscript, Brandeis University, Waltham, Mass., 2002.

23. Alaimo K, Olson CM, Frongillo EA, et al. Food insufficiency, family income and health in preschool and school-aged children. Am J Public Health 2001;91:781–6.

24. Casey PH, Szeto K, Lensing S, et al. Children in food insufficient low-income families: prevalence, health and nutrition status. Arch Pediatr Adolesc Med 2001;155:508–14.

25. Wehler CA, Scott RI, Anderson JJ. Community Childhood Hunger Identification Project. Washington, D.C.: Food Research and Action Center, 1995.

26. Kleinman, RE, Murphy JM, Little M, et al. Hunger in children in the United States: potential behavioral and emotional correlates. Pediatrics 1998;101:E3.

27. Murphy JM, Pagano ME, Nachmani J, et al. The relationship of school breakfast to psychosocial and academic functioning. Arch Pediatr Adolesc Med 1998;152: 899–907.

28. Reid LL. The consequences of food insecurity for child well-being: an analysis of children's school achievement, psychological well-being and health. Joint Center for Poverty Research Working Paper 137. Chicago, Ill.: JCPR, Northwestern University, 2000.

29. Alaimo K, Olson CM, Frongillo EA. Family food insufficiency, but not low family income, is positively associated with dysthymia and suicide symptoms in adolescents. J Nutr 2002;132:719–25.

30. Alaimo K, Olson CA, Frongillo EA. Food insufficiency and American school-aged children's cognitive, academic and psychosocial development. Pediatrics 2001;108: 44–53.

31. Winicki J, Jemison K. Food insecurity and hunger in the kindergarten classroom: its effects on learning and growth (mimeograph). Washington, D.C.: USDA Economic Research Service, 2001.
32. Brown JL, Pollitt E. Malnutrition, poverty and intellectual development. Scientific American 1996;274:38–43.
33. Murphy JM, Wehler CA, Pagano ME, et al. Relationship between hunger and psychosocial functioning in low-income American children. J Am Acad Child Adolesc Psychiatry 1998;37:163–70.
34. Science and Education Administration, Department of Agriculture. Food consumption and dietary levels of low-income households, nationwide food consumption survey, preliminary report, No. 8. Washington, D.C.: USDA, 1991.
35. Martin KS, Cook J. Differences in nutrient adequacy among poor and non-poor children. Waltham, Mass.: Center on Hunger and Poverty, Brandeis University, 1995.
36. Child Health Outcomes Project. Monitoring the health of America's children: ten key indicators. Chapel Hill, N.C.: University of North Carolina, 1984.
37. Franz M. Nutritional requirements of the elderly. J Nutr Elderly 1981;1.
38. Reagan R. President's news conference on foreign and domestic issues. *New York Times*, July 24, 1984.
39. Brown JL. Letter to members of Congress. Waltham, Mass.: Center on Hunger and Poverty, Brandeis University, April 2001.
40. Brown JL, Beeferman L. From new deal to new opportunity. American Prospect February 12, 2001.
41. Beeferman LW, Venner SH. Promising state asset development practices: a resource guide for policymakers and the public. Waltham, Mass.: Asset Development Institute, Center on Hunger and Poverty, Brandeis University, April 2001.

15

CHRONIC DISEASES

Derek Yach

Introduction

When considering health inequalities worldwide, public health professionals tend to focus on infectious diseases, hunger, and poor access to health
services. This focus has become entrenched in the priorities and spending
patterns of international donors and health agencies (box 15-1). In addition, there may have been a further narrowing of the scope of public health
in recent years, leading to serious neglect of major chronic diseases that
kill many people and cause considerable suffering. This neglect is a major
injustice. Differences in morbidity and mortality rates of chronic diseases—
and their risk factors, by sex, race, ethnic group, and socioeconomic status—
account for a significant proportion of overall inequalities in survival and
quality of life within the population. However, these inequalities are amenable to reduction, provided appropriate policies and programs are implemented. This chapter addresses mainly the socioeconomic dimensions of
social injustice and chronic disease risks. Gender aspects have recently been
reviewed elsewhere.[1]

Worldwide, approximately 56 million deaths occurred in 2003. Chronic diseases in adults accounted for 60 percent of them: cardiovascular

(*text continues on p. 257*)

253

BOX 15-1 Selected Actors' Neglect of the Global Burden
of Chronic Diseases

Heads of State

Heads of state of the "G8"—the eight major industrial democracies—recognized
health as a global challenge at the G8 Summit in 2000; acknowledged
that health is the "key to prosperity" and "poor health drives poverty"; and
agreed to mobilize resources, ultimately leading to the establishment of the
Global Fund for HIV/AIDS, Tuberculosis, and Malaria.[1,2] No subsequent commitment has yet been made for chronic diseases.

The World Health Organization

With the important exception of tobacco control, financial resources for
chronic disease control across WHO remains paltry compared with other
major contributors to the global burden of disease. In 2002, the Noncommunicable Disease Cluster spent 7.2 percent of the total headquarters
regular budget expenditure and 9.0 percent of extrabudgetary expenditure, and the six regional offices spent between 2.5 percent (Africa) and
5.0 percent (Europe) of their regular budget expenditure, on noncommunicable disease programs.[3]

Research Institutions

The exponential growth of funding for international research over recent
decades has not been proportionally allocated to the growing burden of
chronic disease.[4,5] Major international research funding portfolios, including the Wellcome Trust in the United Kingdom (UK), the Medical Research
Council (in the UK), and the Canadian Institutes of Health Research continue to focus their research programs almost entirely on infectious disease.[6–8] One notable exception is the Fogarty International Center at the
U.S. National Institutes of Health, which has allocated one-third of its resources for the next several years to chronic disease research and training
programs in developing countries.[9]

Donors

Chronic diseases in developing countries have received substantially less
attention than other health issues. Although official development assistance
for health has increased in the past 5 years, this has been almost entirely
absorbed by HIV/AIDs in sub-Saharan Africa.[10] Bilateral aid agencies rarely
prioritize chronic disease or related risk factors.[11] The Bill and Melinda Gates

(continued)

Foundation does not yet include chronic diseases in its portfolio. Many foundations in the United States support innovative domestic chronic disease research and training programs but not internationally.

The World Bank and Regional Development Banks

The World Bank's Health, Nutrition, and Population Sector Strategy recognizes the increasing burden of chronic diseases on the poor.[12] Yet this is not reflected by investment in chronic disease control, nor is it reflected in the Bank's Poverty Strategy Reduction Papers (PRSPs), which are intended to guide investment priorities to reduce poverty in the poorest countries in the world.

Although all regional development banks have health sector strategies, only one—the Asian Development Bank (ADB)—includes chronic diseases.[13] This has been met by minimal spending commitments. A review of economic analysis of health sector projects carried out for the ADB in 1999 recommends that "reallocating subsidies from chronic diseases to the prevention and treatment of communicable diseases would better target public subsidies to the poor" (p. 8).[14] The rationale for this recommendation was that the cost of treating chronic disease is most likely to accrue to individuals and, as such, should be left to the private market.[14]

Private-Public Partnerships

There are now about 50 private public partnerships that address diseases of poverty on an international basis,[15] but all focus on infectious diseases. The potential for new partnerships with food and related industries to address diet and physical activity remains largely untapped.

Health and Development Initiatives

United Nations health and development reports play a major role in setting priorities for global health. Despite their impact in low- and middle-income countries, chronic diseases are not recognized as a health and development issue. The United Nations Population Fund (UNFPA) does not mention chronic illnesses in its strategy on population and development,[16–18] and the United Nations Children's Fund (UNICEF) recent goal-setting program, A World Fit for Children, excludes risk factors for chronic conditions for children from the 25 action points proposed to "promote healthy lives,"[19] despite strong global evidence that tobacco use and obesity are ubiquitous risks among children in developing countries.

(continued)

BOX 15-1 *(continued)*

References

1. G8 Communique Okinawa 2000. Available at: http://www.g8.utoronto.ca/summit/ 2000okinawa/finalcom.htm. Accessed January 22, 2005.
2. The Global Fund. Available at: http://www.theglobalfund.org/en/. Accessed January 22, 2005.
3. World Health Organization. Financial management report: Expenditure on implementation of objectives in programme budget 2002–2003—all sources of funds, covering the period 1 January 2002—31 December 2002. Prepared for the Meeting of Interested Parties, Geneva, Switzerland, November 3–7, 2003. Geneva, Switzerland: World Health Organization, 2003.
4. Global Forum for Health Research. The 10/90 Report on Health Research 2001–2002. Geneva, Switzerland: Global Forum for Health Research, 2002: 89, 94.
5. Global Forum for Health Research. Monitoring financial flows for health research. Geneva, Switzerland: Global Forum for Health Research, 2002.
6. Wellcome Trust. Available at: http://www.wellcome.ac.uk/en/1/biosfgintpopsu prem.html. Accessed January 22, 2005.
7. United Kingdom Medical Research Council. Available at: http://www.mrc.ac.uk/. Accessed January 22, 2005.
8. Canadian Institutes for Health Research. Available at: http://www.cihr-irsc.gc.ca/ index.html. Accessed January 22, 2005.
9. Fogarty International Center. Available at: http://www.fic.nih.gov/. Accessed January 22, 2005.
10. Michaud C. Development assistance for health (DAH): recent trends and resource allocation. Paper presented at Second High Level Consultation on Macroeconomics and Health, October 28–30, 2003. Geneva, Switzerland: World Health Organization, 2003.
11. World Health Organization. Bilateral aid guide. Geneva, Switzerland: World Health Organization, Department of Government and Private Sector Relations, 2003.
12. World Bank. Health, nutrition, and population sector strategy paper. Washington, D.C.: World Bank, Health Nutrition and Population Division, 1997.
13. Asian Development Bank. Policy for the health sector. Available at: http://www .adb.org/Documents/Policies/Health/health100.asp. Accessed January 22, 2005.
14. Ramesh A, Gertler P, Lagman A. Economic analysis of health sector projects—a review of issues, methods, and approaches. Manila, The Philippines: Asian Development Bank, 1999, p 8.
15. Widdus R. Editorial: Public-private partnerships for health require thoughtful evaluation. Bull WHO 2003;81(4).
16. United Nations Population Fund. International Conference on Population and Development (ICPD). Available at: http://www.unfpa.org/icpd/icpd.htm. Accessed January 22, 2005.
17. United Nations Population Fund. Key actions for further implementation of the programme of action of the ICPD. Available at: http://www.unfpa.org/icpd5/ icpd5.htm. Accessed January 22, 2005.

(continued)

18. United Nations Population Fund. Summary of the ICPD Programme of Action. Available at: http://www.unfpa.org/icpd/summary.htm. Accessed January 22, 2005.
19. World Health Organization/United Nations Children's Fund. Making a difference for the health of children, young people and women. Report of a technical meeting of UNICEF/WHO senior staff. Geneva, Switzerland: World Health Organization, 2002.

disease (CVD), especially coronary heart disease (CHD) and stroke, caused 16.7 million deaths; cancer, 7.0 million deaths; chronic respiratory disease, 5.2 million deaths; and diabetes, almost 1 million deaths.[2] Eighty percent of CVD deaths occur in low- and middle-income countries.[3] Deaths attributable to many chronic diseases rank as major causes of death in developing countries (see fig. 21-2 on p. 387). Mental health problems are leading contributors to the burden of disease in many countries[4] and contribute significantly to the incidence and severity of many chronic diseases, including CVD and cancer. (See chapter 16.)

Cardiovascular Disease

CHD and stroke are the two leading CVD causes of death among both men and women in developed and developing countries.[5] Yet, in absolute numbers, twice as many deaths from CVD occur in developing countries as in developed countries. CVD accounts for 2.8 million deaths a year in China and 2.5 million in India, dwarfing the combined totals of all deaths from infectious diseases in these countries.[3] In developing countries, the age at which people die of CVD is significantly younger than in developed countries, leading to economic and family hardship on a large scale (fig. 15-1). In India and South Africa, for example, CVD death rates in working-age women are higher today than they were in U.S. women in the 1950s.[6]

In rural and urban Tanzania, stroke mortality rates are threefold higher than in the United Kingdom. CVD rates for 30- and 40-year-olds in many developing countries are now the same as for 40- and 50-year-olds in developed countries.[5] While CVD deaths have declined by 50 percent since the 1960s in the United States, the United Kingdom, and many other developed countries, they continue to increase rapidly in most developing countries.[6]

Predictions for the next two decades include a near-tripling of CHD and stroke mortality in Latin America, the Middle East, and even sub-Saharan Africa. Projected CHD mortality for all developing countries is anticipated to increase between 1990 and 2020 by 120 percent for women and 137 percent for

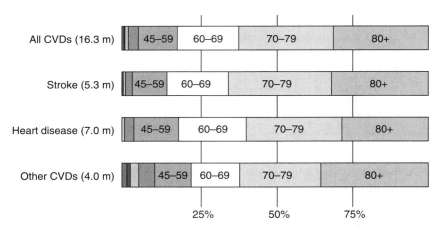

Figure 15-1 Deaths due to cardiovascular diseases, by age, 2000. (From World Health Organization. World health report 2003: shaping the future. Geneva, Switzerland: World Health Organization, 2003.)

men—compared with age-related increases of between 30 percent and 60 percent in developed countries.

Diabetes Mellitus

The global prevalence of diabetes mellitus in adults was estimated to be about 5 percent in 2003. Various projections suggest that it will increase to 5.4 percent in 2025[7] and 6.5 percent in 2030.[8] Virtually all of the projected doubling of global diabetes prevalence over the next 25 years will occur in developing countries. By 2025, an estimated 228 million adults with diabetes, of the 300 million worldwide, will live in developing countries.[7] By 2020, most people with diabetes in developing countries will be between 45 and 64 years of age. In developed countries, by contrast, most people with diabetes will be over 65 years old. These projections consider demographic changes and some aspects of urbanization but not current increases in childhood and adult obesity in most urban settings.[8]

   One example of rapid change and diabetes prevalence comes from the Pacific region. Diabetes was virtually nonexistent in people indigenous to the Pacific who maintained a traditional lifestyle. However, in recent years, fueled by rapid change in diet and a reduction in physical activity, diabetes prevalence has soared. A similar picture is emerging in many island states and even in some of poorest countries of the world.[9] For example, epidemiological data indicate that diabetes prevalence in adults (35 years and over) in urban areas of Tanzania is at least 10 percent.

Cancer

About 10 million people are diagnosed with cancer every year worldwide, and 7 million die of the disease. The International Agency for Research on Cancer (IARC) estimates that cancer incidence increased 19 percent between 1990 and 2000.[10] The major causes of cancer are (a) tobacco use in both developed and developing countries, (b) chronic infections in developing countries, and (c) a complex array of dietary, environmental, and other factors. Lung cancer, the most frequently occurring cancer worldwide and a type of cancer that is primarily due to tobacco use, accounts for 1.2 million deaths a year—about 17 percent of all cancer deaths. Cancers caused by tobacco are increasing in most developing countries and among women in almost all countries. In a few developed countries, tobacco-related cancer incidence has started to decline as men smoke less. In contrast, cancers caused by chronic infections and by food contaminants and food-preparation methods have started to decline in developing countries. There has been little change in the incidence of the two most common cancers in women—breast and cervical cancer—over the past few decades. Survival rates remain very low for lung, liver, and stomach cancers, although they have increased for many other cancers in recent years, due mainly to early detection and increasingly effective treatment.[10]

Chronic Respiratory Diseases

Chronic respiratory diseases include two major groups of diseases: chronic obstructive pulmonary disease (COPD)—comprising chronic bronchitis and emphysema—and asthma. COPD accounts for 4.8 percent of all deaths worldwide (2.7 million annually); 50 percent of COPD deaths occur in China and countries in the Western Pacific and an additional 24 percent occur in India. Major risk factors for COPD include tobacco use, a range of occupational exposures, indoor air pollution from the burning of biomass fuel, and childhood respiratory infections. These risk factors are substantially higher among people living in developing countries and in poor communities in developed countries.

Aging and Risk Factors

The current burden of chronic diseases reflects cumulative lifetime risks. The future burden will be determined by current population exposures to the major chronic disease risk factors. The aging of populations, due mainly to a decline in fertility rates and a higher proportion of children living into adulthood, is an important underlying determinant of chronic disease epidemics.[3] While demographic change has been well described in developed countries, the pace

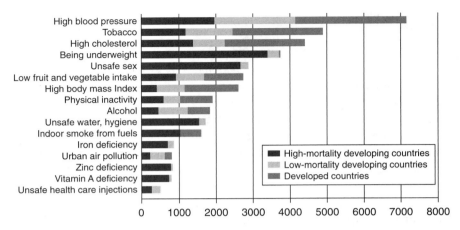

Figure 15-2 Deaths attributable to 16 leading risk factors, worldwide, 2000 (in thousands). (From World Health Organization. World health report 2003: shaping the future. Geneva, Switzerland: World Health Organization, 2003.)

and impact of aging in developing countries are only starting to be recognized. Recent United Nations projections suggest that the proportion of the population over age 60 will rise from about 6 percent to about 15 percent in Algeria, Egypt, Iran, South Africa, and Tunisia. Developed countries are already under pressure to address the pensions and social insurance demands of aging populations; developing countries will soon have to do so, although they will be starting from a base of substantially fewer resources.

Major risk factors explain the incidence of most chronic diseases. Many are common to several chronic diseases. And most are modifiable.[3] In developed countries, seven chronic disease risk factors—tobacco use, high blood pressure, alcohol use, increased cholesterol, increased body mass index, low fruit and vegetable intake, and physical inactivity—are among the 10 leading risk factors contributing to the overall burden of disease. In contrast, in high-mortality developing countries, four chronic disease risk factors—tobacco use, high blood pressure, indoor air pollution, and high cholesterol—are among the 10 leading risk factors contributing to the burden of disease (fig. 15-2).[2]

How Social Injustice Influences Chronic Diseases

Social Class and Chronic Disease Risks and Outcomes

For policy decisions, the rates and potential risks of chronic diseases can be conceptualized by use of a "chronic disease consumption curve" (fig. 15-3). In high-income and some middle-income countries, where risk factors for

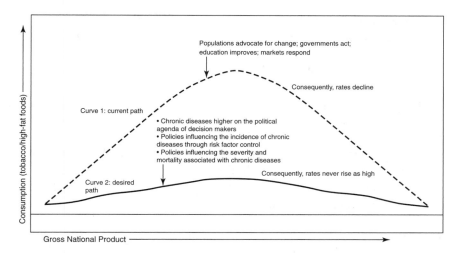

Figure 15-3 Chronic disease consumption curve.

chronic diseases have been established for decades, chronic diseases caused by these risk factors are a major reason for inequalities by social class, ethnicity, and gender.[11–14] In the United States, it is estimated that a few conditions, mainly related to chronic diseases, account for most of the socioeconomic and racial disparities in years of potential life lost: (a) tobacco-related diseases, accounting for much mortality among people with relatively few years of education; and (b) hypertension, HIV, diabetes mellitus, and trauma among blacks.

Socioeconomic inequalities, which are well described for CVD and cancer (and their major risks factors), are present from ages as young as 2 years, even in a politically egalitarian country with a homogeneous population like Iceland.[15] Studies of trends in major risks for chronic diseases in developed countries—smoking, obesity, hypertension, and physical inactivity—have demonstrated that almost all risks are higher among people from the lowest social classes, mirroring trends in morbidity and mortality.[16] A recent study estimated that 14 risk factors—smoking being the most important—explained 73 percent of the social differences in CHD incidence and mortality for men and 77 percent for women.[17] (See chapter 2.)

In most low- and middle-income countries, where risk levels have been high for years, there are much lower risk levels among the more-affluent and more-educated groups but a mixed picture concerning disease morbidity and mortality. This discrepancy is due to the variable and often-long lag period between increased risk levels and increased chronic disease occurrence in a population.

In lower-income countries, risks such as tobacco use, physical inactivity, and obesity are initially higher among those with the highest levels of disposable income. A social class drift occurs as commodities and consumption patterns become available and affordable to the poor at a time when health education and effective government actions have yet to be implemented.

An important recent study comparing the relationship between social class and consumption patterns in the United States and China illustrated these points.[18] Using a composite "lifestyle index" that included data on diet, smoking, alcohol use, and physical activity, there was an inverse relationship between socioeconomic status and the lifestyle index in the United States but a direct relationship in China. (China is on the ascending limb of fig. 15-3, and the United States, on the descending limb.)

This phenomenon suggests that policymakers in low- and middle-income countries should not wait for the appearance of a social class gradient in the occurrence of chronic disease (or chronic disease risk factors) before implementing strong preventive and health-promoting policies. Governments of developing countries, including the very poorest, made this point throughout the negotiations for the Framework Convention on Tobacco Control.[19] They recognize the need for action, but they need international support to make it happen.

Cumulative Exposure to Risks Increases Inequalities

A downward spiral occurs with chronic diseases. As Gunnar Myrdal, the recipient of the Nobel Prize for Economics in 1974, told the World Health Assembly of the World Health Organization (WHO), people are sick because they are poor, and become poorer because they are sick.[20]

The major risks for cancer, CVD, and diabetes accumulate from early in fetal life. Early-life risk factors—such as suboptimal diets, early termination of breastfeeding, exposure to tobacco and alcohol, indoor exposure to biomass fuels, and recurrent respiratory infections—contribute to the development of chronic diseases in adulthood. Increased lifetime cumulative exposure to these risk factors, combined with social and economic risk factors, leads to disparities in chronic disease occurrence in later adult life. Recent birth cohort studies have documented how and when these life-course influences happen.[11,12] The risk of developing CVD or diabetes is influenced by biological and social factors from fetal development to adulthood. Some life course influences are disease specific, whereas others are cohort specific. Major risk factors are firmly established for many major chronic diseases. For example, 80 to 90 percent of patients who develop clinically significant CHD and more than 95 percent of patients who have experienced a fatal CHD event have had at least one of the major cardiac risk factors—smoking, diabetes, hypertension, and hypercholesterolemia.[21]

COPD and lung function decrement in adults are the result of cumulative exposures that start early in life. South African studies have shown that what were assumed to be racial or genetic differences in lung size are probably due to early childhood respiratory infections occurring in crowded homes where biomass fuel is used, combined with tobacco use and adverse occupational exposures.

Trends in risk factors for chronic diseases in developing countries are disturbing. For example, a survey of 1 million 13- to 15-year-olds demonstrated that (a) tobacco use occurs in about 20 percent of children in almost all of the over 100 countries surveyed,[22] and (b) almost as many girls as boys smoke. Furthermore, obesity and overweight have become problems of developing countries. In China in 1995, 8 percent of boys and 12 percent of girls were overweight; it is projected that in 2025, about 24 percent of boys and 37 percent of girls will be overweight.[23]

In most developing countries, chronic disease risk factors have increased over time. Moreover, rapid increases in obesity and tobacco use among children during the past decade, especially in cities of developing countries, portend a massive increase in chronic disease occurrence in future decades that will impose additional strains on already stressed national health systems.

Asymmetrical Access to Healthy Messages

In countries and communities with low health-literacy levels, commercial "messages" have a particularly strong influence on behavior. However, the impact of being functionally illiterate is even more pervasive and undermines many public health efforts to control chronic disease. Low levels of health literacy are associated with reduced comprehension about causes of disease, the value of prevention and health promotion, how and when to seek care, and adherence to therapy—especially therapy that must be taken for several years.[24] Although well-designed advertising and marketing campaigns can help to promote health, they have not been explicitly designed to reach the poorest and most illiterate groups.

Global marketing of tobacco, alcohol, and salty, sugary, and fatty foods now reaches most parts of most countries. Much global marketing is targeted at children under age 14. Marketers use sophisticated means to ensure that their messages "slip below the radar of critical thinking," take advantage of weak regulatory environments, and sometimes use false, misleading, or deceptive advertising to reach their targets.[25] Unopposed commercial messages can increase the consumption of unhealthy products. Meanwhile, the weakness of the government's voice has prevented messages about healthy behaviors and diets from reaching the poorest communities of most countries, making it difficult for the people to make healthy choices.

Attitudes, perceptions, and beliefs are partially shaped by commercial interests, which are especially dominant and pervasive in countries and communities without access to continuous information about (a) public health risks and how to avoid them, and (b) effective treatments and where to obtain them. This asymmetry in access to "healthy information" particularly affects the poorest of the poor.

Aggressive promotional marketing of tobacco products, alcohol, and unhealthy foods exploits the vulnerability of individuals and populations and targets specific population subgroups, including young people, members of ethnic minorities, and low-income populations. Internal tobacco industry documents reveal that cigarette-marketing campaigns have been designed to target young people. Children are exposed to, and respond to, cigarette advertising through their consumption choices. In the United States, alcohol advertisements in magazines and on radio stations popular with young people lead to high youth exposure. By using images popular with youth, such as those focusing on masculine pride, action, and celebrity endorsements, alcohol advertisements reinforce positive attitudes towards alcohol consumption. Young children are also heavily targeted with advertisements—legally—for unhealthy foods, which may be deliberately designed to encourage children to pester their parents to purchase these products. This advertising affects children's food preferences, purchasing behavior, and consumption patterns. Racial and ethnic minority groups are targeted by tobacco, alcohol, and food companies.

In developing countries, companies take advantage of weak regulatory environments to use a wide range of techniques to target populations. In these emerging markets, companies are highly strategic in attempting to reach low-income populations. In China, for example, South African Breweries became profitable by targeting the mass market with locally brewed beer. Other companies take a more targeted approach. In Asian countries, tobacco companies use glamorous images to advertise "light" and "mild" cigarettes specifically to women. In many developing countries, transnational food companies attempt to take "stomach share" away from other foods and drinks, with techniques specifically designed to attract children to eat at fast-food restaurants and consume soft drinks and snacks. Across all commodities and countries, extensive market research is used to better understand the perceptions and desires of the target market. And the results are starting to pay off in terms of increased profits for transnational corporations—with increased prevalence of unhealthy consumption patterns among children in emerging markets.

Increased Comorbidity and Demands for Long-term Care

Not only do poorer communities and countries suffer from a heavier burden of cumulative risk throughout life but, as a consequence, they also suffer from a higher burden of comorbidity. Chronic infectious diseases, such as HIV/AIDS, tuberculosis (TB), and schistosomiasis, have a harsh impact on the poorest countries; so do injuries and chronic noninfectious diseases, such as CVD, cancer, and diabetes. All have serious consequences for the provision of health care, especially long-term care. WHO estimates that developing countries in sub-Saharan Africa, Latin America, and the Eastern Mediterranean will experience threefold to fourfold increases over the next several decades in people requiring long-term care services, which are rudimentary in most developing countries.[26]

The interactive impacts between certain infectious and noninfectious diseases have become clearer. Several infectious agents can cause cancer: for example, hepatitis B virus causes liver cancer; human papillomavirus (HPV), cervical cancer; *Helicobacter pylori*, stomach cancer; HIV infection, several cancers, including Kaposi's sarcoma and non-Hodgkin's lymphoma; and *Schistosoma haematobium*, bladder cancer.[10] All of these cancers are common in the least-developed countries, where resources for treatment are extremely inadequate. Vaccines to prevent these infections and effective drugs to treat them could greatly reduce the cancer burden in these countries.

Tobacco increases the death rate from TB—a classic disease of poverty—in those already infected. In India, smokers are 4.5 times more likely to die of TB than are nonsmokers.[27] Although an estimated 80 percent of TB patients smoke, little progress has been made in helping TB patients to quit. As a result, tobacco is probably the major cause of death in treated TB patients.

Comorbidity between mental and physical disease is also common. The proportion of patients with depression who also have common chronic diseases, such as CVD, diabetes, cancer, and HIV/AIDS, ranges from 22 to 44 percent.[28] Because the burden of these individual diseases falls proportionately on the poor, the combined impact of depression and these diseases is substantial—an observation that is generally ignored from a preventive or therapeutic perspective. (See also chapter 16.)

Decreased Access to Quality Medical Care

The poor generally do not have access to tests for early detection of chronic diseases, such as diabetes, hypertension, and cervical cancer, leading to many cases of these diseases presenting at an advanced stage. In the United States, for example, the widest socioeconomic gradients exist for patients diagnosed at advanced stages with melanoma of the skin, prostate cancer, and female breast cancer. Compared with their counterparts in low-poverty areas, people in high-poverty areas are almost 2.5 times more likely to be diagnosed with advanced-stage melanoma of the skin and almost twice as likely to be diagnosed with advanced-stage cancers of the prostate and female breast.

Patients in low social classes have consistently poorer survival for many forms of cancer than those in high social classes, especially for cancers of the bladder, colon, female breast, and uterus.[13] In addition, chemotherapeutic agents most effective against the 10 leading cancers are not readily available in many developing countries, where they are often subject to high import duties.[10] In addition, inhaled beclomethasone is often not available or affordable in developing countries, placing patients with COPD and asthma at considerable risk for premature death.

Participation in breast cancer screening has been shown to depend on income and education, health insurance, and the type of health service. Women of low social classes tend to have lower screening rates than do those in higher social classes.[29] In both developed and developing countries, women of low socioeconomic status have increased risk of cervical cancer but less participation in cervical cancer screening. Survival by stage of cervical cancer varies little; thus, the major goals in screening programs for cervical cancer—and other chronic diseases—are to reduce barriers to early access and to ensure public resources for long-term sustainability of programs. Socioeconomic differences tend to decrease when participation is promoted, cultural and economic barriers are removed, and social support is offered.

Roots and Underlying Issues

Macroeconomic Influences

The direct and indirect pathways by which global and regional forces influence chronic diseases are complex. The indirect effects are mediated by national economic performance and act mainly through changes in household income, government expenditure, the exchange rate, and prices. National income is especially important because of its effects on public-sector resources available for health and its effects on household health-related behaviors—especially those of low-income households—and costs of health care.[3]

It is often assumed that global economic development increases income and subsequently improves all aspects of health. A more globalized approach to development has resulted in some positive consequences for health in developing countries. Yet while greater economic investment and higher incomes among some groups have eased some of the health challenges in developing countries, chronic diseases have been exacerbated, leading to economic costs. Important drivers here are trade, foreign investment, promotional marketing, and urbanization.

Trade and investment drive economic development and may not encourage healthy behaviors. Conditions for trade and investment that are more open can bring economic benefits but also risks. Expanded global trade of, and foreign direct investment in, tobacco have promoted demand. Among the world's 100 nonfinancial transnational corporations, ranked by foreign assets in 2000, were several associated with noncommunicable disease risks, including tobacco, food, and alcohol companies. These powerful companies often seek to avoid health conditionalities being linked to their investments, which may weaken the regulatory environment that has effectively controlled chronic disease risks in developed countries.

Economic investment in the unregulated marketing of unhealthy products encourages acquisition of the risk factors for chronic diseases. Global tobacco, alcohol, food, and automobile companies all invest heavily in marketing their products, creating an environment where healthy choices are more difficult. Developing countries experience many of the risks associated with globally interconnected economic development, without necessarily receiving the investments found in many high-income countries required to provide protections from these risks.

Certain transnational corporations have played a key role in avoiding regulations and suppressing advocacy by governments and WHO aimed at encouraging healthy consumption patterns. For example, the tobacco industry has asserted that WHO should not focus on "lifestyle issues" of affluent Western countries, such as tobacco. It has also attempted to redirect WHO policies on tobacco and alleged that WHO was misspending its budget "at the expense of more urgent public health needs, particularly in developing countries, such as prevention of malaria and other communicable diseases."[30] Lobbyists for tobacco, sugar, and other food interests have worked hard to keep attention away from the need to address consumption patterns that drive chronic diseases and their views have become the accepted position of many policymakers.

Consumption patterns become increasingly unhealthy in countries and communities where (a) incomes are rising, (b) public health and legislative capacities are weak, and (c) commercial pressures—often hidden from the public—are stronger than government's influence.

In time, most major risks for chronic diseases concentrate among the poor. Economic development is often accompanied by greater political awareness of the benefits of prevention, even if it requires tackling strong commercial interests to implement preventive measures. Thus, countries with the highest levels of both income and education—and a high degree of openness in policy development—seem to have public health policies that encourage reduced levels of unhealthy consumption (fig. 15-3). In countries where the news media are not restricted and the government is democratic, the intensity and quality of the public discourse on how best to address chronic disease risks is far better than elsewhere. The more extensive the discourse, the more likely "healthy" policies will be adopted by governments and supported by the population.

An additional macroeconomic impact of chronic disease is related to the protection of domestic producers by some developed countries and their regional organizations. For example, certain agricultural subsidies in the United States and the European Union restrict imports of fresh produce from developing countries, thereby seriously reducing incomes in these countries.[3] These agricultural subsidies should be removed.

Urban and Rural Factors

Urbanization increases chronic disease risks. These risks increase with rising levels of disposable income, marketing of and better access to certain products, and cultural changes in taste and behavior. Increased tobacco use and consumption of energy-dense foods are occurring in many poor rural areas, with resultant increases in cancer risks and obesity. For example, a recent study of poor rural South Africans over age 30 showed that the prevalence of diabetes was 10 percent in both men and women; tobacco use exceeded 50 percent (mainly snuff in women, mainly cigarettes in men); and the prevalence of hypertension was 25 percent in men and 29 percent in women[31]—all of these rates are similar to those in urban South Africa.

Even obesity rates, which are closely associated with physical inactivity patterns, are not always higher in urban than in rural areas. In Pakistan[32] and South Africa,[33] obesity rates, especially among rural women, exceed 35 percent; in India and China, obesity rates are increasing mainly in cities.[23] *Rates* of all major chronic disease risk factors, except smoking, are worse in urban than rural areas of Thailand[34]; however, the *number* of people with risk factors is highest in rural areas.

Generally Weak Noncommunicable Disease Policies and Programs in Developing Countries

The extent of missed opportunities for both primary and secondary prevention remains very high in most countries. A recent WHO review of the capacity of 185 countries to implement chronic disease control programs provided stark information on the neglect of chronic diseases in many countries.[35] Only about 40 percent of countries had a specific budget line for noncommunicable diseases, and less than 50 percent of countries had a policy or plan for these diseases. In addition, the survey found that essential medicines for chronic disease management were not always available in primary care settings.

Pathways operating at different levels link experiences of disadvantage with their biological impact on a specific chronic disease problem.[36] Six such pathways that lead from disadvantage to end-stage renal disease for indigenous Australians and also apply to many other chronic diseases, are the following:

1. Direct linkage from disadvantage, such as via infections transmitted in crowded housing, to renal damage
2. Indirect linkage via psychosocial factors, particularly chronic stress
3. Indirect and intergenerational linkage via health-damaging behaviors
4. Indirect linkage via factors in the health care system that impede access
5. Indirect cultural factors, including poor understanding of issues related to prevention, diagnosis, and treatment of renal disease
6. Linkage to renal disease via government and corporate polices.

What Needs to Be Done

Institute Comprehensive Prevention, Health Promotion, and Treatment Policies That Reach the Poorest People in All Countries

Myrdal, over 50 years ago, cautioned against quick fixes for complex public health problems. Efforts to reach permanent improvement of health standards, with maximal beneficial effect on the well-being of people, will need to be integrated in a broad economic and social reform policy.[20] Comprehensive, multisectoral approaches over decades are needed. Education, health services, and intersectoral action will be required to reduce socioeconomic and other differences in chronic disease outcomes. In the Netherlands, it is estimated that increased educational levels could counteract increased ill health that is expected to occur due to aging of the population.[37] Increased education is associated with reduced exposure to health risks, increased levels of well-being and wealth, and more effective use of health services. Increased investment in health (and media) literacy in developing countries could potentially slow the demand for expensive tertiary treatment—a demand that already distorts the meager health budgets of developing countries away from prevention.[38]

Place Greater Emphasis on Prevention and Health Promotion

The application of existing knowledge has the potential to make major, rapid, and cost-effective contributions to the prevention and control of chronic disease epidemics. However, there are important constraints on the implementation of effective policies. The global health agenda is dominated by the notion that communicable (infectious) diseases need to be prevented and treated before chronic (noncommunicable) diseases receive attention. However, chronic diseases, such as CVD and diabetes, need to be addressed, in part because of their severe adverse economic impact on poor families and developing countries.[39]

Although chronic disease prevalence has increased markedly in all but the poorest countries, the institutional response to disease prevention and control is still based on the infectious disease paradigm. As a consequence, the global and national capacity to respond to chronic disease is woefully inadequate, and few countries have implemented comprehensive prevention and control policies. Furthermore, several commercial entities involved in the production and promotion of unhealthy products, such as the tobacco industry[40] and some major food companies,[41] exert much adverse influence on the development of health policy.

There is only limited advocacy at the global level for a chronic disease prevention and control agenda. What little advocacy exists tends to be fragmented and specific to certain risk factors or diseases. In addition, CVD, diabetes, and cancer are not generally regarded as major diseases of poverty in developing countries today. In contrast, there is growing dominance of commercial and consumer organizations that have placed treatment of selected diseases at the center of health policy debates and funding priorities. The most effective advocates for prevention, such as national tobacco control advocacy groups, have focused on single issues. Stronger and broader alliances of major health professional organizations, consumer groups, enlightened businesses and industries, and academic institutions are needed to prioritize strategies for the prevention of chronic disease in developing countries.

Strengthen Capacity and Mobilize Resources

Capacity at the national level for chronic disease prevention and control is weak in most developing countries. Donor agencies and governments have been reluctant to invest in national institutions and infrastructure. A global commitment is needed for sustainable progress in chronic disease policy development and implementation. The Tropical Disease Research Program of WHO, funded by a consortium of donors, has developed over the past 20 years an impressive network of communicable disease researchers[42]—a useful model for chronic disease research.

Inadequate support by international donors for chronic disease prevention and control in developing countries, however, is a major impediment to progress. Over the past 5 years, new private foundations and new sources of public development finance have led to many billions of dollars being invested, appropriately, in infectious disease control for HIV/AIDS, malaria, tuberculosis, and vaccine research and field programs. There are no significant new sources of funding anywhere near this magnitude for prevention of chronic disease. Tobacco control has recently received modest increases in support from international donors. In addition, WHO, European Commission, and World Bank representatives have agreed that tobacco control should be financed as part of development funding,[43] as is done for HIV/AIDS control.

Develop Global Norms That Benefit Developing Countries

Many developing countries lack the basic human resources to develop and implement laws and regulations, as well as tax policies, that are important for chronic disease control. For them, international support is often the catalyst for national action, and global norms provide the umbrella of legitimacy that they need to develop and implement national laws. There is also an increasing need to establish global norms in many spheres concerning the influences of transnational corporations on chronic diseases—from marketing and trade to human resource flows. Such norms can balance the otherwise unrestrained influences of powerful interests and can assist countries that have limited national public health and regulatory ability. To do so, public health capacities in trade and political science must be strengthened so as (a) to effectively participate in the World Trade Organization (WTO), where health issues are increasingly considered, and (b) to develop stronger norms that could be used as the basis for resolving trade disputes concerning products associated with adverse health impacts.

The Framework Convention on Tobacco Control (FCTC) is one example of a global norm that can protect developing countries from industry pressures as they introduce effective tobacco control. The FCTC represents the first time that WHO used its treaty-making right to advance public health goals. The FCTC was adopted by all 192 WHO member states in May 2003 and came into force in February 2005. This pioneering convention aims to protect health and save the lives of billions in present and future generations through tobacco advertising bans, larger health-warning labels on tobacco products, measures to protect against secondhand smoke, tobacco tax and price increases, and efforts to eliminate illicit trade in tobacco products. The FCTC could provide a template for policy development for control of diet-related and food-related chronic diseases. Other norms that are important for noncommunicable disease control include the International Code of Marketing of Breast-milk Substitutes and the Codex Alimentarius Commission (with its likely increased focus on food labeling and health claims).

More, however, will be needed. Treaties are probably not the solution to the complex issues related to nutrition or physical inactivity. A combination of multistakeholder and intergovernment codes are better options to pursue, especially in relation to restricting marketing of alcohol and food items to young children. Such approaches are already being used in many ways in many developing countries to improve labor conditions, environmental quality, and protection of human rights. These approaches are cheaper and quicker to implement than traditional legislative approaches but require strong independent oversight to ensure they have the desired impact.

Reorient Health Services to Address Chronic Disease

Many lives are lost prematurely because of inadequate treatment and long-term management of chronic diseases, even though simple and inexpensive approaches exist.[44] Even in wealthy countries, the potential of these interventions is not fully put to use. The situation in both poorer countries—and poor communities within rich countries—is even less satisfactory. In most countries, effective means of preventing, treating, and providing palliative care for cancer exist but are not implemented. There are many opportunities for coordinated risk reduction, care, and long-term management of chronic disease. For example, smoking cessation is a priority for all patients who smoke; dietary and physical activity advice should be provided to most patients in virtually all health care settings. Few efforts have been made to explicitly target poor communities with such interventions. A good example of these are smoking cessation programs in the United Kingdom that have successfully reached poor smokers.

Considerable progress has been made in improving access to, and reducing the price of, antiretroviral drugs for HIV/AIDS, drugs to treat TB, and several vaccines. Similar progress has yet to be made for essential drugs that are required to improve survival for treatable cancers, diabetes, and CVD. A patient with heart disease in a poor nation has the same right to effective drug treatment as a patient with malaria, tuberculosis, or HIV/AIDS.[45] Nongovernmental organizations have yet to advocate as effectively for better access to chronic disease treatment as they have for selected infectious diseases, despite the huge saving in lives and suffering that would result.

Promote Broader Societal Changes

Many aspects of chronic disease prevention require legislative, financial, and engineering approaches. These aspects, often not under the control of health departments, can complement educational programs. Educational programs have a limited impact, especially among the poor and illiterate. Implementation of the following measures can bring about a disproportionately large positive impact for poor populations: infrastructural changes that promote public transport and physical activity, laws that ban tobacco advertising and smoking in public places, tax policies that raise excise taxes on tobacco, and agricultural policies that provide schools and poor communities with easy, government-funded access to fruits, vegetables, and other food staples.

Build on Opportunities to Link Control of Communicable Disease With Control of Noncommunicable Disease

Continued strengthening of certain aspects of infectious disease control, particularly related to chronic infectious diseases such as TB and HIV/AIDS, will benefit the control of CVD, diabetes, and cancer. The same transformation of health care systems is required to address long-term disease management and enhanced compliance to treatment for both infectious and noninfectious chronic diseases.[44] For sub-Saharan African countries, there is an opportunity to ensure that new platforms for health service delivery that are being built to expand access to treatment for HIV/AIDS also address noninfectious chronic diseases. The marginal increased investments required would probably yield substantial gains for public health among poor communities that already suffer from CVD, diabetes, and cancer.

Conclusion

Over the past few years, there have been several initiatives that suggest a growing awareness among public health professionals of the need to act decisively to prevent social injustice in public health. Initially, academics and researchers led the way. Now policymakers in government are responding with new policies and funded projects. Those that explicitly address chronic diseases are mainly based in developed countries, although the approaches used have applications worldwide. Several recommendations that generally apply are as follows[46]:

1. Ensure that a government spending review, performed by the treasury or finance ministry, identifies how government spending—not limited to health department spending—could be directed to reduce health disparities.
2. Ensure better coordination in health service delivery between traditional boundaries.
3. Develop partnerships with the voluntary organization, business, and community sectors.
4. Invest in programs that aim to improve support for young children and families.
5. Improve housing and social services.

6. Identify specific programs that will close life-expectancy gaps, such as by reducing smoking among the poor and among children.
7. Provide better access, including financial support, to poor communities for early detection and long-term treatment of chronic diseases.

At long last, social injustice concerning chronic diseases is being recognized as neither inevitable nor acceptable.

References

1. Brands A, Yach D. Noncommunicable diseases and gender. World Health Organization, 2001. Geneva, Switzerland: World Health Organization, 2001.
2. World Health Organization. World health report, 2002. Geneva, Switzerland: World Health Organization, 2002.
3. Beaglehole R, Yach D. Globalisation and the prevention and control of noncommunicable disease: the neglected chronic diseases of adults. Lancet 2003;362:903–8.
4. World Health Organization. World health report, 2001. Geneva, Switzerland: World Health Organization, 2001.
5. World Health Organization. World health report, 2003. Geneva, Switzerland: World Health Organization, 2003.
6. Leeder S, Raymond S, Greenberg H, et al. A race against time: the challenge of cardiovascular disease in developing economies. Center for Global Health and Economic Development, The Earth Institute, Mailman School of Public Health. New York, N.Y.: Columbia University, 2004.
7. King H, Aubert RE, Herman WH. Global burden of diabetes, 1995–2025: prevalence, numerical estimates, and projections. Diabetes Care 1998;21:1414–31.
8. Wild S, Roglic G, Green A, et al. Global prevalence of diabetes: estimates for 2000 and projections for 2030. Diabetes Care 2004;27:1047–53.
9. Foliaki S, Pearce N. Prevention and control of diabetes in Pacific people. BMJ 2003; 327:437–39.
10. Stewart BW, Kleihaus P, eds. World cancer report. International Agency for Research on Cancer. Lyon, France: IARC Press, 2003.
11. Aboderin I, Kalache A, Ben-Shlomo Y, et al. Life course perspectives on coronary heart disease, stroke and diabetes: key issues and implications for policy and research. Geneva, Switzerland: World Health Organization, 2001.
12. Batty GD, Leon DA. Socio-economic position and coronary heart disease risk factors in children and young people. Eur J Public Health 2002;12:263–72.
13. Kogevinas M, Pearce N, Susser M, et al., eds. Social inequalities and cancer. IARC Scientific publications no. 138. Lyon, France: IARC Press, 1997.
14. Mackenbach JP, Cavelaars AEJM, Kunst AE, et al. Socio-economic inequalities in cardiovascular disease mortality. An international study. Eur Heart J 2000;21:1141–51.
15. Halldorsson M, Cavelaars AE, Kunst AE, et al. Socio-economic differences in health and well-being of children and adolescents in Iceland. Scand J Public Health 1999;27:43–7.
16. Galobardes B, Costanza MC, Bernstein MS, et al. Trends in risk factors for lifestyle-related diseases by socioeconomic position in Geneva, Switzerland, 1993–2000: health inequalities persist. Am J Public Health 2003;93:1302–9.

17. Woodward M, Oliphant J, Lowe G, et al. Contribution of contemporaneous risk factors to social inequality in coronary heart disease and all causes mortality. Prev Med 2003;36:561–8.
18. Kim S, Symons M, Popkin BM. Contrasting socio-economic profiles related to healthier lifestyles in China and the United States. Am J Epidemiol 2004;159(2):184–91.
19. The WHO Framework Convention on Tabacco Control. World Health Assembly Resolution 56.1, May 21, 2003.
20. Myrdal G. Economic aspects of health. Address to the World Health Assembly. Geneva, Switzerland: World Health Organization, 1952.
21. Canto JG, Iskandrian AE. Major risk factors for cardiovascular disease: debunking the "only 50%" myth. JAMA 2003:947–9.
22. Global Youth Tobacco Survey Collaborating Group. Differences in worldwide tobacco use by gender: findings from the Global Youth Tobacco Survey. J School Health 2003; 73:207–15.
23. Popkin BM, Horton S, Kim S, et al. Trends in diet, nutritional status and diet-related noncommunicable diseases in China and India: the economic costs of nutrition transition. Nutr Rev 2001;59:379–90.
24. Zobel E, Rowe K, Gomez-Mandic C. An updated overview of medical and public health literature issues: an annotated bibliography published in 2002 Harvard School of Public Health: Health Literacy Website, 2003. Available at: http://www.hsph.harvard.edu/healthliteracy/literature/lit_2002.html. Accessed Janaury 20, 2005.
25. Walsh D. Slipping under the radar: advertising and the mind. Presented at WHO symposium Marketing to Young People, Treviso, Italy, April 2002.
26. World Health Organization. A long-term care futures tool-kit. Geneva, Switzerland: World Health Organization/Washington, D.C.: The Institute for Alternative Futures, 2002.
27. Gajalakshmi V, Peto R, Kanaka TS, et al. Smoking and mortality from tuberculosis and other diseases in India. Lancet 2003;362:507–15.
28. Saraceno B, Gatti A. Personal communication, 2003.
29. Morgan MA, Behbakht K, Berlin M, et al. Racial differences in survival from gynaecologic cancer. Obstet Gynecol 1996;88:914–8.
30. World Health Organization. Tobacco company strategies to undermine tobacco control activities at WHO. Report of the Committee of Experts on Tobacco Industry Documents. Geneva, Switzerland: WHO, 2000.
31. Alberts M, Urdal P, Steyn NP, et al. Prevalence of common non-communicable diseases and associated risk factors in a rural black population of South Africa. Bull WHO 2005 (in press).
32. Nanan DJ. The obesity epidemic—implications for Pakistan. J Pakistan Med Assoc 2002;52:342–6.
33. Puoane DJ, Steyn K, Bradshaw D, et al. Obesity in South Africa: the South African Demographic and Health Survey. Obes Res 2002;10:1038–48.
34. InterASIA Collaborative Group. Cardiovascular risk factor levels in urban and rural Thailand. Eur J Cardiovasc Prev Rehabil 2003;10:249–57.
35. Alwan A, MacLean D, Mandil A. Assessment of national capacity for noncommunicable disease prevention and control. Geneva, Switzerland: World Health Organization, 2001.
36. Cass A, Cunningham J, Snelling P, et al. Exploring the pathways leading from disadvantage to end-stage renal disease for indigenous Australians. Soc Sci Med 2004; 58:767–85.

37. Joung IMA, Kunst AE, van Imhoff E, et al. Education, aging and health: to what extent can the rise in educational level relieve future health (care) burden associated with populations aging in the Netherlands? J Clin Epidemiol 2000;53:955–63.
38. Commission on Macroeconomics and Health. Macroeconomics and health: investing in health for economic development. Report of the Commission on Macroeconomics and Health. Geneva, Switzerland: World Health Organization, 2001.
39. Steve Leeder, personal communication.
40. Yach D, Bettcher. Globalisation of tobacco industry influence and new global responses. Tobacco Control 2000;9:206–16.
41. Nestle M. Food politics: how the food industry influences nutrition and health. Berkeley, Calif.: University of California Press, 2002.
42. Nchinda T. Research capacity strengthening in the south. Soc Sci Med 2002;54: 1699–711.
43. European Commission. Tobacco and health in the developing world. A background paper for the high level roundtable on tobacco control and development policy. Brussels, Belgium: European Commission, World Bank, and World Health Organization, February 2003.
44. Epping-Jordan JE, Bengoa R, Yach D. Chronic conditions—the new health challenge. South Afr Med J 2003;93:585–60.
45. WTO takes a first step (editorial). Lancet 2003;362:753.
46. Department of Health. Tackling health inequalities—a programme for action. United Kingdom, London 2003. Available at: http://www.doh.gov.uk/healthinequalities/programmeforaction/. Accessed January 23, 2005.

16

MENTAL HEALTH

Carles Muntaner and Jeanne Geiger-Brown

Introduction

Epidemiologists were among the first scientists to document that the poor suffer from a higher rate of mental disorders than the affluent.[1] Investigations of social inequities and mental health have been fueled, in part, by social justice concerns about the need to improve the harsh living conditions to which workers, immigrants, and racial and ethnic minorities have been exposed.[2-5] The absence or poor quality of psychiatric care for poor working class, immigrant, or racial and ethnic minority populations points to a related need.[2]

There is a strong inverse association between socioeconomic privilege—based on class, race, ethnicity, nationality, gender, age, or sexual orientation—and mental disorders.[6] The evidence is particularly strong to support the association between socioeconomic position, measured in terms of income, educational credentials, or occupational social class, and the most frequent forms of psychiatric illnesses, such as depression, anxiety disorders, and substance use disorders.[6] For example, a comprehensive meta-analysis of the prevalence and incidence studies of socioeconomic position and depression indicated that persons with low educational credentials or low income are at higher risk of depression.[7] In the United States, individuals with annual household incomes of less than $20,000 per year were found to have a prevalence of major depression in the past month that was twice as high as that for individuals with annual household incomes of $70,000 or more.[4] Studies of U.S. metropolitan areas have found even stronger associations (with odds ratios of 11 to 16) between high- and low-income respondents and depression.[2] In a 13-year follow-up study that used psychiatric interviews as a method of assessment, poverty was found to increase the risk of depression by 2.5 times.[8] In the same study in East Baltimore, respondents who did not receive income from property were 10 times more likely to have an anxiety disorder than were those who obtained some income from property.[2] (See chapter 2.)

With regard to occupational social class, the prevalence of depression in the past 6 months among those employed in household services was 7 percent, almost three times that of executive professionals (2.4 percent).[5] More recent studies show that blue-collar workers are between 1.5 and 2.0 times as likely to be depressed as white-collar workers.[1] Similar risk increases have been reported with a 1-year follow-up period.[1] Being born to parents employed in manual labor occupations confers almost twice the risk of depression for women and almost four times the risk of depression for men compared with those born to at least one parent not in the working class.[1]

In addition to depression, similar two- to three-fold differences in prevalence between high and low socioeconomic position have been reported in the United States for substance use disorders, alcohol abuse or dependence, antisocial personality disorder, anxiety disorders, and all psychiatric disorders combined.[2,3] Internationally, even larger differences have been found—up to four-fold higher current prevalence of depression among working-class respondents compared with their middle-class counterparts.[3]

Mental disorders, which have a major worldwide impact on disability,[9] are the leading cause of disability among women and, by 2020, are expected to become the main cause of years lost to disability.[9] The relevance of mental disorders to social injustice and public health is both in the strength of association between socioeconomic factors and mental disorders and in the great consequences that this association has for the quality of life of affected individuals and their families.

Underlying the study of social inequalities and mental health are competing notions of what constitutes social injustice. Two opposing views of social justice and mental health are prominent. The first is that behavior is a matter of individual agency or volitional control, accounting for the disproportionate burden of mental illness among workers, women, and minorities. This view holds that most social outcomes, including mental health, reflect personal autonomous choices and that therefore there is little that society, as a whole, is obliged to do for people who are afflicted by mental disorders. In one study, for example, educated "liberals" respected the autonomy and individual rights of homeless persons but felt little obligation to do anything to improve their situation.

In contrast, the "structural" view focuses on the social relations of class, race, ethnicity, and gender inequality as determinants of individual outcomes, including mental disorders. The social justice implications of this view include a collective responsibility for those whose mental health is negatively affected by class, gender, and racial and ethnic inequalities in access to economic, political, and cultural resources. For example, a recent ethnographic study of African-American and white working-class men concluded that African-American men have a greater sense of collective responsibility and are less prone to use individual responsibility as an explanation for personal outcomes than their white counterparts.[10] Western European and U.S. whites are more likely to use individualistic attributions for the outcomes of persons in social situations—personal attributes are seen as the cause of personal outcomes, as opposed to the features of the situation.[11]

We believe that there is sufficient evidence from social science to maintain that social class, gender, and racial/ethnic inequalities in mental health stem from social structures rather than from personal choices. Furthermore, a contemporary definition of public health—as organized efforts by society to improve the health of populations—implicitly acknowledges both social determinants and collective responsibility for the public's health.

The description of social injustice in mental health cannot be separated from the technical knowledge that constitutes normative or prescriptive epidemiology. Public mental health is thus faced with the obligation to improve the health of groups affected by social injustice—that is, public health officials have the responsibility to improve the mental health of populations that due to economic, political, or cultural inequalities have a high rate of mental disorders. For example, a society's unequal distribution of economic, political, or cultural resources will generate worse mental health among the relatively poor, powerless, and less educated. Furthermore, inequalities in property generate an intergenerational transmission of poverty that has disproportionately affected African-Americans in the United States. Political inequalities preclude immigrants from obtaining equal rights, while confining them to economic, political, and cultural subordination. And cultural factors such as racism, patriarchy, or classism can lead to labor market discrimination and residential segregation with negative economic, political, and cultural consequences for people of various races and ethnicities, nationalities, religions, age groups, categories of sexual orientation, gender, medical conditions or disabilities, and social classes.

The Relationship Between Social Injustice and Mental Health

Social Injustice Produces Mental Disorders

Poverty, Inequality, and Workplace Domination

Poverty is a consistent risk factor for multiple mental disorders, including depression, anxiety disorders, antisocial personality, and substance-use disorders.[2,6,7] Cross-sectional and longitudinal studies have found consistent associations between area poverty and mental disorders. About two-thirds of income inequality studies have shown an association between high income inequality and high rates of mental disorders.

Social class inequality, which includes relations of property and control over the labor process, is also associated with mental illness. Social class, understood as a social relation linked to the production of goods and services,[12] is conceptually and empirically distinct from socioeconomic status (SES). Thus, social class is associated with mental disorders over and above SES.[13–18] One study found a small overlap between SES and social class measures, but the association between social class and depression could not be accounted for by SES.[15] Other studies have found initial evidence of a nonlinear relationship between social class and mental health, as would be predicted by social class models but not by SES models.[16,18] Low-level supervisors (who do not have policymaking power but can hire and fire workers) have higher rates of depression and anxiety than both upper-level managers (who have organizational control over policy and personnel) and front-line employees (who have neither). Control over organizational assets is determined by the possibility of influencing company policy (making decisions on number of people employed, products or services delivered, amount of work performed, and size and distribution of budgets) and by sanctioning authority over others in the organization (granting or preventing pay raises or promotions, hiring, and firing or temporally suspending subordinates). The repeated experience of organizational control at work would protect most upper-level managers against mood and anxiety disorders. Low-level supervisors, on the other hand, are subjected to "double exposure": the demands of upper management to discipline the workforce and the antagonism of subordinate workers, while exerting little influence over company policy. This "contradictory class location" may place supervisors at greater risk of depression and anxiety disorders than either upper management or nonsupervisory workers. Nevertheless, the literature on social class and major psychiatric disorders still lacks evidence of pathways linking class position to depression and anxiety disorders.

Does Social Injustice Get Under the Skin?

There is controversy on the relative importance of "neo-material" determinants (contemporary physical or biological risk or protective factors) and "psychosocial" determinants, such as perceptions of relative standing in the income distribution, of socioeconomic position (SEP) gradients in health in wealthy countries.[19,20] Neo-material indicators of SEP, such as owning a car or a house, and indices of deprivation have recently been incorporated in the social epidemiology of mental disorders.[21–23] For example, in a national survey of United Kingdom households, an independent association was found between housing tenure and access to a car, on the one hand, and neurotic disorder (including some anxiety disorders) and depression, on the other.[21,23] Also, an analysis of the British Household Panel Survey found that low material standard of living was associated with risk for depression and anxiety disorders.[21] A geographic area deprivation index, including housing tenure and car ownership, has been associated with the prevalence and persistence of risk for depression. Although deprivation indicators suggest that absence of material goods increases the risk of psychiatric disorders, research has yet to uncover the specific mechanisms linking material factors to depression or anxiety. On the other hand, some studies have provided cross-sectional and prospective evidence of an association between (a) psychosocial factors, such as perceived job demands and perceived financial hardship, and (b) depression, symptoms of depression, and anxiety disorders.[8,21] A common limitation of both "neo-material" and "psychosocial" studies is overreliance on self-report measures of depression and anxiety, and infrequent use of diagnostic interviews to assess mental disorders. Even in prospective studies that take into account reverse causation, it is difficult to rule out the possibility that features of the material environment (physical and biological exposures) are confounded with a respondent's perceptions.[24] However, the reported associations of job insecurity or remaining in a downsized organization with symptoms of anxiety and depression suggest that psychosocial exposures can have independent effects on psychiatric disorders.[25]

Discrimination and Mental Health

Women have at least twice the risk of men for depression and anxiety disorders—in part because of their lower socioeconomic standing and higher exposure to stressors.[26] Low SEP increases the risk of depression. Low-income people have higher rates of depression than do people with higher incomes or the general population.[27,28] Factors such as financial strain and level of debt are associated with higher rates of depression.[8,29] (See chapter 4.)

Women residing in states with the highest levels of income inequality have substantially higher rates of depression than do women living in states with the lowest quintile of income inequality.[30] New mothers of low SEP have higher rates of depressive symptoms 2 months postpartum than do women of high SEP,[31] perhaps due to their social networks being smaller.

Large surveys in psychiatric epidemiology have tended to show small differences in mental health status among races, although the effects of racial discrimination and other forms of racism, such as residential segregation, are just beginning to be examined. One exception seems to be a higher rate of anxiety disorders among black women in the United States. Perceptions of racial and ethnic discrimination are consistently associated with worse mental health.[32] Ageism and discrimination based on sexual orientation adversely affect mental health.[33,34] (See chapters 3, 6, and 7.)

How Mental Disorders Become Problems of Social Injustice

Mental health services vary in quantity and quality across geographic areas. In addition to the natural variation, there are systematic differences in the availability, accessibility, and appropriateness of treatment and in treatment outcomes for racial and ethnic minorities. Other marginalized groups suffer, including those who are homeless or incarcerated, children in foster care, traumatized persons, refugees, those with substance-use disorders, and those with alternative sexual preferences. These disparities in access and quality of care cause minority and marginalized groups—those with limited political power and access to resources—to suffer a disproportionate health burden because of unmet mental health needs. As rates of mental illness are similar despite racial/ethnic background, the disparity in outcomes relates directly to the ability of the mental health service sector to diagnose and appropriately treat individuals from different backgrounds, as well as to differences in the willingness of individuals to submit to treatment by clinicians they mistrust or fear.

A recent report[35] classified the causes of racial/ethnic disparities into patient, provider, and institutional factors.

Patient factors included cultural beliefs about health and medical care by members of the minority group, mistrust of the health care system (based on past discrimination), language barriers and other difficulties in communication, patient "preference" (usually describing patient noncompliance), and other socioeconomic factors associated with race and ethnicity.

Provider factors included a lack of cultural competency, styles of physician practice, atypical symptom presentation, and negative stereotypes and other biases that operate either consciously or unconsciously. All of these provider factors are thought to influence both diagnosis and treatment of racial/ethnic minority patients.

Institutional factors included lack of familiarity with the presenting case mix and failing to treat the uninsured.

These individual, provider, and institutional factors interact with each other to produce poorer treatment for members of racial/ethnic minority groups.

Access to Treatment

The availability of mental health services depends both on having sufficient providers to meet the specialty mental health care needs of a given population and on the available care being culturally relevant to the population. Because most U.S. mental health providers are European-American, most minority consumers cannot find a provider of the same racial/ethnic background.[36,37] For African-Americans, this difficulty is striking; only 2 to 4 percent of mental health professionals are African-American.[36] In addition, many African-Americans live in the urban South, where specialty mental health treatment is less available.[36] Similarly, African-Americans are incarcerated, homeless, in foster care, and uninsured at a disproportionate rate to their relative composition in the U.S. population, and mental health services are far less available to these high-need individuals. The situation is even worse for American Indians and Alaska Natives. The number of mental health care providers available for these groups is much smaller and far less likely to be racially or ethnically similar. In 1998 in the United States, only 29 psychiatrists were of American Indian or Alaskan Native heritage and only a very small fraction of physicians identified themselves as American Indian or Alaska Native.[38] Asian-Americans, Pacific Islanders, and Hispanics often have limited availability of services because of limited proficiency in English.[38]

Affordable care and generous insurance coverage have a strong influence on receipt of services. Members of minority groups are less likely to have health insurance and to be able to pay for mental health care. With insurance, mental health coverage seldom reaches parity with coverage for treatment for somatic disorders, even in states where parity has been legislated. Federal regulations have attempted to improve insurance coverage for children; however, children with mental disorders, even with Children's Health Insurance Program coverage, are often inadequately covered for mental and substance-use disorders. Insurance coverage is often tied to employment, and because many blue-collar jobs have been moved overseas, many blue-collar workers are not able to pay for care.

Feelings of mistrust deter some minority patients from receiving mental health services. Mistrust may be based on a historical legacy of discrimination and maltreatment but may also derive from recent experiences with culturally insensitive clinicians. One study found that 12 percent of African-Americans and 15 percent of Latinos perceived that physicians treated them with disrespect or unfairly compared with 1 percent of whites.[39] Immigrants to the United States from other countries whose governments persecuted their citizens—and American Indians—are unlikely to trust authorities, including those in clinical roles.

Mental health disorders are undeniably stigmatizing. Stigma operates at the individual, family, community, and societal levels. At the individual level, mentally ill persons who fear rejection due to their illnesses are often socially isolated and behaviorally are less likely to seek and be adherent to therapies. At the family and community levels, these prejudices against those with a mental illness affect members of some minority groups more than whites. In some Asian cultures, the shame of having a mentally ill family member adversely influences the potential of other immediate-family members to marry or to work. Stigma by association is also present in other cultures. Asians living in Los Angeles are half as likely as whites to disclose a mental health problem to a friend or relative and are very unlikely to see a psychiatrist for assistance; the basis for these differences is thought to be pervasive stigma. Asians and Hispanics view mentally ill patients with more distrust than do whites.[40] Contact with mentally ill patients—and thus, direct experience with them—decreased perceptions of dangerousness for whites but not for blacks.[40] Such contact also improves the ability of mentally ill patients to integrate into the community.[41] As a society, the United States has reduced discrimination experienced by the mentally ill with the passage of the Americans with Disabilities Act (ADA). However, the stigma of mental illness can still prevent the mentally ill from acquiring housing and employment with accommodations, as required under the ADA—because they must disclose the nature of their disability to prospective employers and may be reluctant to do so for fear of recrimination. The claims outcome for filers under the ADA has not been favorable for most.

Patients with mental disorders often have multiple needs that extend beyond visits to psychiatrists, and they must negotiate their way through a complex physical and mental health system to receive needed care. In addition, they often require income supports, assistance with supported housing and employment, and legal aid. The system of service delivery that supports individuals is fragmented by funding streams, geographic borders, and, to some extent, diagnoses. Because systems of care have difficulty organizing to provide comprehensive care, case-management models have been used to try to reduce the effect of persistently fragmented services on satisfying patients' needs.

The use of mental health services by minorities has been assessed. One study found that African-Americans do not underuse mental health services but are more likely to receive care in a general, rather than a specialty, mental health setting.[37,42] Perhaps African-Americans have unfavorable attitudes toward mental health treatment and may fear being "guinea pigs."

A study of adolescents found that African-American males receive treatment at one-third the rate of African-American females and one-half the rate of white males, suggesting a referral bias based on racial discrimination.[43] Other reasons for racial differences in treatment contacts might be (a) African-Americans having a higher threshold for tolerating symptoms before seeking help, (b) African-Americans having lower expectations that treatment would be helpful, and (c) African-Americans possibly being shunted into the juvenile justice system. African-American children, aged 5 to 14, on Medicaid are less than half as likely to be prescribed psychotropic medication as are white youth, with psychostimulants being prescribed for whites at 2.5 times the rate they are prescribed for African-Americans.[44] In poor inner-city neighborhoods, there are few behavioral pediatricians, less psychiatric follow-up care, and cultural differences in interpretation of symptoms of attention deficit-hyperactivity disorder (ADHD) in the family that reduce referral for care.

Studies using treated prevalence samples suggest racial differences in the amount and type of treatment received. A study at an inpatient treatment facility found that African-Americans have shorter lengths of stay, higher rates of urine drug screens, and higher neuroleptic doses for schizophrenics compared with whites.[45] Whites had a higher rate of one-on-one observation for risk of self-harm, which corresponded to a higher rate of diagnoses of personality disorders.[45]

There may be an unconscious bias about "treatability" for blacks, especially when comorbid substance-use disorders are present.[45] Blacks may receive less close observation because they are reluctant to disclose suicidal thoughts because of cultural mistrust.[45] Administrative claims data from the Los Angeles County mental health system revealed that blacks used fewer sessions with a psychotherapist, Asians and Latinos had more frequent outpatient treatment than those of other racial/ethnic groups, and Asians had the most outpatient sessions. Patients of lower SEP had fewer psychotherapy sessions, more sessions with a nonprofessional therapist, less medication treatment, and less overall treatment.[46] Another study found that the single factor linking ethnicity to "treatment readiness" was having low SEP.[47] Low SEP may inhibit participation in the bureaucratic mental health system but may also create more distress from stressful life events. A secondary analysis of BlueCross/BlueShield claims found no differences in service utilization based on race alone.[48] Thus, there are differences among treated prevalence studies in patterns of service utilization by race, and the reasons for reported differences vary by investigator.

Inequalities in the Quality of Treatment

Once an individual is received into treatment, the outcome of care depends on the clinician making a correct diagnosis, and then using appropriate methods of treatment to ameliorate the presenting symptoms. Treatment guidelines that are based on scientific evidence have been published by several professional organizations and evidence-based reporting organizations and supported by government agencies. The translation of this research into clinical practice is deficient for all races. Few practitioners use evidence-based treatment for patients with mental disorders.[49] Compared with whites, African-Americans are less likely to receive guideline-based treatment for anxiety or depression,[50,51] less likely to receive an antidepressant,[51] less likely to receive a selective serotonin reuptake inhibitor (SSRI) (rather than an earlier-developed antidepressant), and more likely to be overmedicated with antipsychotics.[52,53] Unfortunately, minorities are severely underrepresented in clinical trials where interventions for major mental disorders are tested; thus, the efficacy of these treatments among minority group members is not known.

Populations at Risk for Unjust Treatment

Lesbian, gay, bisexual, and transgender (LGBT) persons living in the community suffer from homophobia and heterosexualism in the broader society (see chapter 7). School-age children can experience teasing, abuse, and violence daily, leading to substance-use disorders, generalized anxiety, and depression. These individuals can suffer from psychological difficulties as they cope with both overt discrimination and internalization of hate messages. For LGBT males, rates of depression and panic attacks are higher than those for heterosexual men.[54] Although psychiatrists formerly pathologized homosexuality as a disorder, recent studies indicate that LGBT individuals who seek psychotherapy are generally satisfied with their experience.[55] Some are reluctant to disclose their gender orientation to therapists, fearing negative reactions to their gender identity or unfamiliarity with the life issues that are associated with same-sex relationships.

Mental disorders and comorbid substance use are common among prisoners (see chapter 9). For youth entering the criminal justice system, these disorders are often unrecognized. Prisoners have often experienced trauma and family disruption during childhood. Treatment during incarceration is often inadequate, and aftercare upon release is generally poor compared with care for somatic disorders. The experience of incarceration is traumatizing for many; stressful daily experiences with other inmates and correctional staff members can induce mental illness in those predisposed to these disorders. "Supermax" prisons have been described as "incubators for psychosis"; sensory deprivation is severe and electroshock instruments are often used to force compliant behavior. The period of incarceration presents an opportunity for focused treatment and rehabilitation; however, this has not been a social priority despite some suggestion that it would reduce rates of re-arrest. To better serve this population, collaboration between the mental health and criminal justice systems is required, as well as a reconceptualization of the role of prisons to be restorative rather than punitive.

Refugees suffer myriad traumas that they bring with them (see chapter 11). Many are fleeing war, famine, or repressive regimes that use torture and intimidation to control the population. Posttraumatic stress disorder (PTSD) is common among those who have been subjected to torture or rape or have witnessed murder. Often refugees are leaving behind relatives with no way to be assured of their safety or ability to contact them. In new countries, refugees have difficulties with language, cultural assimilation, social isolation, and poverty and are often at the bottom of the social strata despite past professional successes in their countries of origin.

When mental health problems are recognized, refugees continue to face problems in treatment. In cultures with traditions of somatization of emotional distress, they may be misdiagnosed with somatic illnesses. Because of the extended period between traumatic event and treatment, the outcomes of therapies are less than optimal. In some cultures, psychotherapy is not culturally acceptable, so different models of treatment must be used to assist refugees; trust is sometimes difficult when medical care providers in countries of origin participated in torture. Systems of care must be coordinated to include somatic and mental health care, as well as housing, social services, language instruction, employment assistance, and income supports.

For the 750,000 children in foster care in the United States, the risk for experiencing mental disorders or developmental delays is high. Many of these children have been abused or neglected just at the time of early brain development. Once in the foster care system, behavioral problems often worsen because of difficulty with attachment to the foster caregiver, separation from siblings, and uncertainty about the relationship with the biological parent. In the worst case scenario, the foster care setting or the social service system increases the stress on the child and can lead to iatrogenic mental disorders. Child welfare workers can be a vital link to appropriate pediatric services but only if the worker's caseload is sufficiently small to be able to screen children for behavioral symptoms over the life of the placement. Older children who have failed to "catch up" emotionally are aged out of the system at 18 and can have difficulties living independently. The child welfare worker must be able to coordinate care across systems while advocating for the child's needs. Successful programs have been developed that integrate intensive mental health treatment at a young age.[56] (See chapter 5.)

On any given night in the United States, more than 700,000 people are homeless, of whom 20 to 25 percent are mentally ill and 50 percent have a substance-use disorder (see chapter 10). Minorities are overrepresented among those with mental disorders, and poverty is an important moderator of the influence between being mentally ill and homeless.[57] Successful independent housing and vocational rehabilitation programs have been developed that are effective in reducing the number of shelter days that are used by consumers and should be promoted. These are more effective when treatment for comorbid substance-use disorders is provided and when there is good coordination between community mental health providers and the shelter care system.[58]

What Needs to Be Done

Social class, gender, race, and ethnic inequalities represent a substantial source of social injustice, but they have been rarely examined in relation to mental health. Studies on policies that alleviate these forms of unjust inequalities and their impact on mental disorders are needed to document the impact of contemporary social policies. For example, there are few studies of the mental health impact of housing policy, child care policy, wage ordinances, and social services among low-income women.

Public health change is multidisciplinary, as it corresponds to any social technology. For example, raising a child not only requires schooling; it also requires economic support—food, clothing, and housing—and emotional support. Similarly, reversing the mental health effects of social injustice will require more than addressing the immediate social determinants of mental illness, such as stigma, lack of access to treatment, and homelessness. The United States, for example, has many social movements—for the elderly, poor, women, minorities, children, homeless, and mental patients—and yet, in many health indicators, it fares worse than countries of comparable wealth.[59,60] Denmark and Sweden do not have so many single-issue social movements, but they do have powerful political organizations and labor movements that address these issues—poverty, gender, aging, children's health, and mental health—simultaneously in an egalitarian manner. Unless we tackle the broader social policies that affect well-being, including mental health, it will not be possible to adequately redress the effects of social injustice on the public's mental health.

The effect of stigma on the quality of life for patients with mental disorders cannot be understated. The only antidote to discrimination is the provision of systematic, repetitive, culturally appropriate public education that paints a realistic picture of mental illness. Media portrayals of individuals with mental disorders stress dangerousness, deviant behavior, and unpredictability. Accurate portrayals that stress the biological basis for the disorder, describe issues of discrimination, and show positive outcomes for those who receive optimal treatment, would challenge discriminatory beliefs. This coupled with an investment in true community-based services, such as Assertive Community Treatment—in model form, not diluted, in which individuals would have meaningful opportunities to reintegrate into their communities—would expose the lay public to real people with mental disorders.

Obtaining justice for persons with mental illness requires that advocates for the mentally ill use a "bottom-up" approach to challenging discrimination. Groups such as the National Alliance for the Mentally Ill have implemented commendable programs to assist consumers and their families and to advocate for health policies that reduce stigma. Each advocacy group, for a category of patients such as those with manic-depression, depression, alcoholism, or childhood ADHD, takes on its own cause with vigor. Yet it would be very appropriate to develop umbrella organizations to assist these groups to leverage their efforts. In addition, changing the focus from illness care to civil rights has the potential to leverage additional change if alliances with powerful civil rights organizations can be developed.

Conclusion

We recommend the following action steps:

1. Reframe the issue of mental health disparities among deprived and victimized populations from a medical to a civil rights issue, and use enforcement as a lever to improve the access and quality of care delivered in all settings where mentally ill persons are treated or housed. This should include examination of federal financing systems for evidence of disparities in clinical care programs that are funded by taxpayers.
2. Collect data systematically on ethnicity, race, socioeconomic position, neighborhood disadvantage, and primary language in all clinical records and health databases.
3. Include stakeholders in a meaningful way in all policy forums where their health services are acted on.
4. Increase the recruitment of socioeconomically, ethnically, and racially diverse physicians, nurses, psychologists, social workers, and other health professionals to provide treatment for the mentally ill. Provide culturally competent education for all professionals who treat people with mental disorders.
5. Insure the uninsured and insist on parity for care of mental disorders. Provide feedback mechanisms to ensure that treatment adheres to evidence-based practices with known efficacy.
6. Focus on primary prevention efforts by strengthening families at risk and reducing adverse conditions, such as poverty, discrimination, and racism.

7. Increase the participation of all ethnic and racial minorities in funded efficacy and effectiveness research studies.
8. Mount public education efforts designed to combat stigma.
9. Include mental health policies aimed at reducing the social injustice that determines mental illness, such as poverty, disparities, stigma, and access to quality care, in the political programs of government and non-governmental organizations, including political organizations and unions, at the local, state, and national levels.

References

1. Eaton WW, Musick Addington A, Bass J, Forman V. Risk factors for major mental disorders. A review of the epidemiologic literature. Baltimore, Md.: Department of Mental Health, Bloomberg School of Public Health, Johns Hopkins University, November 2002. Available at: http://www.jhu.edu/~janthony/share/Environme-II.dbf. Accessed January 24, 2005.
2. Eaton WW. The sociology of mental disorders. 3rd ed. London, England: Praeger, 2001.
3. Regier DA, Farmer ME, Rae DS, et al. One month prevalence of mental disorders in the US and socio-demographic characteristics. Acta Psychiatr Scand 1993;88:35–47.
4. Blazer DG, Kessler RC, McGonagle KA, et al. The prevalence and distribution of major depression in a national community sample: the national comorbidity survey. Am J Psychiatry 1994;151:979–86.
5. Roberts RE, Lee ES. Occupation and the prevalence of major depression, alcohol and drug abuse in the US. Environ Res 1993;61:266–78.
6. Eaton WW, Muntaner C. Socioeconomic stratification and mental disorder. In: Horwitz AV, Scheid TL, eds. A handbook for the study of mental health: social contexts, theories and systems. New York, N.Y.: Cambridge University Press, 1999.
7. Lorant V, Deliege D, Eaton WW, et al. Socio-economic inequalities in mental health: a meta-analysis. Am J Epidemiol 2003;157:98–112.
8. Eaton WW, Muntaner C, Bovasso G, et al. Socioeconomic status and depression. J Health Soc Behav 2001;42:277–93.
9. Murray CJ, Lopez AD. Evidence-based health policy—lessons from the Global Burden of Disease Study. Science 1996;274:740–3.
10. Lamont M. The dignity of working men. New York, N.Y.: Russell Sage Foundation, 2002.
11. Nisbett RE. The geography of thought. New York, N.Y.: The Free Press, 2003.
12. Krieger N, Williams DR, Moss NE. Measuring social class in U.S. public health research: concepts, methodologies, and guidelines. Annu Rev Public Health 1997;18:341–78.
13. Wohlfarth T, Winkel FW, Ybema JF, et al. The relationship between socio-economic inequality and criminal victimisation: a prospective study. Soc Psychiatry Psychiatric Epidemiol 2000;36:361–70.
14. Wohlfarth T, van den Brink W. Social class and substance use disorders: the value of social class as distinct from socioeconomic status. Soc Sci Med 1998;47:51–8.
15. Wohlfarth T. Socioeconomic inequality and psychopathology: are socioeconomic status and social class interchangeable? Soc Sci Med 1997;45:399–410.

16. Muntaner C, Eaton WW, Diala C, et al. Social class, assets, organizational control and the prevalence of common groups of psychiatric disorders. Soc Sci Med 1998; 47:243–53.

17. Muntaner C, Eaton W, Diala CC. Socioeconomic inequalities in mental health: a review of concepts and underlying assumptions. Health 2000;4:82–106.

18. Muntaner C, Borrell C, Benach J. The association of social class and social stratification with patterns of general and mental health in a Spanish population. Int J Epidemiol 2003;32:950–8.

19. Pearce N, Davey Smith G. Is social capital the key to inequalities in health? Am J Public Health 2003;93:122–9.

20. Lynch J, Due P, Muntaner C, et al. Social capital—Is it a good investment strategy for public health? J Epidemiol Community Health 2000;54:404–8.

21. Weich S, Lewis G. Material standard of living, social class, and the prevalence of the common mental disorders in Great Britain. J Epidemiol Community Health 1998; 52:8–14.

22. Lewis G, Bebbington P, Brugha T, et al. Socioeconomic status, standard of living, and neurotic disorder. Lancet 1998;352:605–9.

23. Lewis G, Bebbington P, Brugha T, et al. Socio-economic status, standard of living, and neurotic disorder. Int Rev Psychiatry 2003;15:91–6.

24. MacLeod J, Davey Smith G, Heslop P, et al. Psychological stress and cardiovascular disease: empirical demonstration of bias in a prospective observational study of Scottish men. Br Med J 2002;324:1247–51.

25. Ferrie JE, Shipley MJ, Stansfeld SA, et al. Future uncertainty and socioeconomic inequalities in health: the Whitehall II study. Soc Sci Med 2003;57: 637–46.

26. Kessler R, Berglund P, Demler O, et al. National Comorbidity Survey Replication. The epidemiology of major depressive disorder: results from the National Comorbidity Survey Replication (NCS-R). JAMA 2003;289:3095–105.

27. Ritter C, Hobfoll SE, Lavin J, et al. Stress, psychosocial resources, and depressive symptomatology during pregnancy in low-income, inner-city women. Health Psychol 2000;19:576–85.

28. Danziger SK, Carlson MJ, Henly JR. Post-welfare employment and psychological well-being. Women Health 2001;32:47–78.

29. O'Campo P, Eaton WW, Muntaner C. Labor market experience, work organization, gender inequalities, and health status: results from a prospective study of US employed women. Soc Sci Med 2004;58:585–94.

30. Kahn R, Wise PH, Kennedy BP, et al. State income inequality, household income, and maternal mental and physical health: cross sectional national survey. Br Med J 2000;321:1311–5.

31. Seguin L, Potvin L, St-Denis M, et al. Socio-environmental factors and postnatal depressive symptomatology: a longitudinal study. Women Health 1999;29:57–72.

32. Noh S, Kaspar V. Perceived discrimination and depression: moderating effect of coping, acculturation, and ethnic support. Am J Public Health 2003;93:232–8.

33. Mays VM, Cochran SD. Mental health correlates of perceived discrimination among lesbian, gay, and bisexual adults in the United States. Am J Public Health 2001;91: 1869–76.

34. Ory M, Kinney Hoffman M, Hawkins M, et al. Challenging aging stereotypes: strategies for creating a more active society. Am J Prev Med 2003;25(3 suppl 2): 164–71.

35. Physicians for Human Rights. The right to equal treatment: an action plan to end racial and ethnic disparities in clinical diagnosis and treatment in the United States, 2003. Available at: http://www.phrusa.org/research/domestic/race/race_report/other.html. Accessed January 24, 2005.
36. Manderscheid RW, Henderson MJ, eds. Mental Health, United States, Chapter 20, Mental Health Practitioners and Trainees. Rockville, MD: Center for Mental Health Services, 2000. Available at: http://www.mentalhealth.org/publications/allpubs/SMA01-3537/chp20table2.asp. Accessed January 24, 2005.
37. Cooper-Patrick L, Gallo JJ, Gonzales JJ, et al. Race, gender, and partnership in the patient-physician relationship. JAMA 1999;282:583–9.
38. Manderscheid RW, Henderson MJ, eds. Mental health, United States. Rockville, Md.: Center for Mental Health Services, 1998.
39. Brown ER, Ojeda VD, Wyn R, et al. Racial and ethnic disparities in access to health insurance and health care [report]. Los Angeles, Calif.: UCLA Center for Health Policy Research and the Henry J. Kaiser Family Foundation, 2000.
40. Whaley AL. Ethnic and racial differences in perceptions of dangerousness of persons with mental illness. Psychiatr Serv 1997;48:1328–30.
41. Prince PN, Prince CR. Perceived stigma and community integration among clients of assertive community treatment. Psychiatric Rehabil J 2002;25:323–31.
42. Cooper-Patrick L, Gallo JJ, Powe NR, et al. Mental health service utilization by African Americans and whites: the Baltimore Epidemiologic Catchment Area Follow-Up. Med Care 1999;37:1034–45.
43. Cuffe SP, Waller JL, Cuccaro ML, et al. Race and gender differences in the treatment of psychiatric disorders in young adolescents. J Am Acad Child Adolesc Psychiatry 1995;34:1536–43.
44. Zito JM, Safer DJ, dos Reis S, et al. Racial disparity in psychotropic medications prescribed for youths with Medicaid insurance in Maryland. J Am Acad Child Adolesc Psychiatry 1998;37:179–84.
45. Chung H, Mahler JC, Kakuma T. Racial differences in treatment of psychiatric inpatients. Psychiatr Serv 1995;46:586–91.
46. Flaskerud JH, Hu LT. Racial/ethnic identity and amount and type of psychiatric treatment. Am J Psychiatry 1992;149:379–84.
47. Briones DF, Heller PL, Chalfant HP, et al. Socioeconomic status, ethnicity, psychological distress, and readiness to utilize a mental health facility. Am J Psychiatry 1990;147:1333–40.
48. Padgett DK, Patrick C, Burns BJ, et al. Ethnicity and the use of outpatient mental health services in a national insured population. Am J Public Health 1994;84:222–6.
49. Lehman AF, Steinwachs DM. Patterns of usual care for schizophrenia: initial results from the Schizophrenia Patient Outcomes Research Team (PORT) Client Survey. Schizophr Bull 1998;24:11–22.
50. Wang PS, Berglund P, Kessler RC. Recent care of common mental disorders in the United States. J Gen Intern Med 2000;15:284–92.
51. Young AS, Klap R, Shebourne CD, et al. The quality of care for depressive and anxiety disorders in the United States. Arch Gen Psychiatry 2001;58:55–61.
52. Melfi CA, Croghan TW, Hanna MP, et al. Racial variation in antidepressant treatment in a Medicaid population. J Clin Psychiatry 2000;61:16–21.
53. Walkup JT, McAlpine DD, Olfson M, et al. Patients with schizophrenia at risk for excessive antipsychotic dosing. J Clin Psychiatry 2000;61:344–8.

54. Cochran SD, Mays VM, Sullivan JG. Prevalence of mental disorders, psychological distress, and mental health services use among lesbian, gay, and bisexual adults in the United States. J Consult Clin Psychol 2003;71:53–61.
55. Jones MA, Gabriel MA. Utilization of psychotherapy by lesbians, gay men, and bisexuals: findings from a nationwide survey. Am J Orthopsychiatry 1999;69:209–19.
56. Zeanah CH, Larrieu JA. Intensive intervention for maltreated infants and toddlers in foster care. Child Adolesc Psychiatr Clin North Am 1998;7:357–71.
57. Draine J, Salzer MS, Culhane DP, et al. Role of social disadvantage in crime, joblessness, and homelessness among persons with serious mental illness. Psychiatr Serv 2002;53:565–73.
58. Gonzales G, Rosenheck RA. Outcomes and service use among homeless persons with serious mental illness and substance abuse. Psychiatr Serv 2002;53:427–46.
59. Muntaner C, Lynch JW, Hillemeier M, et al. Economic inequality, working-class power, social capital, and cause-specific mortality in wealthy countries. Int J Health Serv 2002;32:629–56.
60. Navarro V, Borell C, Benach J, et al. The importance of the political and the social in explaining mortality differentials among the countries of the OECD, 1950–1998. Int J Health Serv 2003;33:419–94.

17

ASSAULTIVE VIOLENCE AND WAR

James A. Mercy

Introduction

Violence can be both a consequence of social injustice and a tool used to perpetrate it. Intimate partner violence, for example, can stem to some degree
from customs that support gender inequality.[1] Genocide, as was evidenced in
Nazi Germany and more recently in Rwanda, is the most extreme example of
using violence as a tool to perpetrate social injustice by attempting to deny an
entire population group of its right to exist.[2] Public health has a fundamental
role to play in preventing violence by promoting social justice.

Violence is now viewed as a leading public health problem worldwide.[3]
The involvement of the public health community in violence prevention has
expanded with heightened awareness that violence is a major contributor to
premature mortality, morbidity, and disability.[4]

Public health professionals have helped develop and implement strategies
to prevent violence from occurring in the first place (primary prevention).[5] In
addition, they have brought a multidisciplinary, scientific approach to violence prevention aimed at identifying effective measures. The evidence base
for preventing some forms of violence has been substantially strengthened
since the entry of public health professionals into this field.[6] They have also
emphasized the need for collective action to prevent violence, involving

collaboration among different scientific disciplines, organizations, and communities.

Efforts to address violence as a public health problem have increased dramatically since the late 1970s.[7] In 1979, the Surgeon General's Report, *Healthy People*, documented the dramatic gains made in the health of Americans during the previous century and identified 15 priority areas in which, with appropriate action, further gains could be expected.[8] Among those areas was the control of stress and violent behavior. A variety of violence prevention activities within the public health sector followed. In 1983, for example, the Centers for Disease Control and Prevention established a Violence Epidemiology Branch, and in 1985 the Surgeon General held a workshop on violence and public health.[9] In 1996, the World Health Assembly—the annual gathering of all ministers of health—adopted a resolution stating that violence is a global public health priority.[3]

Defining Violence

The World Health Organization (WHO) defines violence as "the intentional use of physical force or power, threatened or actual, against oneself, another person, or a group or community that either results in or has a high likelihood of resulting in injury, death, psychological harm, maldevelopment, or deprivation"(p. 5).[10] Under this definition, suicidal behavior is considered an important type of violence, and violence can be wielded through threats or intimidation as well as physical force. The definition includes outcomes that go beyond physical injury and death, such as psychological harm, maldevelopment, and deprivation. It defines violence as it relates to the health and well-being of individuals—not in cultural terms.[10] This is an important feature because some people who intend to harm others may not perceive their acts to be violent because of prevailing cultural norms within their societies. Physical violence toward spouses or children, for example, is regarded as an acceptable practice in some societies, even though these acts may have serious health consequences for the victims.[11,12]

Three general types of violence are encompassed by the WHO definition: interpersonal, self-directed, and collective. Interpersonal violence includes forms perpetrated by an individual or small group of individuals, such as child abuse and neglect by caregivers, youth violence, intimate partner violence, sexual violence, and elder abuse.[10] Self-directed violence includes suicidal behavior as well as acts of self-abuse, where the intent may not be to take one's own life. Collective violence is the use of violence by groups or individuals who identify themselves as members of a group, against another group or set of individuals, to achieve political, social, or economic objectives. It includes war, terrorism, and state-sponsored violence toward its own citizens.[2]

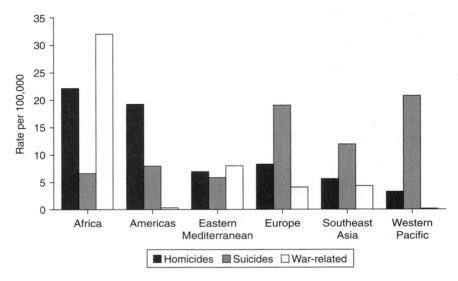

Figure 17-1 Rate of violent death by type and World Health Organization region, 2000. (From World Health Organization. Global Burden of Disease Project [2000]. Available at: http://www3.who.int/whosis. Accessed June 13, 2005.)

The Public Health Burden of Violence

Worldwide, more than 4,500 people each day, on average, die violent deaths.[4] More than 90 percent of these deaths occur in middle- and low-income countries. About one-half of the estimated 1.7 million violent deaths that occurred worldwide in 2000 were suicides, about one-third were homicides, and one fifth were due to war-related injuries. Rates of violent death vary considerably by region, country, and area within countries (fig. 17-1).

The data on violent deaths, however, reflect only a small part of the health and social burden of violence. Violent behaviors, such as suicide attempts, physical and psychological abuse, sexual assault, neglect, acts of war, terrorism, and political violence, are very prevalent in many parts of the world. For example, in some countries nearly 50 percent of children report they have been hit, kicked, or beaten by their parents,[13] and about 20 percent of women and 5 to 10 percent of men report having suffered sexual abuse as children.[14] Similarly, between 10 and 69 percent of women worldwide report that they have been physically assaulted by their male partners at some point.[11]

The physical and mental health consequences of these violent behaviors can persist long after the violence has stopped. These consequences are cumulative as victims experience different types of violence and multiple episodes over time.[11,15,16] Permanently disabling spinal cord and brain injuries, burns, and the losses of limbs, eyesight, and hearing are not uncommon consequences of war, terrorism, and other forms of violence where highly lethal weapons are used.[2,17] Victims of child maltreatment, sexual violence, and intimate partner violence suffer a variety of immediate and long-term health consequences that can profoundly affect their quality of life.[11,12,15,18] Women abused by their partners, for example, are at higher risk of physical injury, depression, suicide attempts, chronic pain syndromes, psychosomatic disorders, gastrointestinal disorders, infertility, sexually transmitted infection, and other consequences.[11] Exposure to maltreatment and other forms of violence during childhood contribute to (a) high-risk behaviors and conditions, such as depression, smoking, obesity, high-risk sexual behaviors, unintended pregnancy, and alcohol and drug use and (b), as a consequence, causes of death, disease, and disability such as heart disease, cancer, suicide, and sexually transmitted diseases.[15] Wars have many of the same consequences as interpersonal violence for the physical and mental health of combatants.[2,19] Modern warfare, however, has had a increasingly devastating effect on civilians, who are specifically targeted or caught in its wake through its adverse impact on nutrition, crowding, sanitary conditions, and availability of medical care[19,20] (box 17-1).

In those nations and communities most heavily affected, violence can have a substantial economic impact.[21] Estimates of the economic impact of violence between acquaintances and strangers in six Latin American countries have ranged from about 5 percent of the 1997 gross domestic product in Peru to almost 25 percent in El Salvador.[22] The subcategories of these costs (table 17-1 on p. 301), although not entirely exclusive or exhaustive, serve to illustrate the magnitude of the economic burden associated with violence. High rates of violence can severely limit the economic growth of countries and regions by increasing the costs of health and security services, diverting funds from socially beneficial activities to nonproductive ones, and threatening the establishment and viability of business.[21]

Social Injustice as a Cause of Violence

The forms of social injustice that often spawn violence can be subdivided into three general categories: (a) the unequal access, distribution, or concentration of economic resources; (b) the influences of cultural norms, beliefs, or attitudes; and (c) the policies and practices of criminal justice, education, social welfare, and political institutions. Empirical research on the links between social injustice and violence is largely derived from cross-sectional and cross-national research, ecological studies, and longitudinal studies. Historical, ethnographic, and qualitative research is a valuable adjunct to these empirical analyses. It is difficult, however, to reach firm conclusions about the

(*text continues on p. 301*)

BOX 17-1 War and Public Health
Barry S. Levy and Victor W. Sidel

An estimated 191 million people died directly or indirectly as a result of conflict during the twentieth century, more than half of whom were civilians.[1] During some wars in the 1990s, as many as 90 percent of the people killed were noncombatants.[2] Many of them were innocent bystanders, caught in the crossfire of opposing armies; others were civilians who were specifically targeted during wars. During each year of the 1990s, there were about 30 to 50 wars, mainly civil wars that are infrequently reported by the news media in the United States. Most of these civil wars have taken place in developing countries. For example, more than 3.8 million people have died during the civil war in Congo in the past several years—and troops from six other African countries have participated in this war.[3] As another example, over 30 years of civil war in Ethiopia have led to the deaths of 1 million people, about half of whom were civilians.[4]

Many people survive wars, only to be physically scarred for life. Millions of survivors are chronically disabled from injuries sustained during wars or the immediate aftermath of wars. Landmines are a particular threat. For example, in Cambodia, 1 in 236 people is an amputee as a result of a landmine explosion.[5] Approximately one-third of the soldiers who survived the civil war in Ethiopia were injured or disabled and at least 40,000 individuals lost one or more limbs during the war.

Millions more are psychologically impaired from wars, during which they have been physically or sexually assaulted; forced to serve as soldiers against their will; witnessed the death of family members; or experienced the destruction of their communities or entire nations. Psychological trauma may be demonstrated in disturbed and antisocial behavior, such as aggression toward others, including family members. Many soldiers suffer from post-traumatic stress disorder (PTSD) on return from military action.[6]

Rape has been used as a weapon in many wars—in Korea, Bangladesh, Algeria, India, Indonesia, Liberia, Rwanda, Uganda, the former Yugoslavia, and elsewhere. As acts of humiliation and revenge, soldiers have raped the female family members of their enemies. For example, at least 10,000 women were raped by military personnel during the war in Bosnia and Herzegovina. The social chaos brought about by war also creates situations and conditions for sexual violence.[7]

Children are particularly vulnerable during and after wars. Many die as a result of malnutrition, disease, or military attacks. Many are physically or psychologically injured. Many are forced to become soldiers themselves or sexual slaves to military officers. Their health suffers in many other ways as

(continued)

well, as reflected by increased infant and young-child mortality rates and decreased rates of immunization coverage.[8]

The infrastructure that supports social well-being and health is destroyed during many wars, so that many civilians do not have access to food, clean water, medical care, or public health services. For example, during the Gulf War in 1991 and in the 12 years of economic sanctions that followed, an estimated 350,000 to 500,000 children died, with most of these deaths due to inadequate nutrition, contaminated water, and shortages of medicines, all of which may be indirectly related to destruction of the infrastructure of civilian society: health care facilities, electricity generating plants, food supply systems, water treatment and sanitation facilities, and transportation and communication systems.[9] The 2003 attack on Iraq by the United States and United Kingdom left much of the infrastructure of the country devastated.

In addition, during wartime many civilians flee to other countries as refugees or become internally displaced persons within their own countries, where it may be difficult for them to maintain their health and safety (see chapter 11). Refugees and internally displaced persons are vulnerable to malnutrition, infectious diseases, injuries, and criminal and military attacks. A substantial number of the approximately 37 million refugees and internally displaced persons in the world today were forced to leave their homes because of war or the threat of war.[10]

War and the preparation for war divert huge amounts of resources from health and human services and other productive societal endeavors.[11] This is true in many countries, including the United States, which ranks first among nations in military expenditures and arms exports but forty-second among nations in infant mortality. In some developing countries, national governments spend the equivalent of US$10 to US$20 per capita on military expenditures but only US$1 per capita on all health-related expenditures. The same type of distorted priorities also exist in more developed countries. For example, in early 2003, at a time when federal, state, and local governments in the United States were experiencing substantial budgetary shortfalls and it was difficult for them to find monies to maintain adequate health and human services, the U.S. Congress allocated more than $70 billion for the war in Iraq.

War often creates a cycle of violence, increasing domestic and community violence in the countries engaged in war. War teaches people that violence is an acceptable method for settling conflicts. Children growing up in environments in which violence is an established way of settling conflicts often choose violence to settle conflicts in their own lives. Teenage gangs mirror the activity of military forces. Men, sometimes former military servicemen who have been trained to use violence, commit acts of violence against women.

Finally, war and the preparation for war have profound impacts on the environment. The disastrous consequences of war for the environment are

(continued)

BOX 17-1 (*continued*)

often clear. Examples include (a) bomb craters in Vietnam that have filled with water and provide breeding areas for mosquitoes that spread malaria and other diseases; (b) destruction of urban environments by aerial carpet bombing of major cities in Europe and Japan during World War II; and (c) the more than 600 oil well fires in Kuwait, which were ignited by retreating Iraqi troops in 1991, that had a devastating effect on the ecology of the affected areas and caused acute respiratory symptoms among those exposed, sometimes many miles away. Less obvious are the environmental impacts of the preparation for war, such as the huge amounts of nonrenewable fossil fuels used by the military before (as well as during and after) wars and the environmental hazards of toxic and radioactive wastes, which can contaminate air, soil, and both surface water and groundwater. For example, much of the area in and around Chelyabinsk, Russia, the site of a major nuclear weapons production facility, has been determined to be highly radioactive and residents there have been evacuated.[12]

In the early twenty-first century, new geopolitical, tactical, and technological issues concerning war are arising that have an impact on health, law, and ethics. These issues include the use of new weapons; the increasing use in guerilla warfare (and terrorism) of suicide, or "homicide," bombers; the use of drone (unmanned) aircraft and high-altitude bombers; and newly adopted United States policies on "preemptive" wars and on "first-use" of nuclear weapons.

References

1. Rummel RJ. *Death by Government: Genocide and Mass Murder since 1900*. New Brunswick, NJ, and London: Transaction Publications, 1994.
2. Ahlstram C. *Casualties of Conflict: Report for the Protection of Victims of War*. Uppsala, Sweden: Department of Peace and Conflict Research, Uppsala University, 1991.
3. Coghlan B, Brennan R, Ngoy P, et al. Mortality in the Democratic Republic of Congo: results from a nationwide survey. New York, N.Y.: International Rescue Committee and Burnet Institute, 2004.
4. Kloos H. Health impacts of war in Ethiopia. Disasters 1992;16:347–354.
5. Stover E, Keller AS, Cobey J, et al. The medical and social consequences of land mines in Cambodia. JAMA 1994;272:331–336.
6. Kanter E. Post-traumatic stress disorders. In: Levy BS, Wagner GR, Rest KM, Weeks JL, eds. *Preventing Occupational Disease and Injury*. 2nd ed. Washington, DC: American Public Health Association, 2005:410–413.
7. Ashford MW, Huet-Vaugn Y. The impact of war on women. In: Levy BS, Sidel VW, eds. *War and Public Health*. New York, NY: Oxford University Press, 1997:186–196.
8. Machel G. *Impact of Armed Conflict on Children*. New York, NY: UNICEF, 1996.
9. Hoskins E. Public health and the Persian Gulf War. In: Levy BS, Sidel VW, eds. *War and Public Health*. New York, NY: Oxford University Press, 1997:254–278.

(*continued*)

10. Cranna M, ed. *The True Cost of Conflict.* London: Earthscan and Saferworld, 1994.
11. Levy BS, Sidel VW. The impact of military activities on civilian populations. In: Levy BS, Sidel VW, eds. *War and Public Health.* New York, NY: Oxford University Press, 1997:149–167.
12. Levy BS, Sidel VW. War. In: Frumkin H, ed. *Environmental Health: From Global to Local.* San Francisco, Calif: Jossey-Bass, 2005:269–287.

relationship between social injustice and violence because violent behavior, in whatever form it takes, is caused by a complex interaction among a broad range of biological, psychological, social, economic, and political factors. Moreover, research into some of these dimensions of social injustice is very limited.

The Influence of Economic Forms of Social Injustice

To varying degrees, economic resources are unequally distributed in every nation, but the mere presence of this unequal distribution does not constitute social injustice. Social injustice arises when an individual or a group takes advantage of their power to economically exploit another individual or group, or when the unequal distribution of resources interferes with the ability of individuals or groups to meet their basic human needs.

Economic Exploitation

Economic exploitation is associated with violence when an individual (or a group) uses force or his or her (its) greater power to (1) misappropriate the funds

TABLE 17-1   Economic Costs of Social Violence* in Six Latin American Countries (Expressed as Percentage of 1997 Gross Domestic Product)

	Brazil	Columbia	El Salvador	Mexico	Peru	Venezula
Health losses[†]	1.9	5.0	4.3	1.3	1.5	0.3
Material losses[‡]	3.6	8.4	5.1	4.9	2.0	9.0
Intangibles[§]	3.4	6.9	11.5	3.3	1.0	2.2
Transfers[¶]	1.6	4.4	4.0	2.8	0.6	0.3
Total	10.5	24.7	24.9	12.3	5.1	11.8

*For the purposes of this table, social violence is defined as violence that occurs between acquaintances and strangers.
[†]Expenditures on health services incurred as a result of the violence.
[‡]Private and public expenditures on police, security systems, and judicial services.
[§]Amount that citizens would be willing to pay to live without violence.
[¶]Value of goods lost in robberies, ransoms paid to kidnappers, and bribes paid as a result of extortion.

(From Buvinic M, Morrison A, Shifter M. Technical study: violence in Latin America and the Caribbean: a framework for action. Washington, D.C.: Inter-American Development Bank, 1999.)

or resources of another person or group, or (2) force another person or group to engage in behavior that economically benefits the perpetrator of the violence.

Robbery is taking, or attempting to take, anything of value from another person by force, by the threat of force, or by putting the victim in fear.[23] It is an example of using violence to misappropriate the economic resources of another person. In the early 1990s, the annual prevalence of robbery victimization was about 7 percent for residents of cities in sub-Saharan Africa, about 5 percent in Latin-American cities, and almost 1.5 percent in Asian cities.[24] In 1999, the prevalence of robbery victimization in industrialized countries was highest in Poland (1.8 percent), Australia (1.2 percent), England and Wales (1.2 percent), Portugal (1.1 percent), and France (1.1 percent), and lowest in Japan and Northern Ireland (0.1 percent).[25]

Sexual trafficking is a graphic example of economic exploitation associated with violence. Every day, women and girls throughout the world are bought and sold into prostitution and sexual slavery.[18] The U.S. Central Intelligence Agency estimated that 45,000 to 50,000 women and children are trafficked to the United States each year.[26] Women and children are often forced into participation through physical assaults, rape, and threats of violence; working as a prostitute is associated with a high risk of violence-related injury.[27] The estimated annual occurrence of violence to prostituted children throughout the world is 2.5 million physical assaults, 2.5 million rapes, and 6,900 homicides.[27] Fifty percent of persons trafficked out of Kyrgyzstan reported being physically abused or tortured by their employers.[28] (See box 21-1 on p. 382.)

Poverty and Relative Deprivation

Poverty is consistently found to have a strong and positive correlation with interpersonal violence, especially homicide.[29] However, when other community factors distinct from, but related to, poverty are controlled, this association is substantially weakened, suggesting that the effect of poverty on interpersonal violence may be conditional on other factors. These factors include community change associated with high residential mobility, concentrations of poverty, family disruption, high population density, and community disorganization, as reflected in weak intergenerational family and community ties, weak control of peer groups, and low participation in community organizations.[30,31] Poorer communities and their residents appear to be most vulnerable to interpersonal violence when exposed to fundamental economic and population changes that lead to community disorganization that, in turn, undermines their ability to exert social control over violent behavior. In the United States, for example, the shift from goods-producing industries to service-producing industries—and the associated relocation of manufacturing industries out of the inner cities—is a fundamental change that has been linked to the problem of inner-city violence.[32] Similarly, rapid population growth and related economic tensions in Algeria, Senegal, and elsewhere in Africa have been found to be associated with increases in youth violence.[33–35]

Relative deprivation, which refers to the magnitude of the gap between the rich and the poor in a society or community, is typically measured by examining economic inequality. Income inequality is strongly related to homicide rates.[36,37] Extreme social and economic inequalities, especially those between—rather than within—distinct population groups have also been hypothesized to be risk factors for collective violence.[2]

An extension of this concept involves the geographic concentration of economic deprivation. It has been argued that in the United States, beginning in the 1960s, many inner-city communities became increasingly isolated islands of poverty as middle- and working-class residents moved out of ghetto communities into areas with better housing and job opportunities.[32] The exodus of more economically stable families from inner cities undermined the viability of basic community institutions, such as churches and schools, that served as social buffers against violence. The resulting concentration of poverty isolated primarily African-American, inner-city residents from job networks, a pool of available marriage partners, quality schools, and conventional role models. This form of relative deprivation has led to a high concentration of those very factors that are highly associated with poverty and strongly related to interpersonal violence—residential instability, family disruption, and community disorganization.[29–31] Recent research has supported the theory that the concentration of poverty and the imbalance between concentrations of affluence and poverty in a neighborhood are important predictors of community variations in interpersonal violence.[38]

The Influence of Cultural Forms of Injustice

Culture embodies the shared beliefs, values, customs, symbols, and behaviors that members of a society "use to cope with the world and with each other, and that are transmitted from generation to generation through learning" (pp. 3–4).[39] The cultural context plays an important role in both contributing to and protecting people from violent behavior. Cultural sources of injustice are often very entrenched in societies because they are rationalized by a body of shared knowledge and beliefs that most members of a society accept, sometimes without question. Several aspects of culture contribute toward unjust and violent treatment of specific social groups, such as women, children, and members of racial and ethnic minority groups.

Hate-Motivated Violence

Hate-motivated violence consists of acts of interpersonal or collective violence that are directed toward other people, property, or organizations because of the group to which they belong or identify with.[40] These forms of violence are most commonly perpetrated against individuals or groups based on race, ethnicity, religion, and sexual orientation. Motivations for hate-related violence often emerge from cultural beliefs and attitudes that foster negative stereotypes. However, these beliefs and attitudes are often supported or exacerbated by political or economic conflicts between or among groups, such as between the Palestinians and Israelis or among immigrant groups competing in tight job markets.

Hate-related violence has a long tradition in the United States. It is perhaps best exemplified by the lynching of African-Americans by both organized groups, such as the Ku Klux Klan, and unorganized lynch mobs, which escalated following the Civil War and Reconstruction.[41] Other groups have also been targets of hate-related violence in the United States. Surveys conducted between 1988 and 1991 indicated that from 9 to 24 percent of gay respondents reported that they had been punched, hit, or kicked because of their sexual orientation.[42] Moreover, between 37 and 45 percent of gay respondents reported they had received threats of physical violence because of their sexual orientation.[42] In the 10 days following the terrorist attacks on New York and Washington on September 11, 2001, violent attacks on people of Middle Eastern descent or those perceived to be of Middle Eastern descent escalated dramatically in the United States (fig. 17-2).[43]

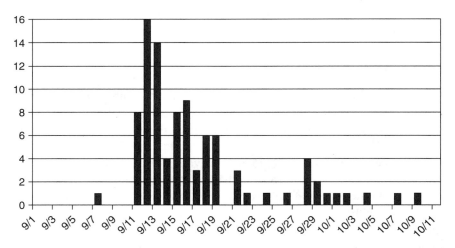

Figure 17-2 Hate-related violent attacks on Middle Easterners, United States, September 1–October 11, 2001. (From Swahn MH, Mahendra RR, Paulozzi LJ, et al. Violent attacks on Middle Easterners in the United States during the month following the September 11, 2001 terrorist attacks. Injury Prevent 2003;9:187–189. Reproduced with permission from the BMJ Publishing Group.)

Military actions whose primary purpose is to forcefully displace groups from their homelands based on their religious, ethnic, or national identity are a collective manifestation of hate-related violence. The wars and associated "ethnic cleansing" in the former Yugoslavia and Rwanda are recent examples. In these conflicts, the tools of ethnic cleansing were the torture and murder of noncombatant men, women, and children; the systematic use of rape to terrorize communities; the destruction of residences, farms, industries, and basic infrastructures that supply water, power, food, sanitation, and other necessities; denial of medical care; and interference with humanitarian relief efforts.[44] Other examples of "ethnic cleansing" that have received less public attention have occurred in Sri Lanka, East Timor, Armenia and Azerbaijan, Ossetia and Georgia, China and Tibet, and Iraq and Kurdistan.[44] (See box 17-2.)

Gender Inequality

Gender inequality has many faces. For example, cultural traditions that favor male over female children, early marriage for girls, male sexual entitlement, and female "purity" place women and girls in a subordinate position relative to men and make them highly vulnerable to violent victimization.[45,46] More subtle cultural attitudes and beliefs about female roles may also contribute to violence and exist, to varying degrees, in every part of the world.[47] An ethnographic study of wife-beating in 90 societies concluded that it occurs most often in societies where men hold the household economic and decision-making power, where divorce is difficult for women to obtain, and where violence is a common conflict resolution tactic.[48] Rape is also more common in societies where cultural traditions favoring male superiority are strong[49] (see chapter 4).

Maintaining the sexual "purity" of girls is a powerful cultural value that is associated with violence in many parts of the world. Female genital mutilation, for example, is a practice usually performed on girls before puberty in many parts of Africa, some Middle Eastern countries, and immigrant communities around the world.[50] An estimated 80 to 135 million women and girls worldwide have undergone female genital mutilation.[50,51] Within the societies that practice it, female genital mutilation is considered essential to make a woman eligible for marriage because it is believed to reduce her desire for sex and, therefore, the likelihood that she will have sex before she is married or later outside of marriage.[51] "Honor killings," another extreme outcome of cultural traditions found mainly in Middle Eastern and south Asian countries, occur when a female is killed by her own family after her virginity or faithfulness has been brought into question because of, for example, infidelity or rape.[45,52] Data on this phenomenon are very limited, but a study of homicides in Alexandria, Egypt, found that 47 percent of female victims were killed by a relative after they had been raped by another person.[52]

Genocide, also known in recent years as ethnic cleansing, is by far the most far-reaching and despicable form of social injustice. In one of its first actions after its formation, the General Assembly of the United Nations on December 11, 1946, declared that genocide is a crime under international law.[1] The term was defined in 1948 in the Convention on the Prevention and Punishment of the Crime of Genocide: "Genocide means any of the following acts committed with intent to destroy, in whole or in part, a national, ethnical, racial or religious group, as such:

1. Killing members of the group;
2. Causing serious bodily or mental harm to members of the group;
3. Deliberately inflicting on the group conditions of life calculated to bring about its physical destruction in whole or in part;
4. Imposing measures intended to prevent births within the group;
5. Forcibly transferring children of the group to another group."[2]

Examples of events that are widely considered to constitute genocide include the killing of an estimated 1 million Armenians in Turkey in 1915; the killing of 6 million Jews in Germany and occupied countries during World War II; the killing of 800,000 Tutsis and Hutus in Rwanda and Burundi in 1944; the "ethnic cleansing" of ethnic Albanians in Kosovo in 1999; and the killing of an estimated 80,000 Muslims in Darfur in the Sudan in 2004. In Kosovo, military intervention authorized by the United Nations was used to stop the killing. In Rwanda, there was no effective intervention. As this box is being prepared, it is not clear whether military intervention will be used in Darfur.

   The United Nations has permitted intervention in extraordinary humanitarian emergencies, including the use of armed force. Intervention in Kuwait in 1991 to force the withdrawal of Iraqi troops and in Kosovo in 1999 to prevent ethnic cleansing of ethnic Albanians are examples of military intervention authorized by the United Nations that have been widely accepted. On the other hand, the United States and other developed countries, as well as the United Nations itself, have been criticized for not intervening in Rwanda in 1994. Beginning in 2003, as Human Rights Watch reported in 2004, the government of Sudan has been responsible for ethnic cleansing and other crimes against humanity in Darfur, one of the world's poorest and most inaccessible regions on Sudan's western border with Chad. The Sudanese government and the Arab militias it arms and supports have committed numerous attacks on the civilian population. Government forces have

(continued)

directly participating in massacres; summary executions of civilians, including women and children; burning of towns and villages; and the forcible de-population of wide areas long inhabited by Muslim populations.[3] Other groups have alleged that the reports have been exaggerated and that the presence of oil reserves in the region would be the driving force for outside military intervention.[4]

Debate continues not only about the clear documentation of genocide or ethnic cleansing but also about the authority of United Nations or of individual countries to intervene when a government that is involved in or has permitted severe, life-threatening, social injustice refuses to permit outside intervention to protect the population threatened. The question those concerned with response to social injustice of this magnitude must consider is whether military intervention is acceptable when the injustice is so great that the dangerous consequences of armed intervention pale in comparison. One of the problems lies in the "preemptive" attack on Iraq by the United States and the United Kingdom, which may have created such a backlash against unwarranted and unauthorized military interven-tion that no effective response to severe humanitarian emergencies will be possible. Military intervention may be justified under emergency circum-stances if there were strict adherence to certain conditions, such as prompt use of nonmilitary intervention to attempt to correct the problem; preauthorization of military intervention by the United Nations Security Council; imposition of a strict deadline and conditions for the withdrawal of the interveners; and a plan for prompt restoration of representative government.

References

1. The crime of genocide. United Nations General Assembly Resolution. 1946:96, December 11, 1946.
2. Convention on the prevention and punishment of the crime of genocide, article 2, General Assembly resolution 260A(III). New York, N.Y.: Office of the UN High Commissioner for Human Rights, December 9, 1948. Available at: http://www.unhchr.ch/. Accessed January 25, 2005.
3. Darfur destroyed: ethnic cleansing by government and militia forces in western Sudan. Human Rights Watch, 2004. Available at: http://www.hrw.org/reports/2004/sudan0504. Accessed January 25, 2005.
4. Laughland J. The mask of altruism disguising a colonial war: oil will be the driving factor for military intervention in Sudan. The Guardian (UK), August 2, 2004.
5. Power S. A problem from hell: America and the age of genocide. New York, N.Y.: Basic Books, 2002.

The cultural preference for male children is associated with high levels of female infanticide in China, some Middle Eastern countries, and India.[53] In China, the preference for sons is particularly strong in rural areas, where traditional cultural beliefs have their strongest hold.[54] It has also been suggested that the "one couple, one child" policy in China may have exacerbated the problem of female infanticide.[54,55]

Suicidal behavior can be both a direct and an indirect consequence of cultural traditions that support male dominance. As an indirect consequence, women exposed to intimate partner violence are at greater risk of suicidal behavior.[11] The subordination of women has also been more directly linked to high rates of suicidal behavior, particularly among women in their childbearing years.[53] In India and Nepal, for example, culturally related phenomena, such as dowry disputes and arranged marriages, have been linked with suicidal behavior among young women.[45] In China, young rural women are at particularly high risk of suicide; their rates are 66 percent higher than rates among young rural men.[56] Low status, limited opportunities, and exposure to various forms of domestic violence may partially explain their elevated rates.[57]

The Influence of Institutional Forms of Social Injustice

Social injustice often becomes incorporated into the policies and operations of key social institutions. Legal institutions, for example, can become tools of social injustice when a society creates laws that deny human rights or civil liberties to a specific social group. Violence can erupt as a response to institutionalized injustice or may be used to suppress opposition to it.

Political Repression

History is replete with examples of governments that have used their military and police powers to systematically repress their own citizens. El Salvador provides a graphic illustration of the devastating effects that violent political repression can have on a nation's population. After coming to power through a military coup in 1979, the Salvadoran government began to use its military forces to violently suppress efforts on the part of peasants and labor activists to improve living and working conditions.[58] During a civil war that lasted from 1980 through 1992, about 70,000 (mostly unarmed) people were killed by government forces and their allied death squads.[59] Torture was an officially sanctioned policy of the Salvadoran government forces and was widely used on rebel combatants and their suspected supporters.[58] The political repression and associated war in El Salvador have had broad and long-lasting effects on the health and welfare of the population.[58] Similar scenarios have played out in many other places over the past few decades, including

Argentina, Brazil, Chile, Colombia, Ethiopia, Guatemala, Haiti, Kashmir, Nicaragua, the Philippines, and South Africa.[44]

There may be a relationship between the type of government and violent political repression that is affected by the ability of a government to respond to threats to its regime by opposition groups.[60] Democratic governments are less prone to repression because threats can be politically channeled through the more widely available official and legitimate avenues for voicing and organizing dissent and the greater accountability of political leaders to voters.[60,61] Moreover, the system of checks and balances in democracies makes it difficult to organize institutions of the state for repression. In general, autocracies also have low levels of violent political repression because demands by opposition groups are muted by the existence of state institutions that can be easily mobilized to carry out repressive actions. Governments that have intermediate levels of democracy are the most likely to engage in violent political repression because they tend to lack the institutional mechanisms for (a) addressing demands by those in opposition that exist in mature democracies, or (b) deterring opposition, as in the case of autocracies.[60]

The Unfair Distribution of Justice

Criminal justice institutions—police, courts, and correctional agencies— in any society are responsible for apprehending, adjudicating, and punishing people who break the law. As part of this responsibility, they also enforce the norms of social justice that are encoded into the law. In many ways, criminal justice institutions, therefore, are a society's first line of defense against social injustice. The manner in which these institutions carry out these responsibilities has important implications for both social injustice and violence.

The ability of a state to provide social protection to its citizens is associated with violence. The presence of strong national institutions for social protection is negatively associated with homicide.[62] Having inefficient—or even corrupt—criminal justice institutions may not constitute social injustice, but these inefficiencies can contribute to situations in which citizens take the responsibility for justice into their own hands. In Brazil, for example, support for efforts to have "undesirable" children and adolescents eliminated through death squads, lynchings, and other forms of violence is related to widespread perceptions that the justice system does not work and that police are inefficient and corrupt.[63] Similarly, in postapartheid South Africa, impunity from human rights abuses and the inability of police to change their methods may have contributed to generalized feelings of insecurity and an increasing number of extrajudicial actions involving violence.[64] Another way in which criminal justice institutions may contribute to social injustice and violence is through the use of force by police. Over the past century, most civil disturbances occurring in the United States were initiated or exacerbated by the perception that police had inappropriately used deadly force.[65,66]

What Needs to Be Done

The relationship between social injustice and violence is embedded within the broader issues of political and economic development and the clash between traditional and modern culture. Interventions to reduce social injustice that contribute to violence will necessitate that public health professionals extend their attention and influence far beyond what has traditionally been considered their appropriate realm. To prevent violence, we must become more creative than simply calling for reductions in poverty, for greater democracy, and for the enforcement of human rights. While these are all laudable goals, their attainment requires strategies that are grounded in science and that are practical, given the clear constraints and obstacles to progress in these areas. Fortunately, there are some promising directions toward which public health efforts could be directed that have health and social benefits extending beyond violence prevention. These directions all require more thorough scientific assessment, engagement with partners in other sectors, and a sustained effort.

Increasing the Cost of Injustice

Where behavior is influenced, even, in part, by economic considerations, increasing the cost of that behavior may be an effective primary prevention strategy. Increases, for example, in the price of beer and alcohol have been found to be associated with lower consumption and small decreases in wife abuse (3.1 to 3.5 percent) and child maltreatment (1.2 percent).[67,68] Because the primary motivation for sexual trafficking is economic gain, strategies to increase the cost of trafficking may be useful in reducing its profitability and, hence, its frequency. Public health professionals, working together with human rights organizations, could be of help by conducting research to make the case for more effective law enforcement intervention and use of media advocacy or social marketing strategies to bring greater attention to the problem and greater pressure on policymakers to address it.

An innovative approach to media advocacy on the issue of trafficking of women and children is illustrated by WITNESS, an organization that uses video and other communication technology, in partnership with local activists, to expose human rights abuses and mobilize public concern.[69] Its advocacy has been used in Thailand, Malaysia, Indonesia, the Philippines, Taiwan, the United States, and Vietnam to encourage policymakers to enact legislation based on human rights standards that will help to increase the costs and reduce the frequency of trafficking by, among other things, fully engaging law enforcement agencies in bringing those that engage in this business to justice.

Deconcentrating Poverty

The high geographic concentration and social isolation of poor people compound many problems that contribute to interpersonal and, potentially, collective violence. Interventions and policies that seek to deconcentrate poverty by dispersing poor people within more economically and socially heterogeneous communities may help to reduce their isolation from jobs, positive role models, marriage partners, and good schools. For example, one evaluation of a housing voucher program in the United States, in which public housing tenants are given vouchers they can use to rent housing in the private market in any location, found that enabling families to move from public housing complexes into neighborhoods with lower levels of poverty substantially reduced violence by adolescents.[70] A systematic review of evaluations of the effects of housing voucher programs found them to also be effective in reducing violent victimization and property crime.[71] Efforts to reduce the inequalities that are exacerbated by extreme concentrations of poverty may be among the most powerful strategies for preventing violence and the economic injustice that underlies it.

Reducing Social Distance

Hate-motivated violence appears to flourish in societies and communities where racially or ethnically distinct groups hold dearly to negative beliefs and stereotypes about each other. The occurrence of this type of violence may be associated with the social distance that separates such groups.[72] The greater the social distance, as reflected, for example, in the frequency of interaction, the level of functional independence, and degree of cultural disparity between two groups, the greater is the frequency and severity of collective violence.[73] One study attempting to explain the presence and absence of communal violence between Hindus and Muslims in India provides support for this theory.[74] The findings suggest that the presence of strong associational forms of civic engagement, such as integrated business organizations, trade unions, political parties, and professional associations, appears to protect against outbreaks of ethnic violence. In relatively peaceful communities, the existence of these forms of association created a context that essentially reduced the social distance between these ethnic groups. In those settings, violence came to be seen as a threat to business and political interests that were shared across ethnic groups, thereby increasing the motivation to nip in the bud rumors, small clashes, and tensions, rather than to let them fester.[74] Consequently, interventions and policies that support the creation and maintenance of formal mechanisms of association between social groups, otherwise at odds with one another, may be a useful tool in the prevention of collective violence, particularly where conflicting groups are in close geographic proximity.

Redefining Harmful Cultural Norms

Cultural norms undergo change, which can be promoted and even accelerated. Norms associated with smoking and drunk driving in the United States, for example, have undergone substantial changes over the past several decades. Although harmful traditions associated with gender inequality are, in many ways, qualitatively different from smoking- and drinking-related norms, efforts to alter them are nevertheless possible. For example, the Reproductive, Education, and Community Health Program in the Kapchorwa District of Uganda has reportedly been successful in reducing rates of female genital mutilation by enlisting the support of elders in incorporating alternatives to this practice that are consistent with their original cultural traditions.[75] Approaches to influencing social norms that are based on reinforcing sentiments or beliefs within a population that run counter to a harmful norm have been successful in reducing alcohol abuse on some college campuses and have been suggested for addressing sexual assault.[76,77] Public health programs along these lines in traditional societies must be approached with extreme sensitivity, given the passionate attachment to traditions that often exists.[10] However, these programs, which can be implemented in ways that are sensitive to cultural traditions and are likely to reduce harm, may be met with broader support than anticipated.

Strengthening Democratic Institutions

Given the possible horrendous public health impact of political repression, public health professionals and organizations should have a greater voice in preventing it. Primary prevention in this realm should include the creation and support of stable democratic institutions. Cross-national research suggests that the probability of violent political repression is greatest in nations that are in transition from autocratic to democratic regimes—that is, in "semi-democracies" (p. 120).[60] An important reason for this finding may be that in these semi-democracies, the institutional framework for responding to public demands and addressing threats from opposition groups is typically insufficient.[61] A focus on assisting semi-democracies in the development of institutions, such as political party systems, mechanisms for the peaceful transfer of power, and service systems that address basic human needs, may be the most useful for preventing repression.[60] Public health professionals, in collaboration with political scientists, can play an important role in using science to further understand how best to prevent political repression and bringing these strategies to the attention of policymakers. Furthermore, assistance to semi-democracies in strengthening public health services may help to forestall conditions that could contribute to political repression.

Conclusion

Social injustice is fundamentally related to the problem of violence. Although we can only guess at the proportion of the health burden of violence attributable to social injustice, it is clearly enormous. Yet public health has been reluctant to address social determinants of health.[78] If public health professionals are to have a tangible and sustained impact on violence worldwide, they must begin to more forthrightly address social injustice as a root of violence. The science of public health has much to contribute. New partnerships will be critical to the success of these efforts.[78] Most exciting of all, explicit recognition of the role that social injustice plays in violence opens up many new frontiers for prevention. All of this should be no surprise to those of us who work in public health because, as Dr. William Foege, former director of the Centers for Disease Control and Prevention, observed, "At its base, the practice of public health is the search for social justice" (p. 11).[79]

References

1. Heise L. Violence against women: an integrated ecological framework. Violence Against Women 1998;4:262–90.
2. Zwi AB, Garfield R, Loretti A. Collective violence. In: Krug E, Dahlberg LL, Mercy JA, et al, eds. World report on violence and health. Geneva, Switzerland: World Health Organization, 2002:213–9.
3. World Health Assembly. Prevention of violence: public health priority (WHA 49,25). Geneva, Switzerland: World Health Organization, 1996.
4. Krug E, Dahlberg LL, Mercy JA, et al., eds. World report on violence and health. Geneva, Switzerland: World Health Organization, 2002.
5. Mercy JA, Rosenberg ML, Powell KE, et al. Public health policy for preventing violence. Health Affairs 1993;12:7–29.
6. U.S. Department of Health and Human Services. Youth violence: a report of the Surgeon General. Rockville, Md.: U.S. Department of Health and Human Services, Centers for Disease Control and Prevention, National Center for Injury Prevention and Control, Substance Abuse and Mental Health Services Administration, Center for Mental Health Services, and National Institutes of Health, National Institute of Mental Health, 2001.
7. Abad GH. Violence requires epidemiological studies. Trib Med 1962;2:1–12.

8. U.S. Department of Health, Education, and Welfare. Healthy people: the Surgeon General's report on health promotion and disease prevention. Washington, D.C.: U.S. Government Printing Office (DHEW [PHS] publication no. 79-55071).

9. Mercy JA, O'Carroll PW. New directions in violence prediction: the public health arena. Violence Victims 1988;3:285–301.

10. Dahlberg LL, Krug EG. Violence—a global public health problem. In: Krug E, Dahlberg LL, Mercy JA, et al, eds. World report on violence and health. Geneva, Switzerland: World Health Organization, 2002:3–21.

11. Heise L, Garcia-Moreno C. Violence by intimate partners. In: Krug E, Dahlberg LL, Mercy JA, et al, eds. World report on violence and health. Geneva, Switzerland: World Health Organization, 2002:213–39.

12. Runyan D, Wattam C, Ikeda R, et al. Child abuse and neglect by parents and other caregivers. In: Krug E, Dahlberg LL, Mercy JA, et al, eds. World report on violence and health. Geneva, Switzerland: World Health Organization, 2002:213–39.

13. Hahm HC, Guterman NB. The emerging problem of physical child abuse in South Korea. Child Maltreatment 2001;6:169–79.

14. Finkelhor D. The international epidemiology of child sexual abuse. Child Abuse Neglect 1994;18:409–17.

15. Felitti VJ, Anda RF, Nordenberg D, et al. Relationship of childhood abuse and household dysfunction to many of the leading causes of death in adults. The Adverse Childhood Experiences (ACE) Study. Am J Prevent Med 1998;14:245–58.

16. Follete V, Polusny MA, Bechtle AE, et al. Cumulative trauma: the impact of child sexual abuse, adult sexual assault, and spouse abuse. J Traumatic Stress 1996;9:25–35.

17. Cukier W, Chapdelaine A. Small arms, explosives, and incendiaries. In: Levy BS, Sidel VW, eds. Terrorism and public health. Oxford, England: Oxford University Press, 2003:155–74.

18. Jewkes R, Sen P, Garcia-Moreno C. Sexual violence. In: Krug E, Dahlberg LL, Mercy JA, et al, eds. World report on violence and health. Geneva, Switzerland: World Health Organization, 2002:213–39.

19. Garfield RM, Neugut AI. The human consequences of war. In: Levy BS, Sidel VW, eds. War and public health. Washington, D.C.: American Public Health Association, 2000:27–38.

20. Levy BS, Sidel VW. The impact of military activities on civilian populations. In: Levy BS, Sidel VW, eds. War and public health. Washington, D.C.: American Public Health Association, 2000:149–67.

21. Mercy JA, Krug EG, Dahlberg LL, et al. Violence and health: the United States in a global perspective. Am J Public Health 2003;93:256–61.

22. Buvinic M, Morrison A, Shifter M. Technical study: violence in Latin America and the Caribbean: a framework for action. Washington, D.C.: Inter-American Development Bank, 1999.

23. Federal Bureau of Investigation. Crime in the United States 2000. Washington, D.C.: U.S. Department of Justice, 2001.

24. Zvekic U, Alvazzi del Frate A. Criminal victimization in the developing world. Rome, Italy: United Nations Interregional Crime and Justice Research Institute, 1995 (publication no. 55).

25. van Kesteren J, Mayhew P, Nieuwbeerta P. Criminal victimization in seventeen industrialized countries: key findings from the 2000 International Crime Victims Survey. The Hague, Netherlands: Research and Documentation Centre of the Dutch Ministry of Justice, 2001 (publication no. 187).

26. Richard AO. International trafficking in women to the United States: a contemporary manifestation of slavery and organized crime. Washington, D.C.: Center for the Study of Intelligence, 1999.

27. Willis BM, Levy BS. Child prostitution: global health burden, research needs, and interventions. Lancet 2002;359:1417–22.

28. Chauzy JP. Kyrgyz Republic: trafficking. Geneva, Switzerland: International Organization for Migration, January 20, 2001 (press briefing notes).

29. Sampson RJ, Lauritsen JL. Violent victimization and offending: Individual-, situational-, and community-level risk factors. In: Reiss AJ, Roth JA, eds. Understanding and preventing violence, vol 3, social influences. Washington, D.C.: National Academy Press, 1994:1–114.

30. Reiss AJ, Roth JA, eds. Understanding and preventing violence. Washington, D.C.: National Academy Press, 1993.

31. Sampson RJ, Raudenbush S, Earls F. Neighborhoods and violent crime: a multilevel study of collective efficacy. Science 1997;277:918–24.

32. Wilson WJ. The truly disadvantaged: the inner city, the underclass, and public policy. Chicago, Ill.: University of Chicago Press, 1987.

33. Lauras-Loch T, Lopez-Escartin N. Jeunesse et démographie en Afrique. [Youth and demography in Africa]. In: d'Almeida-Topor H, et al., eds. Les Jeunes en Afrique: Évolution et rôle (XIXe-XXe siècles) [Youth in Africa: its evolution and role (19th and 20th centuries)]. Paris, France: L'Harmattan, 1992:66–82.

34. Diallo Co-Trung M. La crise scolaire au Sénégal: crise de l'école, crise de l'autorité? [The school crisis in Senegal: a school crisis or crisis of authority]. In: d'Almeida-Topor H, et al, eds. Les Jeunes en Afrique: Évolution et rôle (XIXe-XXe siècles) [Youth in Africa: its evolution and role (19th and 20th centuries)]. Paris, France: L'Harmattan, 1992:407–39.

35. Rarrbo K. L'Algérie et sa Jeunesse: Marginalisations sociales et désarroi culturel. [Algeria and its youth: social marginalization and cultural confusion]. Paris, France: L'Harmattan, 1995.

36. Fajnzylber P, Lederman D, Loayza N. Inequality and violent crime. J Law Economics 2002;45:1–40.

37. Gartner R. The victims of homicide: a temporal and cross-national comparison. Am Sociol Rev 1990;55:92–106.

38. Morenoff J, Sampson RJ, Raudenbush SW. Neighborhood inequality, collective efficacy, and the spatial dynamics of urban violence. Criminology 2001;39:517–60.

39. Bates DG, Fratkin EM. Cultural anthropology. New York, N.Y.: Allyn and Bacon, 2003.

40. American Psychological Association. Hate crimes today: an age-old foe in modern dress. Washington, D.C.: American Psychological Association, 1998.

41. Brown RM. The American vigilante tradition. In: Graham HD, Gurr TR, eds. Violence in America: historical and comparative perspectives. Beverly Hills, Calif.: Sage Publications, 1979:153–85.

42. Berrill KT. Anti-gay violence and victimization in the United States: an overview. In: Herek GM, Berrill KT, eds. Hate crimes: confronting violence against lesbians and gay men. Newbury Park, Calif.: Sage Publications, 1992:19–45.

43. Swahn MH, Mahendra RR, Paulozzi LJ, et al. Violent attacks on Middle Easterners in the United States during the month following the September 11, 2001 terrorist attacks. Injury Prevent 2003;9:187–9.

44. Geiger HJ. The impact of war on human rights. In: Levy BS, Sidel VW, eds. War and public health. Washington, D.C.: American Public Health Association, 2000:39–50.

45. Hayward RF. Breaking the earthenware jar: lessons from South Asia to end violence against women and girls. Kathmandu, Nepal: UNICEF, 2000.

46. Bennet L, Manderson L, Astbury J. Mapping a global pandemic: review of current literature on rape, sexual assault and sexual harassment of women. Melbourne, Australia: University of Melbourne, 2000.

47. Dobash RE, Dobash RP. Violence against wives: a case against the patriarchy. New York, N.Y.: Free Press, 1979.

48. Levinson D. Family violence in a cross-cultural perspective. Thousand Oaks, Calif.: Sage Publications, 1989.

49. Sanday P. The socio-cultural context of rape: a cross-cultural study. J Soc Issues 1981; 37:5–27.

50. Hosken F. The Hosken report: genital and sexual mutilation of females. Lexington, Mass.: Women's International Network, 1993.

51. Walker A, Parmar P. Warrior marks: females genital mutilation and the sexual blinding of women. New York, N.Y.: Harcourt Brace & Company, 1993.

52. Mercy JA, Abdel Megid LAM, Salem EM, et al. Intentional injuries. In: Mashaly AY, Graitcer PL, Youssef ZM, eds. Injury in Egypt. Cairo, Egypt: United States Agency for International Development, 1993 (PASA no. 263-0102-P-HI-1013-00; project no. E-17-C).

53. Reza A, Mercy JA, Krug EG. The epidemiology of violent deaths in the world. Injury Prevent 2001;7:104–11.

54. United Nations Centre for Human Rights. Harmful traditional practices affecting the health of women and children. Geneva, Switzerland: United Nations High Commission for Human Rights, 1996 (fact sheet no. 23).

55. Johnson K. The politics of the revival of infant abandonment in China, with special reference to Hunan. Population Dev Rev 1996;22:77–99.

56. Phillips MR, Xianyun L, Yanping Z. Suicide rates in China, 1995–99. Lancet 2002; 359:835–40.

57. Heise L, Raikes A, Watts CH, et al. Violence against women: a neglected health issue in less developed countries. Soc Sci Med 1994;39:1165–71.

58. Braveman P, Meyers A, Schlenker T, et al. Public health and war in Central America. In: Levy BS, Sidel VW, eds. War and public health. Washington, D.C.: American Public Health Association, 2000:238–53.

59. Instituto de Derechos Humanos de la Universidad de Centroamerica. La Salud en tiempos de guerra. Estudios Centroamericanos 1991;46:653–71.

60. Regan PM, Henderson EA. Democracy, threats and political repression in developing countries: are democracies internally less violent? Third World Q 2002;23:119–139.

61. Davenport C. Multi-dimensional threat perception and state repression: an inquiry into why states apply negative sanctions. Am J Polit Sci 1995;39:683–713.

62. Pampel FC, Gartner R. Age structure, socio-political institutions, and national homicide rates. Eur Sociol Rev 1995;11:243–60.

63. Scheper-Hughes N, Hoffman D. Kids out of place: street children of Brazil. In: Disposable children: the hazards of growing up in Latin America. New York, N.Y.: North American Congress on Latin America, 1994;27:16–23.

64. Aitchinson J. Violencia e juventude na Africa do Sul: causas, licoes e solucoes para uma sociedade violenta [Violence and youth in South Africa: causes, lessons and solutions for a violent society]. In: Pinheiro PS, ed. Sao Paulo sem medo: um diagnostico de violencia urbana (Sao Paulo without fear: a diagnosis of urban violence]. Rio de Janeiro, Brazil: Garamond, 1998:121–32.

65. Loftin C, Wiersema B, McDowell D, et al. Underreporting of justifiable homicides committed by police officers in the United States. Am J Public Health 2003;93: 1117–21.
66. Report of the National Advisory Commission on Civil Disorders. Washington, D.C.: National Advisory Commission on Civil Disorders, 1968.
67. Markowitz S. The price of alcohol, wife abuse and husband abuse. South Econ J 2000;67:279–303.
68. Markowitz S, Grossman M. Alcohol regulation and domestic violence towards children. Contemp Econ Policy 1998;16:309–21.
69. WITNESS. Available at: http://www.witness.org. Accessed January 23, 2005.
70. Ludwig J, Duncan GJ, Hirschfield P. Urban poverty and juvenile crime: evidence from a randomized housing-mobility experiment. Q J Econ 2001;16:655–80.
71. Centers for Disease Control and Prevention. Community interventions to promote healthy social environments: early childhood development and family housing. MMWR 2002;51:RR-1.
72. Black D. Violent structures. Paper prepared for a Workshop on Theories of Violence. Washington, D.C.: National Institute of Violence, 2002.
73. Senechal de la Roche R. Why is collective violence collective? Sociol Theory 2001;19:126–44.
74. Varshney A. Ethnic conflict and civic life: Hindus and Muslims in India. New Haven, Conn.: Yale University Press, 2002.
75. Reproductive health effects of gender-based violence. In: United Nations population fund. Annual Report 1998;1998:20–1. Available at: http://www.unfpa.org/about/report/report98/ppgenderbased.htm. Accessed January 23, 2005.
76. Perkins HW, Craig DW. A multifaceted social norms approach to reduce high-risk drinking. Newton, Mass.: The Higher Education Center for Alcohol and Other Drug Prevention, 2002.
77. Berkowitz AD. How can we prevent sexual harassment and sexual assault? Educator's Guide to Controlling Sexual Harassment 6, no. 1 (October 1998):1–4.
78. Mann JM. Society and public health: crisis and rebirth. West J Med 1998;169:118–21.
79. McKenna MAJ. The public health beat: what is it? why is it important? Nieman Reports Spring 2003:10–11.

18

ENVIRONMENTAL HEALTH

Colin D. Butler and Anthony J. McMichael

Introduction

Modern environmental health evolved from the concept of "miasmas," or noxious vapors seeping from unhealthy environments and causing diverse illnesses that we now identify as including cholera, bronchitis, and malaria. Although the miasmatic paradigm was discredited by the microbiological and toxicological discoveries of the nineteenth and twentieth centuries, miasmatic thinking still surfaces when novel illnesses appear in proximity to novel environmental phenomena.

Not all miasmas were invisible. London was called the "big smoke" for centuries, and those with means have long tried to live upwind of the worst air pollution, attempting to also escape invisible vapors.

In the course of the twentieth century, many polluting industrial processes in high-income countries were reformed, whereas others were moved, both to rural locations and increasingly to developing countries, which often have large and growing populations and cheap, compliant, nonunionized, vulnerable workforces. Prices and wages in these economies have been depressed due, in part, to low environmental and occupational safety standards, as well as to family-provided—as opposed to state-provided—safety nets. Ancient, widespread, and visible poverty depresses individual and community expectations of affluence. Low wage and price structures permeate the economies, so that life—although rarely health—is maintained on incomes absurdly low by Western standards.

In developing countries, these factors combine to promote extreme poverty for large, but powerless, groups. Their hardship helps to benefit relatively affluent people within these countries as well as populations in developed countries, who are unknown and unknowable to the poor in developing countries.[1,2]

This is how this happens. Globalization has increased the proportion of goods and services consumed by wealthy populations in developed countries. A major reason for the low price of goods and services in developing countries is that these economies are characterized by an environment of cheap labor and high risk. The wages and conditions of the workforce making and providing these goods and services are poor in comparison to similar workers in developed countries. But even if the wages and conditions of the workforce are comparatively good for a developing country, existence at this wage level is enabled by an even poorer stratum of workers who provide goods and services to the workforce that supplies markets in developed countries. Thus a kind of economic food chain exists. Consequently, the price of many consumer items is lowered in developed as well as developing countries, and much pollution and other environmental hazards are sequestered among poor populations, who have little recourse to legal, media, or political countermeasures. Costs that are not incorporated into the price of goods and services are called "externalities." These externalities, such as a greater exposure to environmental and other forms of risk, are generally higher in developing countries. Examples of these hazards include toxic wastes and localized air pollution. Some hazards, such as greenhouse gases, mercury (for example, fumes released by burning coal), and hazardous chemicals embedded in food, are not sequestered.

Scale and Distribution of Environmental Health Hazards

The most quantitatively important environmental causes of ill health are from microbiologically contaminated water and indoor air pollution.[3] Almost the entire burden of these hazards is carried by poor populations in developing countries. Within developed countries, the largest environmental risks are also experienced by the poor.

The importance of environmental health hazards has been questioned, but skepticism is totally unjustified if contaminated food, water, and air are included in environmental health. Doubt is also cast on the hazards of exposure to low levels of persistent pollutants.[4] However, many studies suggest a causal relationship between disease and pollutants, especially those that bioaccumulate in tissue. These include lead, asbestos, mercury, fine airborne particulates, and persistent organic pollutants (POPs), such as organochlorines. Ionizing radiation and electrical fields also harm health. While the burden of disease from these hazards cannot now be reliably determined, in the aggregate it may approach the burden of disease from unsafe water.

Downplaying the scale of environmental hazard has philosophical and political dimensions. There are many cases in which defenders of industry have used deceit, public relations, pragmatism, and corrupted scientific research to obfuscate the need for and delay the progress of reform.[5–7]

Pollution is a tradeoff for the material and economic benefits of urban centers—cooking, heating, and industrial production. However, as understanding, technology, and aspirations have evolved, many individuals and groups have sought to minimize their exposure to the known and perceived risks of environmental hazards. Sometimes the invisibility of these hazards has heightened concern, making the risk more uncertain and difficult to avoid; however, for uneducated and unaware populations, invisibility and ignorance probably contribute to exposure.

Those who are skeptical about environmental hazards also understate the health risk of future climate and ecosystem change,[8] which may cause an enormous burden of future disease—perhaps rivaling that attributed to existing environmental hazards.[9] Again, these costs are likely to be borne mainly by the poor in developing countries, such as low-lying Bangladesh and countries in sub-Saharan Africa.

New Environmental Health Problems

One hundred years ago, POPs had not been synthesized. Greenhouse gases were accumulating in the atmosphere and ecosystems were then becoming degraded, but neither climate change nor ecosystem change would be recognized as a legitimate environmental health issue until the late twentieth century. The synthetic, halogen-based chemicals that damage the stratospheric ozone layer did not exist.

What Is Not Discussed in This Chapter

Vector-borne diseases, once also considered miasmatic, could also be considered environmental, but this use has declined, and they are not discussed in this chapter, except in the context of climate change. Asthma and atopy are not discussed in detail, nor are nutrition, tobacco, and environmental deficiency diseases, such as from lack of iodine. Occupational exposures are discussed in chapter 19.

The Relationship Between Social Injustice and Environmental Health

Water

Unlike many aspects of environmental health, the health burden of microbially contaminated water is established. Although the water and sanitary revolution within developed countries largely occurred more than a century ago,[10] this has not yet been extended to the poorest and most vulnerable quarter of humanity—a population larger than the entire global population in 1900.

More than 1 billion people lack access to microbiologically safe water, and 2.4 billion lack access to improved sanitation. The major cause of disease and death from feces-contaminated water is diarrhea, which particularly affects poor children living in slums and rural areas of developing countries. Chronic or repeated diarrhea in children is not just unpleasant but also a potent cause of physical stunting and reduced cognitive development, perhaps because of malabsorption.[11] Hence, the disability adjusted life-years lost (DALYs) from dirty water is higher than mortality rates alone suggest. The global burden of disease study attributes 2 million deaths annually to this cause (the tenth most important cause), leading to 4 percent of the total DALYs (the sixth most important cause).[3] In both numbers of cases and DALYs, contaminated water is higher than the next leading environmental cause for ill health, indoor air pollution.

The United National Development Program (UNDP) claims that one of the few Millennium Development Goals (see chapter 28) within reach is to halve the proportion of people without access to safe drinking water and improved sanitation.[12] To achieve this goal would involve providing clean water to an additional 50,000-plus people per day, every day, until 2015. More encouragingly, the annual number of deaths due to diarrhea is thought to have fallen by almost one-third during the 1990s, from 2.9 million to 2.1 million, mainly because of improved medical treatment.[3]

Access to water, even of poor quality, is also important for health. Beyond a threshold, the cost of carting water limits its use for washing the hands and face, with consequent adverse health effects.[13]

Indoor Air Pollution

The regular breathing of smoky air from cooking fires is almost entirely confined to poor populations in developing countries. Indoor air pollution is the eighth leading cause of attributable DALYs, responsible for about 3 percent of the global burden. Indoor air pollution increases the risk of acute respiratory infections in childhood—the most important cause of death among children—and of chronic obstructive pulmonary disease. There are also associations between indoor air pollution and pulmonary tuberculosis, nasopharyngeal and laryngeal cancer, cataract, and, when coal is burned, lung cancer.[14]

Outdoor Air Pollution

Outdoor air pollution, from motor vehicles, industry (fig. 18-1), and home heating, is a major human health issue in urban areas. Globally, outdoor air pollution is thought to cause approximately 1 million deaths annually, of which two-thirds occur in low- and middle-income countries. However, because most deaths occur in adults, the burden of disease in DALYs is not as high as that from indoor air pollution.[3]

Since the 1970s, evidence has accumulated that air pollution in developed countries still represents a health problem for health. In the Netherlands, for example, cars are thought to cause more deaths from air pollution than from trauma. Air pollution has also been linked to atopy and cardiac disease.[15] Air is also the main carrier of lead pollution (see below).

Urban air pollution is worst in the megacities of developing countries, exacerbated by the growing use of motor vehicles, dust from construction,

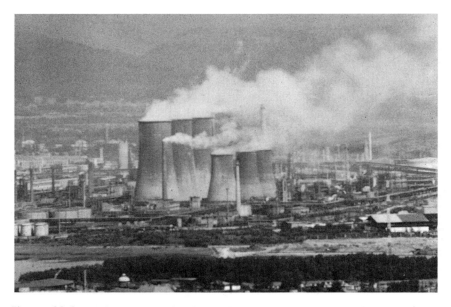

Figure 18-1 Ambient air pollution in the Czech Republic. This chemical plant in the northern part of the Czech Republic has accounted for much air pollution in the surrounding area. (Photograph by Barry S. Levy.)

and smoky fuels used for manufacturing and domestic purposes.[16] Some cities, such as New Delhi and Dhaka, have passed, and are enforcing, legislation to encourage the limited use of cleaner fuels, such as compressed gas. Beijing is also trying to improve its air quality in preparation for the 2008 Olympic Games.

Continental Air Pollution

Haze on a continental scale has recently been recognized as a third category of air pollution. Over South Asia, this haze is called the "Asian Brown Cloud." It is caused mainly by the burning of biofuels, such as firewood, dung, and agricultural waste, by the enormous rural population that lives there.[17]

These polluted air masses affect agriculture (by changing precipitation patterns and reducing the penetration of sunlight), modify climate, and possibly adversely affect health in other ways that distinguish it from the better studied mechanisms of indoor and outdoor air pollution.[18] For example, sulfate-rich air released mainly from Eastern Europe during the 1970s and 1980s has been linked with reduced precipitation over the eastern Sahel during those decades.[19] Hence, the famine and conflict experienced by the poor and vulnerable populations that inhabit that part of the world may be inadvertent consequences of European action.

Soil Contamination

Several parasitic diseases, again mostly affecting poor populations in developing countries, are transmitted by contact with soil and water contaminated by human wastes. The most important of these are schistosomiasis and hookworm. Although hookworm infestation causes few deaths, it contributes to anemia and, thus, reduced economic output and probably cognitive impairment.[11,20,21] Guinea worm is another parasite, which enters the body through contact with contaminated water. Madura foot, caused by a subcutaneous fungus, is also transmitted by prolonged contact with infected soil. Both conditions are confined to developing countries.

Food

Microbial contamination of food, other than through contaminated water, is not discussed in this chapter. However, there is increasing recognition that food is a source of chemical contamination, such as heavy metals in fish and marine mammals, organochlorines in breast milk and farmed fish,[22] and arsenic in crops irrigated by arsenic-contaminated water. Pesticides and other chemicals, such as polychlorinated biphenyls (PCBs), also contaminate food.[23]

Lead

On the basis of lost DALYs, after indoor air pollution, lead exposure is the most important environmental health problem, causing about 1 percent of the global burden of disease.[3] Debate continues about what is a "safe" level of lead, but it is discomforting to realize that the average body lead burden of today's population is estimated to be more than 500 times that of preindustrial populations.[24]

At high exposures, lead is a systemic poison, particularly affecting the central nervous system, kidneys, and hematopoietic system.[24] A problem since Roman times, the main current environmental exposures to lead are from its use as an additive to gasoline, in paint, and in ceramics. Lead exposure has been lowered in most developed countries but remains high in most developing countries. Chronic exposure to low levels of lead is an important cause of reduced cognitive development[25,26] and thus serves to reinforce the disadvantage experienced by poor populations. In the past several years, more than 20 developing countries, such as Thailand, have phased out leaded gasoline or substantially reduced the levels of lead in gasoline.[24]

Asbestos

In developed countries, the health hazards of asbestos exposure are widely appreciated—not only in the workplace but also in the ambient environment. Safer alternatives exist. As a consequence, asbestos use is highly regulated or banned in most developed countries.[27]

The tactics of the asbestos industry have been compared with that of the tobacco industry. As markets in developed countries contract, the industry has aggressively transferred its commercial activities—and hazard—to developing countries.[28,29] In developing countries, the myth that asbestos is safe is aided by the inadequate number of in-country studies and is reinforced by political and industry opposition to regulation.[29,30] The epidemic in most developing countries is less advanced, so mortality is not yet as obvious.

Mercury

Like lead, mercury contamination is a global problem, caused mainly by the burning of coal,[31,32] gold mining, waste incineration, and various industrial processes. Mercury bioaccumulates in the food chain, especially in carnivorous fish and marine mammals.[33] The inadvertent consumption of mercury in marine creatures has been problematic since the Minimata epidemic in Japan in the 1950s, in which birth defects and neurological disorders occurred as a result of industrial dumping of mercury into a bay and its subsequent incorporation into the food chain.[34]

There is debate over the minimum safe mercury exposure, especially for unborn children. Studies from the Seychelles[35] and New Zealand[36] support different interpretations, but a recent review by the U.S. National Academy of Sciences favored the more cautious conclusions of the New Zealand study.[37]

The population at the greatest risk of mercury exposure probably comprises indigenous peoples of the Arctic who mainly eat fish and marine mammals. This population also absorbs disproportionately high concentrations of heavy metals and chemicals, such as PCBs and organochlorines.[38] However, these hazards in this population are associated with only subtle adverse health outcomes, disputed and largely ignored by more powerful groups.[39]

Persistent Organic Pollutants

POPs include a range of synthetic, long-lived chemicals, including many pesticides. One class of POPs, organochlorines, have been especially suspected of having adverse health effects, because of their propensity to bioaccumulate, their long half-lives, and, in some cases, their capacity to mimic estrogen. There is also concern that multiple POP exposures may have synergistic effects, especially to genetically vulnerable subgroups.[40]

Farmers have been repeatedly found to have higher-than-expected rates of lymphoma, possibly due to their exposure to pesticides.[41] In the Seveso accident in Italy in 1976, large quantities of dioxin were released into the environment. Higher concentrations of dioxin and other POPs are still present in the local population more than 25 years later.[42] Female survivors of Seveso have been shown to bear a reduced number of male children than expected.[43] While definite conclusions cannot be drawn from studies of people exposed at Seveso, long-term investigations have indicated increases in the occurrence of certain malignancies, increases in cardiovascular and respiratory deaths early after the incident, and an increase in diabetes.

Organochlorines have also been claimed to contribute to the causation of breast cancer.[44] One study linked dieldrin to breast cancer.[45] While a recent review of this putative relationship concluded that evidence in favor of this hypothesis is weak,[46] this review itself erroneously claimed that a follow-up study by the Danish group[47] found conflicting results.

In the region of the former Aral Sea in Russia, a high rate of respiratory disease has been preliminarily attributed to the inhalation of dust contaminated by pesticides and other chemicals.[48] However, as with many such anecdotes from developing countries, there is no convincing evidence to support a causal association.

Global Climate and Ecosystem Change

The focus of the debate on global climate change is shifting from whether it is occurring to what will be its magnitude and consequences.[49] Predictions that may have seemed far-fetched a decade ago are now coming to pass. As examples, the European heat wave in 2003 caused the deaths of at least 20,000 people,[50] and the entire population of Niue (a small island state in the Pacific) may be dislocated because of an extreme weather event.

Climate change is likely to adversely affect human health through five main mechanisms:

1. From increased heat stress, especially affecting populations neither acclimatized nor technologically adapted
2. Through a change in the distribution of disease-transmitting insects, including mosquitoes and ticks, with probable increases especially for malaria[51] and dengue fever[52]
3. Through an increased frequency of infrastructure- and morale-damaging extreme weather events, including storms, winds, floods,[53] droughts, and fires
4. By interacting with ecosystem change, potentially contributing to food insecurity,[54] loss of biodiversity, and armed conflict
5. By more-drastic effects, such as destabilizing the Western Antarctic and Greenland ice shelves—thus substantially elevating global sea level and disrupting the Gulf Stream, causing paradoxical cooling in Europe—although probably not until the next century.[55,56]

Ecosystem change, even without climate change, can also adversely affect development and health.[57] For example, Hurricane Mitch, which, in 1999, caused extensive devastation in Central America, had a far more severe impact on human health than did Hurricane Andrew, which struck Florida several years earlier. The effects of Mitch, such as huge mudslides that killed many people, were exacerbated by the extent of deforestation on steep hills that had occurred. Bridges collapsed and a considerable amount of infrastructure was damaged. In contrast to Andrew, very few people affected by Mitch were insured. The lack of insurance and emergency services, combined with factors such as poor building standards and mismanagement of relief funds, reinforced conditions of poverty for many people. But wealthy populations are also vulnerable to a collapse of the global insurance industry due to climate change and terrorism.[58]

Environmental Disasters and the Erosion of Trust

Disasters have magnified public suspicion of chemicals and radiation. Chernobyl and Bhopal[59,60] provide two notorious cases in which feared hazardous materials were released and adversely affected the health of thousands of people. Characteristic of many disasters, these events were marked by initial attempts to downplay harm, by claimant victims being denied compensation, and by a trickle of admissions—sometimes over decades—that the damage was greater than originally thought.[61] Collectively, these tactics have eroded public trust, domestically and globally.

The world's worst industrial accident occurred in December 1984 in Bhopal, India, in and around a pesticide-manufacturing factory owned by the multinational company Union Carbide. It mainly affected thousands of people living near the plant. Estimates of the mortality and morbidity are contested, but probably more than 3,800 people died and 350,000 have had chronic sequelae. Some studies into the health effects of Bhopal have been prematurely terminated; others were allegedly suppressed. Many victims have never been properly registered or compensated. As late as 1996, as many as 50,000 survivors still had partial or total disability as a consequence of the disaster. A class-action lawsuit against Union Carbide, filed by victims of the disaster in a U.S. court, was dismissed. The former head of Union Carbide was pronounced a "proclaimed absconder" due to his failure to appear at hearings for a criminal case filed in India.[59]

The Bhopal disaster illustrates both how the poor are trapped and why polluting and risky industries are moved, when possible, to developing countries. Had the Bhopal disaster occurred in the United States, its victims would probably have eventually achieved compensation greater by orders of magnitude. However, it is also likely that, had the plant been in the United States, the incident would never have happened. In fact, Union Carbide operated a similar plant in the United States with greater safety precautions—a reflection of the double standard that exists.

Globalization and Environmental Health

Globalization has many definitions, but two of its widely recognized characteristics are relevant to global environmental health: (a) the continuing driving by trade, technology, and ideology of a single global economic community, with an unprecedented sharing of culture; and (b) market deregulation.[1]

Previously, market forces dictated that the poorest fraction of domestic populations experienced the highest environmental risk. Increasingly, it is the poorest fraction of the global population that experiences this risk.

National Implications

The widespread attempts to restrain capitalism that followed the Depression and accompanied the peak of the Soviet Union's and China's international appeal have weakened substantially in the past three decades, leading to a resurgence of market forces. Increasingly, pockets of impoverished, nonempowered, and vulnerable populations are appearing in high-income countries, especially the United States.[62]

Ascendancy of the free market has helped to promote, and even to celebrate, this inequality. This has fueled the environmental justice movement, which so far has had little success (see below). Because environmental inequality is only one manifestation of multiple, interlocking kinds of inequality, this is not surprising.

What Needs to Be Done

Achieving Environmental Justice

Work linking poverty, disadvantage, and environmental health is often known as the environmental justice movement (EJM).[63–67] The most egregious exposures to environmental health risk clearly occur among the poor populations of developing countries. An evidence-based approach to environmental health at a global scale would thus accord prominent place to this. Unfortunately, this is not reflected in the EJM literature.

Most of this literature is concerned with health inequalities within high-income countries, especially the United States. A partial exception is provided in a report by the Institute of Medicine, entitled *Toward Environmental Justice*.[68] Investigators for this report visited Nogales and reported critically about this maquiladora center on the Mexican–United States border. At its margins, the EJM is also concerned with international issues, such as climate change, tropical deforestation, and the dumping of toxic waste in developing countries.[67]

The fairly narrow focus of the EJM means that few of its suggested remedies are likely to have much effect on either the distribution of global environmental risk or the health burden experienced by the global poor. However, the failure of the EJM to adequately consider global health issues does not necessarily stem from its contributors' ignorance or lack of concern for global issues of fairness. Many interlocking causes combine to depress awareness of the environmental risk experienced by poor populations in developing countries. These include inadequate data and researchers with poor resources within developing countries. In addition, the populations most at risk have many other concerns. The poor cannot lobby effectively, especially in developing countries. Few are literate, and, by definition, they have little power. Many suffer a degree of cognitive impairment—often a result of the environmental and other hazards with which they live. As a result, their voice is muted, especially in proportion to the risk that they face.

In developed countries, and even among privileged populations of developing countries, a publication and readership bias exists in the scientific literature, which depresses interest and concern for the health risk of poor populations. In short, there are few incentives to reward, and many barriers to penalize, those who try to raise the issue of global environmental justice.[69,70]

Creating Greater Awareness of the Costs of Environmental Hazards

The environmental hazards described in this chapter belong to a class of costs called "externalities" by economists. While real, these costs are poorly measured and, by definition, never incorporated into the price of items. Creating greater awareness of externalities is one way to create pressure to reduce them. However, internalizing externalities would reduce profits and increase prices, especially in the short term. And the population that would disproportionately benefit from this action would be those who are currently the poorest and most vulnerable.

Market forces, if unrestrained by legislation and other institutions, are therefore unlikely to reduce externalities. Reforms are likely to be bitterly resisted, not only by those who profit from the creation and maintenance of environmental risk but also by those who consume the material fruits of this risk.

Harnessing Sufficient Political and Economic Will

The world is increasingly unequal, particularly with regard to the distribution of international economic power.[1,70] Although the Millennium Development Goals (see chapter 28) were announced with great fanfare, there is as yet little evidence that many, or even any, will be achieved. The U.S. invasion of Iraq in 2003, counter to the approval of the global community through the United Nations,[71] casts further doubt over our collective capacity to reduce the disproportionate exposure to environmental hazards of the global poor.

It is human to hope for a better future, and it is possible to argue cogently that humans can find a way to intelligently and fairly balance their limited resources with the demand placed upon them.[72] However, the fact that so much progress has been made to reduce the exposures of comparatively privileged populations to known and suspected environmental hazards and so little has been done for the poorest fraction of humanity points to deeper causes than technical ones—and perhaps even deeper than political or economic causes.

While it is unlikely that technology can reduce the concentrations of the harmful substances discussed in this chapter to their preindustrial levels, it is not technologically impossible to provide clean water or, within a lifetime, to reduce global lead, mercury, particulates, and greenhouse gas emissions.

What is lacking is sufficient global will. Although a dramatic change of global consciousness[73] is utopian, major changes in global thinking have occurred before, such as in the birth of the United Nations in 1945, the adoption of the Universal Declaration of Human Rights in 1948, and the World Health Organization's commitment to "Health for All" in 1978.

Reducing Exposure to Hazardous Chemical Exposures

In the late nineteenth century, the Sanitary Revolution spread throughout industrialized England.[74] It could provide a model for the Sustainability Transition to come.[75] The Sanitary Revolution arose from a mix of reformers, enlightened leadership, "noblesse oblige," improving technology, gradually increasing expectations, and, after a while, competition among reforming cities.

The costs undertaken to achieve the Sanitary Revolution did not cripple wealthy economies. Instead, many economic benefits accrued, not only from the stimulus given to new industries but also from reduced sickness. Similarly, cleaner technologies could stimulate new industries. Human productivity could improve if health improved. Agricultural productivity could be enhanced by reduced air pollution.

Other signs that environmental hazards can be alleviated are provided by the reduced use, in developed countries, of lead and asbestos. Acid rain has lessened, as has the use of stratospheric ozone-depleting substances. In some developed countries, such as Germany and Spain, measures are being taken to reduce greenhouse gas emissions.

These examples provide a model for how humanity could avert irreversible environmental damage, improve global public health, and even generate vast numbers of new jobs, especially in developing countries.

Performing Epidemiological Research

The proper investigation of environmental and other health hazards in most developing countries is rudimentary, due to a combination of inadequate local and international resources and access. Many vested interests oppose such investigation, including by the denial of adequate research funds.

James Lavery and colleagues[76] have suggested an additional obstacle. While accepting that environmental health research (EHR) is inappropriately and disproportionately performed, mainly in developed countries, they propose that EHR is unethical among populations "restricted in their ability to avoid environmental hazards by economic or political repression." One could quibble over what this means, but a liberal interpretation would exclude EHR from almost all disadvantaged populations in developing countries. One could argue that research among repressed populations, were it actually possible, is highly ethical, provided that the purpose of the research is to alleviate the repression, such as by drawing global attention to this injustice. For this reason, of course, such research is unlikely to be encouraged.

Nigel Bruce and colleagues[14] have pointed to new research into indoor air pollution as a worthwhile goal, especially in relation to tuberculosis and acute lower respiratory infections. They also argue for a more systematic approach to the development and evaluation of interventions, with clearer recognition of the interrelationships between poverty and dependence on polluting fuels.

As globalization advances, enlightened funding bodies and philanthropists may increase their support for research projects in developing countries. This support could increase local capacity and public awareness, and eventually facilitate legal and social reform. Advocacy for these goals by epidemiologists based in developed countries would go a long way toward answering those who have criticized epidemiology for its loss of public health relevance.[77]

Reforming Organizations and Institutions

Bodies such as the World Bank have long proclaimed their desire to foster genuine development, yet repeatedly these efforts have failed. However, blaming corporations for environmental ill health may be as fallacious as blaming the World Bank and the International Monetary Fund (IMF).

Consumers and shareholders support corporations because the goods they supply are the cheapest and the profits they deliver are the highest. Citizens in high-income countries largely support, implicitly, the policies of the World Bank and the IMF because they feel their own lives are made richer and more secure by so doing.

It follows, then, that it is the attitudes and values of the global middle class that really need to be changed. Is this a pipe dream? It may not be, if middle class people globally could be convinced that their current acquiescence to unsustainable and socially and environmentally exploitative policies places the future of their grandchildren—and perhaps even their children—at serious risk. The force of this conviction could then release an unstoppable wave, driving changes in global values, technologies, advertising campaigns, and new economics. This would not guarantee a sustainable future, but civilization would at least have a fighting chance.

Conclusion

Reducing the health risks of environmental hazards is an important part of fostering the Sustainability Transition. Inequality, overconsumption of natural resources, population growth, and outmoded economic theories and policies[78] are driving civilization farther along a slippery tightrope.

The global problem of poor environmental health, together with non-sustainability, requires ambitious and global strategies, on the scale of a new Manhattan Project, to develop and disseminate the environmentally friendly technologies that are required.[78,79] Demographers and economists need to rediscover the negative economic effects of rapid population growth[80] to stimulate the political will to reduce illiteracy and to promote family planning. A fairer world will lead to a more genuine attempt to achieve the Millennium Development Goals and thus further reduce the human cost of the most important current environmental health issue, that of feces-contaminated water.

This world of value changes sounds utopian. Yet so did the near-global abolition of slavery, space travel, and Internet communication. The panic induced by the SARS epidemic in 2003 illustrates a deep residual fear of epidemics among the educated, global middle class, which can lead to profound behavioral change. Could this instinct for self-preservation be harnessed to change behavior in ways that promote sustainability? Can we hope for a reprise of the response by the London middle class to the malodorous Thames? This might be possible in regard to coping with climate change and even over-consumption.

To effectively address these challenges also requires better education, fairer trade, and more genuine global democracy—all of which is in our collective self-interest. Much more discussion of these ideas is required if the middle class is to be motivated.

References

1. Butler CD, Douglas RM, McMichael AJ. Globalisation and environmental change: implications for health and health inequalities. In: Eckersley R, Dixon J, Douglas B, eds. The social origins of health and well-being. Cambridge, U.K.: Cambridge University Press, 2001:34–50.
2. Raina V, Chowdhury A, Chowdhury S, eds. The dispossessed: victims of development in Asia. Hong Kong: ARENA Press, 1997.
3. Ezzati M, Lopez AD, Rodgers A, et al. Selected major risk factors and global and regional burden of disease. Lancet 2002;360:1347–60.
4. Ames B, Gold LS. Paracelsus to parascience: the environmental cancer distraction. Mutat Res 2000;447:3–13.
5. Stauber JC, Rampton S. Toxic sludge is good for you: lies, damn lies and the public relations industry. Monroe, Me.: Common Courage Press, 1995.

6. Beder S. Global Spin: The corporate assault on environmentalism. Melbourne, Australia: Scribe Publications, 1998.

7. Warren C. Brush with death: A social history of lead poisoning. Baltimore, Md.: Johns Hopkins University Press, 2000.

8. Lomborg B. The skeptical environmentalist. Cambridge, U.K.: Cambridge University Press, 2001.

9. McMichael AJ, Beaglehole R. The changing global context of public health. Lancet 2000;356:495–9.

10. Szreter S. Economic growth, disruption, deprivation, disease and death: on the importance of the politics of public health. Popul Dev Rev 1997;23:693–728.

11. Dillingham R, Guerrant RL. Childhood stunting: measuring and stemming the staggering costs of inadequate water and sanitation. Lancet 2004;363:94–5.

12. United Nations Development Program. Human development report 2003. New York, N.Y.: Oxford University Press, 2003.

13. White GF, Bradley DJ, White AU. Drawers of water: domestic water use in East Africa. Chicago, Ill.: The University of Chicago Press, 1972.

14. Bruce N, Perez-Padilla R, Albalak R. Indoor air pollution in developing countries: a major environmental and public health challenge. Bull WHO 2000; 78: 1078–92.

15. Pyne S. Small particles add up to big disease risk. Science 2002;295:1994.

16. Brunekreef B, Holgate ST. Air pollution and health. Lancet 2002;360:1233–42.

17. Lelieveld J, Crutzen PJ, Ramanathan V, et al. The Indian Ocean experiment: widespread air pollution from South and Southeast Asia. Science 2001;291:1031–6.

18. Ahmad K. Pollution cloud over South Asia is increasing ill health. Lancet 2002; 360:549.

19. Lelieveld J, Berresheim H, Borrmann S, et al. Global air pollution crossroads over the Mediterranean. Science 2002;298:789–91.

20. Couper RTL, Simmer KN. Iron deficiency in children: food for thought [editorial]. Med J Austra 2001;174:162–3.

21. Walgate R. African children talk faster with iron. Bull WHO 2002;80:174.

22. Hites RA, Foran JA, Carpenter DO, et al. Global assessment of organic contaminants in farmed salmon. Science 2004;303:226–9.

23. Neuberger M, Grossgut R, Gyimothy J, et al. Dioxin contamination of feed and food. Lancet 2000;355:1883.

24. Tong S, Prapamontol T, Schirnding YV. Environmental lead exposure: a public health problem of global dimensions. Bull WHO 2000;78:1068–77.

25. McMichael A, Baghurst P, Wigg N, et al. Port Pirie cohort study: Childhood blood lead history and neuropsychological development at age four years. N Engl J Med 1988;319:468–75.

26. Canfield RL, Charles R. Henderson J, et al. Intellectual impairment in children with blood lead concentrations below $10\,\mu$g per deciliter. N Engl J Med 2003;348: 1517–26.

27. LaDou J, Landrigan P, Bailar JC III, et al. A call for an international ban on asbestos. Can Med Assoc J 2001;164:489–90.

28. Harris L, Kahwa I. Asbestos: old foe in 21st century developing countries. Sci Total Environ 2003;307:1–9.

29. Joshi T, Gupta R. Asbestos-related morbidity in India. Int J Occup Environ Health 2003;9:249–53.

30. Braun L, Greene A, Manseau M, et al. Scientific controversy and asbestos: making disease invisible. Int J Occup Environ Health 2003;9:194–205.

31. Glick P. The toll from coal: power plants, emissions, wildlife, and human health. Bull Sci Technol Soc 2001;21:482–500.
32. Zhang MQ, Zhu YC, Deng RW. Evaluation of mercury emissions to the atmosphere from coal combustion, China. Ambio 2002;31:482–4.
33. Bjerregaard P, Hansen JC. Organochlorines and heavy metals in pregnant women from the Disko Bay area in Greenland. Sci Total Environ 2000;245:87–102.
34. Watts J. Mercury poisoning victims could increase by 20,000. Lancet 2001;358: 1349.
35. Myers G, Davidson PW, Cox C, et al. Prenatal methylmercury exposure in the Seychelles. Lancet 2003;361:1686–92.
36. Crump K, Kjellstrom T, Shipp A, et al. Influence of prenatal mercury exposure upon scholastic and psychological test performance: benchmark analysis of a New Zealand cohort. Risk Analy 1998;18:701–13.
37. Kaiser J. Mercury report backs strict rules. Science 2000;289:371–2.
38. Simonich SL, Hites RA. Global distribution of persistent organochlorine compounds. Science 1995;269:1851–4.
39. Webster P. For precarious populations, pollutants present new perils. Science 2003; 299:1642–3.
40. Menegon A, Board PG, Blackburn AC, et al. Parkinson's disease, pesticides, and glutathione transferase. Lancet 1998;352:1344–6.
41. De Roos A, Zahm S, Cantor K, et al. Integrative assessment of multiple pesticides as risk factors for non-Hodgkin's lymphoma among men. Occup Environ Med 2003;60 (http://www.occenvmed.com/cgi/content/full/60/9/e11).
42. Weiss J, Papke O, Bignert A, et al. Concentrations of dioxins and other organochlorines (PCBs, DDTs, HCHs) in human milk from Seveso, Milan and a Lombardian rural area in Italy: a study performed 25 years after the heavy dioxin exposure in Seveso. Acta Paediatr 2003;92:467–72.
43. Clapp R, Ozonoff D. Where the boys aren't: dioxin and the sex ratio [commentary]. Lancet 2000;355:55.
44. Davis DL, Bradlow HL. Can environmental estrogens cause breast cancer? Sci Am 1995;273:144–9.
45. Høyer AP, Grandjean P, Jørgensen T, et al. Organochlorine exposure and risk of breast cancer. Lancet 1998;352:1816–20.
46. Calle E, Frumkin H, Henley S, et al. Organochlorines and breast cancer risk. Cancer J Clinicians 2002;52:253–5.
47. Høyer AP, Jorgensen T, Grandjean P, et al. Repeated measurements of organochlorine exposure and breast cancer risk (Denmark). Cancer Causes Control 2000;11: 177–84.
48. O'Hara SL, Wiggs GFS, Mamedov B, et al. Exposure to airborne dust contaminated with pesticide in the Aral Sea region. Lancet 2000;355:627.
49. Alley RB, Marotzke J, Nordhaus WD, et al. Abrupt climate change. Science 2003; 299:2005–10.
50. World Health Organization. Climate change and human health: risks and responses. Geneva, Switzerland: World Health Organization, 2003.
51. Patz JA, Hulme M, Rosenzweig C, et al. Regional warming and malaria resurgence. Nature 2002;420:627–8.
52. Hales S, de Wet N, Maindonald J, et al. Potential effect of population and climate changes on global distribution of dengue fever: an empirical model. Lancet 2002; 360:830–4.

53. Palmer TN, Räisänen J. Quantifying the risk of extreme seasonal precipitation events in a changing climate. Nature 2002;415:512–4.
54. Fischer G, Shah M, Velthuizen HV, et al. Global agro-ecological assessment for agriculture in the 21st century. Laxenburg, Austria: International Institute of Applied Systems Analysis, 2001.
55. Hasselmann K, Latif M, Hooss G, et al. The challenge of long-term climate change. Science 2003;302:1923–5.
56. O'Neill BC, Oppenheimer M. Dangerous climate impacts and the Kyoto Protocol. Science 2002;296:1971–2.
57. Epstein PR, Chivian E, Frith K. Emerging diseases threaten conservation [editorial]. Environ Health Perspect 2003;111:A506–7.
58. Tucker M. Climate change and the insurance industry: the cost of increased risk and the impetus for action. Ecol Econ 1997;22:85–96.
59. Anonymous. Has the world forgotten Bhopal? [editorial]. Lancet 2000;356:1863.
60. Sharma DC. Bhopal's health disaster continues to unfold. Lancet 2002;360:859.
61. Smith JT, Comans RNJ, Beresford NA, et al. Pollution: Chernobyl's legacy in food and water. Nature 2000;405:141.
62. Ehrenreich B. Nickel and dimed: on (not) getting by in America. New York, N.Y.: Metropolitan Books, 2001.
63. Westra L, Wenz PS, eds. Faces of environmental racism. Confronting issues of global justice. Lanham, Md.: Rowman & Littlefield Publishers, 1995.
64. Faber D, ed. The struggle for ecological democracy: environmental justice movements in the United States. New York, N.Y.: Guilford Press, 1998.
65. Nichols P. From the ground up: environmental racism and the rise of the environmental justice movement [book review]. Ecosystem Health 2001;7:127–9.
66. Lloyd-Smith M, Bell L. Toxic disputes and the rise of environmental justice in Australia. Int J Occup Environ Health 2003;9:14–23.
67. Coughlin S. Environmental justice: the role of epidemiology in protecting unempowered communities from environmental hazards. Sci Total Environ 1996;184:67–76.
68. Clay R. Still moving toward environmental justice. Environ Health Perspect 1999; 107:A303–10.
69. Hornborg A. Towards an ecological theory of unequal exchange: articulating world system theory and ecological economics. Ecol Econ 1998;25:127–36.
70. Butler CD. Inequality, global change and the sustainability of civilisation. Global Change Hum Health 2000;1:156–72.
71. McKee M, Coker R. Politics and science. Lancet 2003;362:1159.
72. Dietz T, Ostrom E, Stern PC. The struggle to govern the commons. Science 2003; 302:1907–12.
73. Raskin P, Gallopin G, Gutman P, et al. Great transition: the promise and lure of the times ahead. Boston, Mass.: Stockholm Environment Institute, 2002.
74. Hamlin C. Public health and social justice in the age of Chadwick: Britain 1800–1854. Cambridge, U.K.: Cambridge University Press, 1998.
75. McMichael AJ, Smith KR, Corvalan CF. The Sustainability Transition: a new challenge [editorial]. Bull WHO 2000;78:1067.
76. Lavery J, Upshur R, Sharp R, et al. Ethical issues in international environmental health research. Int J Hygiene Environ Health 2003;206:453–63.
77. Taubes G. Epidemiology faces its limits. Science 1995;269:164–9.
78. McMichael AJ, Butler CD, Folke C. New visions for addressing sustainability. Science 2003;302:1919–20.

79. Lubchenco J. Entering the century of the environment: a new social contract for science. Science 1998;279:491–7.
80. Birdsall N, Kelley AC, Sinding SW, eds. Population matters: demographic change, economic growth, and poverty in the developing world. New York, N.Y.: Oxford University Press, 2001.

19

OCCUPATIONAL SAFETY AND HEALTH

Andrea Kidd Taylor and Linda Rae Murray

Introduction

Historical Overview and Scope of the Problem

Work offers significant life-sustaining benefits. Throughout human history, it has been a basic requirement of human survival. How work is organized, who does what, and who reaps the benefits of the work largely determine the nature and level of social justice in a society.

Social injustice in the workplace is not just an issue of health disparities or disproportionate representation of workers of color in the most hazardous jobs. It encompasses the lack of workplace democracy and the lack of workers' democratic ability to control their work environment and to shape their own lives. It also reflects the absence of justice in other spheres of society. To appreciate the impact of social injustice on occupational safety and health, we must consider the critical role of work in the entire society.

The nature of work has a profound impact on the social status, well-being, and health of individuals and populations. Wages, economic inequality, working conditions, the structure of the workforce, and occupational segregation—which, in the United States, exacerbates and perpetuates class, racial/ethnic, and gender inequalities—help form the underlying social determinants of health.[1]

The very foundation of our nation is based on historic expropriation of the land from Native Americans, the practice of indentured servitude among new colonists, and development of the Southern economy based on slavery. The lack of workplace democracy in the United States can be traced back to the time of slavery or earlier, where every aspect of some individuals' existence was overshadowed by compulsory labor.[2] When slavery ended after the Civil War, sharecropping became an economic surrogate for slavery; through indebtedness, the former slaves—now tenant farmers—became as tied to the land as they were under slavery.[3]

Waves of immigrants continued to supply cheap labor to industry in the United States. Whether the immigrant workforce was composed of Irish immigrants in steel mills or Asian immigrants in the building of railroads, denial of basic rights and exposure to extreme hazards remained hallmarks. Racism against Asians, Mexicans, Native Americans, and African-Americans led to inhumane treatment and dangerous occupational exposures.

Job discrimination starts when people are denied the right to freely compete for the kind of jobs to which they aspire and for which they are qualified. It continues in the workplace. Historically, within manufacturing, there was (a) discrimination in applying seniority rules and in denying opportunities for in-plant training and industrial courses and (b) "Jim Crow" barriers* in many unions.[4]

The industrial boom of World War II forced a temporary breach in the bastion of Jim Crow with the federal government's establishment of the Fair Employment Practice Committee (FEPC) in 1942. The FEPC, established by executive order of President Franklin D. Roosevelt, was created to promote the fullest employment of all available persons and to eliminate discriminatory employment practices. During this period, the "job ceiling" was slightly raised and thousands of African-American men and women entered areas of skilled employment from which they had traditionally been barred. However, a report issued by the FEPC indicated that (a) nearly two-thirds of all African-American women workers remained in service occupations, (b) close to one-half still held domestic service jobs, and (c) almost one-half of the African-American men continued working as unskilled laborers or as farm workers. While African-Americans gained a foothold in industry, this foothold has always been a precarious one. And the overall strategy of the U.S. free-market enterprise system has been designed to hold poor workers, African-Americans, and other workers of color in perpetuity as a special

---

*After the U.S. Civil War, in most Southern states, "Jim Crow" laws discriminated against African-Americans by prohibiting their attendance together with whites in public schools and facilities, such as restaurants, theaters, hotels, cinemas, and public baths. Even water fountains were segregated.

reserve of cheap and underprivileged labor—an instrument for undercutting the standards of their white brothers and sisters and a deterrent to working class unity.[4]

In the 1930s and 1940s, the traditional tactic of the employing class for any major American industry was to use the African-American sharecroppers of the South and the poorest peasantry of Europe, Mexico, and Asia as "wage-cutters" and "strike-breakers"—thereby limiting workplace democracy. As a result, white workers resented and fostered prejudice against these groups of workers, splitting them from the main body of American labor. In addition, white workers were persuaded to accept the fact that these "inferior" groups had wages and living standards that undercut their own.[4]

During the youth rebellions of the 1960s, young factory workers reacted against the contrast between their civil rights in society and authoritarianism of their workplaces. A free market economy, as a social system, could not survive with the rise in security and equality for workers. Working-class victories and concessions from business were raising expectations and threatening profits, class power, and class rule. Thus, what were viewed as earlier measures of progress, such as better wages, better social programs, and greater security, were redefined as barriers that blocked the needs of a free market system.[5] This drive for the success and stability of free trade led, over time, to a decline in social justice in the workplace and to poor health, particularly for those workers who have remained in low-wage and high-hazard jobs.

Work-related injuries and occupational exposure to toxic chemicals, physical hazards, and poor and risky working conditions are, in general, related to low wages and are increased among workers of low socioeconomic status and racial and ethnic minorities.[6,7] Historically, each group that arrived in the United States worked in the most dangerous jobs in industry and was followed in these jobs by the next immigrant group. Discriminatory hiring and employment patterns that were racially motivated in many industries have been used to prevent many workers of color from moving out of entry-level jobs, in contrast to the job promotion of white immigrant groups.[7]

During the post–World War II economic boom, expanding membership made organized labor a powerful political constituency, but much of the leadership remained white and male, with little inclination to broaden the labor movement to underrepresented workers. Although some unions made significant gains in organizing female workers and workers of color, most of these workers remained unorganized through the 1950s. Among the unions' rank and file and the unions' leadership, racial and sexual discrimination and discriminatory hiring and employment patterns in many industries prevented African-Americans, Latino-Americans, Asian-Americans, and Native

Americans from moving out of entry-level, low-wage, and hazardous jobs.[8,9] In the 1960s, unions mobilized to support national legislation, which led Congress to adopt the Occupational Safety and Health Act in 1970 that established the Occupational Safety and Health Administration (OSHA). In an attempt to create better workplace democracy, the most important consequence of the OSHA was to place workplace health and safety issues on the agenda of unions, workers, health professionals, and the general public. With increasing pressure from their membership, unions formed health and safety committees to teach their members how to identify and control workplace hazards.[10]

Since OSHA was enacted, OSHA regulations have been promulgated very slowly, and in recent years, very few new regulations at all have been adopted. The existing OSHA laws have been weakened by lack of strict enforcement, layers of government bureaucracy, and very influential industry lobbyists. Employers were never very enthusiastic about the prospect of oversight by a centralized government bureaucracy; therefore, it was no surprise when attacks began on OSHA not long after it started promulgating and enforcing standards in the 1970s. Since then, OSHA enforcement and promulgation of new standards have been principally guided by electoral politics.[11]

Although substantial gains have occurred in many workplaces since the passage of OSHA, many disparities remain, due to unchecked hazardous working conditions. One example of such a disparity was the devastating fire that occurred in 1991 at a poultry plant in Hamlet, North Carolina, a poor rural community. Twenty-five workers were killed when locked safety doors prevented them from escaping the fire (fig. 19-1).[12] Today, in the age of the World Trade Organization and the North American Free Trade Agreement (NAFTA)—when manufacturing jobs are being exported to China, Indonesia, Mexico, and elsewhere—many U.S. workers believe that many existing OSHA standards are neither adequately protective of workers' health and safety nor adequately enforced. In this climate, some unions are reluctant to press for better working conditions because, if they do, they believe that employers would threaten to close their workplaces.

The up-and-down pattern in OSHA's effectiveness, regulatory policies, and practices has continued to recent years. For example, in 2001—soon after President George W. Bush took office—the OSHA ergonomics standard, which had been promulgated during the previous Clinton administration, was overturned by Congress. In the current anti-regulatory climate, OSHA is leaning more and more toward appealing to corporate and other big-business interests by developing more voluntary initiatives, including compliance-assistance programs and consultations. OSHA's partnerships with workers and organized labor have virtually disappeared.

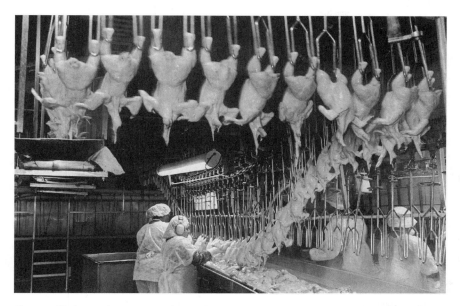

Figure 19-1 Workers processing chickens on an assembly line. Minority workers and women are overrepresented in entry-level jobs like this one, in which safety and health hazards are prevalent. Twenty-five workers in a similar chicken-processing plant died in Hamlet, North Carolina, in 1991, when few workers were able to escape a fire that swept through the plant because the employer had locked most of the exit doors. (Photograph by Earl Dotter.)

Income Inequalities in the United States

Income inequalities in the United States are a reflection, at least in part, of structural factors in the workforce and the general economy. Personal income in the United States peaked twice during the twentieth century—just before World War I and just before the Great Depression. Between the end of World War II and 1970, the average U.S. worker made significant gains in income, with those on the bottom rungs making greater progress. During the 1970s, these trends stagnated.

Since the 1980s, the United States has experienced a steady and significant increase in income inequalities. Structural changes have helped to exacerbate these income inequalities. Possible explanations for the increasing income inequalities have been (a) changes in workforce composition, such as the impact of workers of the "Baby Boom" generation (78 million Americans who were born between 1946 and 1964), more women participating in the wage economy, and new waves of immigrants, especially immigrant workers of color; (b) a decline in the manufacturing sector; (c) an increase in the service sector; and (d) globalization. These income inequalities, in combination with poverty, discrimination, and other factors, have had a profoundly negative impact on the morbidity and mortality of populations.[13]

Social Injustice and Occupational Safety and Health

Occupational safety and health provides an essential basis for worker satisfaction and commitment. The level of concern for safety and health in the workplace is an important indicator of a society's commitment to the overall health and well-being of its workers. Two dynamics have been identified as having a strong impact on worker health: (a) poor working conditions, including little career mobility; and (b) the lack of access to work, including unemployment. Working and living in an environment of physical and social disadvantage—being low in the social hierarchy, being poor, working under adverse conditions, or being unemployed—are major risk factors for ill health.[14] Several studies on unemployment link job loss with elevations in blood pressure, adverse changes in mental health, and excess morbidity and mortality.[15–18]

Workers of color have been, and continue to be, concentrated in jobs with relatively low status, low pay, and high risk. A greater percentage of African-American workers have been exposed to the highest levels of toxic substances, resulting in their having a disproportionate percentage of chronic occupational diseases and premature deaths, such as the following[7,19,20]:

- The landmark silicosis disaster at the construction of the Hawk's Nest Tunnel near Gauley Bridge, West Virginia, in the 1930s
- Toxic and carcinogenic chromate dust exposures in the chromate industry in the 1940s
- Exposure to carcinogenic aromatic hydrocarbons among coke oven workers in the 1950s
- Hazardous exposures in the textile and rubber industries in the 1970s.

Today, in workplaces described as "virtual ghettos," workers are exposed to a range of hazards, from agricultural-industry settings to modern-day sweatshops. Farm work is one of the most dangerous occupations; 71 percent of seasonal farm workers are Hispanic (Latino) and 95 percent of migrant workers are Hispanic. Over 13 percent of workplace fatalities occur in farm work. Between 1993 and 2002, there were over 12,000 case reports of pesticide illness in California, the state with the most comprehensive surveillance program for pesticide illnesses.[21] Illness due to pesticide exposure accounts for many more deaths in developing countries, often as a result of exposure to pesticides that

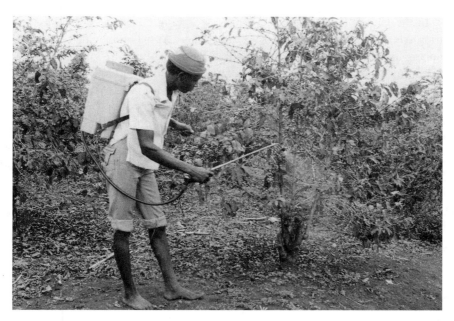

Figure 19-2 Pesticide applicator in Kenya. Workers in developing countries are often exposed to pesticides that have been banned or restricted for use in developed countries, where these pesticides are manufactured. This worker is exposed, both by inhalation and skin absorption, to captafol, a fungicide that has been banned in the United States and in the United Kingdom, where it is produced. (Photograph by Barry S. Levy.)

have been banned or restricted in developed countries (fig. 19-2). Sweatshops are labor-intensive workplaces that violate not only safety and health laws but also child labor laws. Most sweatshop workers are Hispanics, Asians, and African-Americans, and many are immigrants. Repetitive forceful movements, poor lighting, overcrowding, and abusive work conditions are hazards frequently reported among sweatshop workers.[22]

Employment data in the United States for children and adolescents under the age of 16 are not used in official Bureau of Labor Statistics (BLS) estimates or included in published BLS tables. The BLS reports, however, that 34.5 percent of 16- and 17-year-olds—more than 2.6 million adolescents—are employed at any given time during the year.[23] Young people—children and adolescents—in the United States are exposed to many occupational hazards. Annually, approximately 100,000 young people seek treatment in emergency departments for occupational injuries and at least 70 die from occupational injuries. The annual injury rate for adolescents is 4.9 per 100 full-time equivalent workers, compared with 2.8 for all workers. The most dangerous work for young people in the United States is in agriculture (on family farms), retail trade, and construction.[23]

In the United States today, most jobs are being created in service industries, where union membership is very low. Workers of color are more likely to be employed in those service occupations that pay relatively low wages. The "contingent workforce" of part-time, temporary, and contract employees has significantly increased in the past decade. Workers of color, women workers, young people, and older people are overrepresented in this contingent workforce.[24] Rather than creating new permanent jobs, more than a decade of corporate restructuring—downsizing, franchising, and outsourcing—has allowed many companies to reengineer their workplaces, shift to "lean production," and seek flexibility by lowering labor costs. This trend has had a significant impact on worker health and on occupational safety and health, in general. Areas of concern related to the microelectronics industry and technologies are musculoskeletal disorders (MSDs), chemical hazards, job stress, and use of video display terminal hazards (associated with MSDs, eye strain, headaches, and other problems). Repetitive strain injuries have had the highest incidence and fastest growth rate among categories of occupational injuries and diseases. The outsourcing of maintenance work in the U.S. petrochemical industry has caused an increase in occupational safety and health problems, including fatalities, in that industry, particularly among small firms; this outsourcing may have been an indirect cause of several catastrophic explosions that have occurred in recent years, such as those that killed contract and other workers at the Tosco Oil Refinery in California and the Equilon Refinery in the State of Washington.[25,26]

Health Care Access

In addition to poor worker health, lower pay, and fewer benefits, other adversities exist for workers in the contingent workforce, including (a) the stress of not knowing when and for how long they will work; (b) the absence of job security; (c) inadequate protection by laws and regulations, including workers' compensation laws, and occupational safety and health, unemployment insurance, and pension regulations[1]; (d) inadequate or no health insurance; and (e) limited or no access to health care. Language barriers, cultural insensitivity, and the lack of health care providers in communities where contingent workers live compound these problems. These workers are less likely to have a regular source of medical care and less likely to receive occupational health services and clinical preventive services, such as cancer screening. They are also less likely to participate in voluntary worksite health promotion programs. Contingent workers are more likely to die, and die earlier of diseases affecting them[19]; however, there is no documentation that this pattern extends to occupational illnesses and injuries.

Workers of color appear to be less likely than white workers to receive workers' compensation benefits for work-related injuries, even though workers of color, as a group, experience higher rates of occupational injury and disease.[7] Workers with severe job-related disabilities are more likely to receive welfare benefits than disability payments from workers' compensation programs—suggesting that all workers find it difficult to receive adequate compensation for work-related injury and illness.[7]

Unemployment in the United States during the 1990s was at historic lows. The current unemployment rate for African-Americans, however, is 10.2 percent, higher than rates in the 1990s and 2000. The black unemployment rate in the United States remains about twice that of whites (5.2 percent), with Latino unemployment intermediate (7.4 percent).[27] Female workers usually have unemployment rates substantially higher than those of male workers.[28] Unemployed people have higher risks of disease, with documented physiological changes in blood pressure and other health outcomes. The health risks of unemployment increase in areas where the general unemployment rate is higher. Job insecurity and unemployment can result in increased stress, higher blood pressure, heart disease, and adverse mental health outcomes.[29,30]

Education

On average, workers of color have less education, lower income levels, inferior housing, poorer health status, and less access to health care compared with white workers. In 2000, in the civilian labor force 18 years and older, the proportion of workers who had not completed high school was 7 percent for whites, 12 percent for African-Americans, and 36 percent for Latino-Americans. Similarly, the proportion of workers who had completed college was 22 percent for whites, 14 percent for African-Americans, and 8 percent for Latino-Americans.[31]

Due mainly to the low levels of education and on-the-job training that they require, hazardous jobs generally pay low wages. Wages earned by workers tend to rise with their levels of education and experience. However, the wage rates earned by African-Americans rise much less quickly with increases in education and experience than those of whites.[32] One study found that more-educated and more-experienced workers were employed in substantially safer jobs, on average, than less-educated and less-experienced workers. Even after education and job experience are accounted for, black and Latino workers in the United States face, on average, more occupational hazards than their white counterparts.[32] (See box 19-1 for an account of these forms of social injustice.)

Of all of the OSHA regulations, the 1983 OSHA Hazard Communication ("Right-to-Know") Standard (HazComm) is the regulation most often cited

BOX 19-1 Epidemic of Toxic Liver Disease

A Spanish-speaking worker from Puerto Rico presented to a hospital's emergency department with nausea, abdominal pain, and headache. The physician's assistant, suspecting work-related liver disease, took an occupational history and referred the worker to the nearby occupational medicine clinic. The worker and an additional 58 of the 66 workers of a fabric-coating factory were evaluated. Sixty-two percent of them had abnormally elevated liver function tests. Toxic liver disease was diagnosed and the probable causative agent was identified as dimethylformamide (DMF), a solvent used at the factory. Almost 76 percent of the production workers had abnormally elevated liver function tests compared with 8 percent of the nonproduction workers. Literacy was not required of the production workers, of whom 93 percent were Hispanic—most spoke only Spanish; in contrast, English literacy and a high-school education were required of the nonproduction workers, most of whom were white. The long delay in recognizing the epidemic at this factory was largely due to inadequate training provided by the employer, language barriers, the workers' lack of knowledge about the hazards associated with the job, and their lack of access to resources. Fear of job loss also contributed.[33]

by OSHA and violated by employers. Under this standard, employers are required to train workers about hazards related to their jobs and to provide material safety data sheets (MSDSs) that supply essential health and safety information for workers who must handle hazardous chemicals or work around them. Since the promulgation of the standard in 1983, OSHA has required employers to keep MSDSs at their facilities and to make them freely available to workers. At many worksites, HazComm training is inadequate and, in some cases, nonexistent. For workers who speak little or no English or who speak English as a second language, the training conducted may not be well understood or may be incomprehensible. Without knowledge of their rights under the law, many workers do not (a) request health and safety information, (b) complain of hazardous working conditions, or (c) know how or where to file a complaint if such conditions exist.[22]

Globalization and International Occupational Health

Globalization is defined as the increased movement of people, goods, services, production processes, and capital across international borders. If one agrees that a minimum precondition for any notion of social justice is people's ability to shape their own lives, skepticism about globalization's compatibility with social justice might be reinforced. This is especially true if globalization is viewed as largely establishing global rules that act as a constitution for investor rights, which are beyond any parliamentary challenges. If a socially just world is defined as one that supports the full and mutual development of the potential capacity of every individual, many would judge globalization to be inconsistent with that ideal. Globalization has been integral to a free-market economy and free-trade system; ensuring its long-term stability has fallen short of the social justice ideal for workers[5] (box 19-2).

A prime example of globalization and its impact on the social justice ideal for workers has been the implementation of NAFTA. Since the ratification of NAFTA in the early 1990s, approximately 1 million Mexicans have worked in over 4,000 assembly plants, known as *maquiladoras*, on the United States–Mexico border. The plants are owned by foreign corporations or subcontracted by them to produce parts or perform final assembly of products for export. Products that are produced vary from plant to plant; but violations of workers' human, labor, and health rights are consistent among plants—a tragic byproduct of free trade. Such violations are also becoming more apparent in countries like Indonesia and China, where many of the maquiladora industries and jobs have now moved. A growing number of workers will find themselves in the position of Mexican maquiladora workers as more export processing zones (EPZs) are established around the world. EPZs are located intentionally where labor is cheap and plentiful, and people are desperate for jobs. Substantial tax breaks are offered to foreign corporations by governments, sweetening the deal with loose regulations and active repression of unions.[34]

Faced with an impossible choice between safety and livelihood, maquiladora workers often submit to dangerous working and living conditions, while communities are forced to subsidize corporations by absorbing their social and environmental costs. Most maquiladora workers are women, who comprise 50 to 60 percent of the workforce in Mexico and over 70 percent in Guatemala and Honduras. Workplace hazards, such as toxic chemicals, poor workstation design, excessive heat and cold, poor ventilation and lighting, and harmful noise levels, and high production quotas cause a wide range of health problems. Toxic substances, such as organic solvents, paints, acids, glues, and dyes, are common in maquiladoras that produce auto parts, electronics, and furniture. However, workers are rarely informed about the risks, MSDSs are not provided, and there is inadequate labeling of chemicals.

Many maquiladora workers, especially assembly-line workers, also experience MSDSs caused by performing repetitive machine-paced motions and/or standing or sitting in awkward positions for long periods without

BOX 19-2 Economic Globalization
Ellen R. Shaffer and Joseph E. Brenner

Economic globalization refers to the increasing pace and volume of (a) international trade in goods and services among interconnected multinational corporations, (b) the flow of capital across borders, and (c) the related migration of populations, facilitated by technological changes in communication and transportation. It also includes changes in policy favoring the privatization of public enterprises, and reducing government's right to regulate corporate activity in the public interest. While increasing wealth for some corporations, these policies contribute to social inequality and instability. Public health professionals can help ensure that the world's economy supports social justice and sustainable development. The most effective modes of action are through formal organizations or looser networks of like-minded colleagues. Meetings and publications sponsored by professional organizations—as well as relevant listservs and websites—can stimulate thinking and facilitate interactions among individuals and groups with similar concerns.

Basic to any action is analysis of policies, principles, and institutions that shape economic globalization—and their implications for population health and for health care services—as well as an understanding of where opportunities exist to address problems created by globalization.

International financial institutions (IFIs)—the World Trade Organization (WTO), the International Monetary Fund (IMF), and the World Bank—play an important role in establishing policies that govern the global economy. The IMF and the World Bank, which orchestrate loans and enforce economic policies on such matters as interest rates and public budget deficits, also fund programs and set policies in health. The WTO, established in 1995, sets the framework for multinational trade agreements.

Drawing on the wealth, power, and influence of developed countries, the IFIs have prescribed for developing countries controversial measures that rely on (a) market forces to regulate all economic activity, (b) fiscal discipline by states, (c) privatization, (d) deregulation, and (e) liberalization of rules restricting foreign trade. Policies of the IFIs aim to

- Reduce the role of governments by restricting their ability to regulate
- Encourage competition from private companies to own and produce services and goods
- Reduce public funding and allocate public subsidies to private corporations
- Shift the burden of raising revenues for services from public subsidies to individuals, through cost recovery, user fees, or co-payments

(continued)

- Target remaining public subsidies to the poorest, which generally creates a two-tiered system in which people who can afford to pay receive a higher level of services than those who cannot
- Decentralize administrative and financial procedures to the state and local level, thereby weakening control at the national level.

Trade agreements impose these rules and curtail the right and ability of nations to determine whether they wish to abide by them, challenging the role that democratically elected public officials and civil society leaders play in determining the rules of trade and their own policy priorities. The WTO is empowered to impose substantial financial penalties on member nations that it determines do not comply with its rules. Disputes about compliance are adjudicated by tribunals that deliberate without public scrutiny. Government intervention in trade in the interests of social, environmental, and health policy objectives can be disallowed by WTO tribunals. For example, the WTO has overridden prohibitions against importing tuna caught with a method that also snares dolphins.

These policies and the commercialization of vital human services, such as health care and provision of water, adversely affect population health. While the stated goal of privatization and deregulation is to increase prosperity through trade, analysts increasingly contend that they contribute to the rise in global poverty and economic inequality and instability, and therefore to increased preventable illness and death.

For many years, liberalization of trade meant reducing barriers to international trade, such as tariffs and other measures that discouraged competitive trade from foreign producers, relating primarily to goods. Recently, however, agreements such as the General Agreement on Trade in Services (GATS) apply trade rules to vital human services, including health care, education, and provision of water and sanitation, for all 148 member nations of the WTO. Including services broadens the range of public health protections that can be struck down by trade panels.

These agreements could limit the ability of federal, state, or local governments to adopt and enforce public health standards concerning, for example, health care facilities, health insurance, health professional training and licensing, access to medications, environmental protection, occupational health and safety, tobacco, alcohol, firearms, and provision of water and sanitation.

Public health professionals can influence international trade agreements and their adverse impacts on health, by taking actions, such as the following:

1. *Write a journal or a newspaper article exploring the tensions between commercial and health interests.* What rules regulate tobacco companies, the

(continued)

BOX 19-2 *(continued)*

health insurance industry or hospitals? How do those rules contribute to economic productivity and human well-being? How do human rights treaties, international environmental agreements, and trade agreements address the value of life?

2. *Promote assessments of the impact of international trade agreements on population health.* One could examine why trade rules on intellectual property protect pharmaceutical companies from price competition, which would make essential medicines affordable to people with HIV/AIDS and other diseases.

3. *Write a resolution for your professional association explaining the role of trade rules in determining health protections.* Establish a committee to develop and implement an advocacy program that brings the public health perspective to policymakers. (See item 6.)

4. *Ask your member of Congress to designate you and your colleagues as her public health advisory committee.* In this way, you could provide a public health perspective on proposed trade agreements and on the implementation of existing ones. You could hold public hearings to inform your community and the news media. Ask her to recommend that the U.S. Trade Representative establish a similar committee.

5. *Support enforceable commitments to advancing population health and to achieving universal access to health care, affordable medications, and safe, affordable water in the United States and internationally.* Link your daily work with advocacy campaigns to ensure that safe and affordable health care, medicines, and water are not eroded by trade agreements.

6. *Participate in the network of the Center for Policy Analysis Trade and Health (CPATH) (www.cpath.org).* Enroll in the CPATH listserv to stay informed and to participate in campaigns to contact policymakers regarding pending decisions in Congress and at trade summits. Enroll by sending a blank email (nothing in the "subject" line or in the body of the message) to globalizationandhealth-subscribe@topica.com. Ask your professional association to endorse CPATH's Call for Public Health Accountability in Trade. To explore volunteer opportunities and other issues, email at cpath@cpath.org.

breaks.[34] Stress is blamed for a growing number of illnesses and deaths, because maquiladora workers are under constant pressure to work quickly to meet high production quotas. Breaks—even for using the restroom—are permitted infrequently or not at all. Wage and job insecurity may also exacerbate the stress. These workers also have increased rates of reproductive health problems, such as menstrual irregularities and abnormal pregnancy outcomes, including miscarriages and children born prematurely or with birth defects.[34]

For several years, labor advocates, public health practitioners, and scholars have recognized that increasing international trade would threaten worker health and safety. Concern grew that industries from developed countries were relocating to plants in developing countries because of lower labor costs, more lax regulatory environments, and, in some cases, proximity to raw materials and/or markets. These industries failed to follow the same workplace safety and health standards in developing countries that were required in their countries of origin, thereby exposing workers to greater risks.[35]

Concurrent changes in macroeconomic policy among many European and North American nations have also had an impact on occupational safety and health policies; however, workers in developing countries remain a high-risk population, facing a range of workplace hazards at levels not seen in developed countries for decades and in patterns that seem to be accelerating with the growth of global trade.[35] In developing countries, governments often place economic development ahead of worker protection, and independent labor unions, when functional, often focus on wages and job security, rather than on working conditions.

The growth in globalization has also influenced worker safety and health in the United States in recent years, with very few new OSHA standards adopted and many existing ones not being as strictly enforced.[36] Many local government officials and groups of workers, perceiving the same dilemma, refrain from pressing for safer workplaces, fearing job loss from companies closing workplaces and moving to lower-wage areas.

What Needs to Be Done

Educating Workers and Empowering Communities

Worker education is the greatest tool available in creating stronger workplace democracy and worker empowerment. This includes education for workers, not only in occupational safety and health but also on electoral politics, labor union organizing, and coalition building. Recognizing that language and cultural barriers might exist, worker education programs must be designed appropriately and in a language understood by the workers involved, and they also must be designed to specifically address the workers' needs. Worker education can be instrumental in helping to build effective leadership and active participation of workers who otherwise might feel disenfranchised in addressing poor working conditions and health and safety concerns at their worksites.

Community empowerment is defined as a social action process by which individuals, communities, and organizations gain a mastery over their lives in the context of changing their political and social environment to improve equity and quality of life.[14] Hence, if there is workplace democracy, the community would then also have a seat at the table. Such community empowerment would emphasize partnership and collaboration—not a top-down approach.

Preventing Discrimination

Greater workplace democracy and social justice depends on preventing discrimination against workers of color, immigrant workers, women workers, child laborers, and older workers. Institutionalized racism, sexism, and job discrimination are major obstacles to workers and communities in strategizing, organizing, and forming coalitions to fight together for better workplace protections and to establish mechanisms to prevent corporate negligence and indifference. Acknowledging, understanding, and recognizing these obstacles can be useful for identifying and resolving issues that may be the root causes of hostility among different racial and ethnic populations.

Promoting Workplace Democracy and Environmental Justice

Occupational safety and health are linked to the struggle for better workplace democracy—workers' democratic ability to control their work environment and to shape their own lives. The shared principles include equity and empowerment of workers, individuals, and communities. To improve the overall health of workers and promote healthier communities, labor unions, public interest groups, community activists, and public health practitioners should join forces to (a) organize workers and members of the community to fight for equal justice and protection under occupational and environmental laws and regulations, and (b) rally together against corporate interests. Achieving workplace democracy and environmental justice will be more likely with sharing of expertise and resources.[11]

Improving Surveillance and Research

Improved surveillance of occupational exposures and work-related injuries and illnesses, along with systemic development of reliable data sources, needs to be a national priority.

Surveillance systems and research studies should gather and analyze data not only on occupation but also on socioeconomic class and race/ethnicity to help develop hypotheses about the interactions between (a) occupational exposures, and (b) class and race/ethnicity.[20]

Reforming OSHA

In the early 1990s, labor unions organized campaigns promoting OSHA reform. The legislation they proposed, which was not passed by Congress, would have mandated (a) joint labor-management health and safety committees at all worksites, (b) more OSHA compliance officers, (c) more targeted inspections of hazardous workplaces, (d) criminal arrests for employers who willfully violate OSHA standards and cause employee deaths, and (e) the worker's right to refuse hazardous work. Such OSHA reform legislation is still needed today. It could substantially enhance workplace democracy by providing workers with direct participation and a voice "at the table" on health and safety matters at their workplaces.

Public health professionals and students should join with labor leaders in calling for OSHA reform by lobbying Congress and holding their elected officials accountable for protecting the health and safety and rights of all workers. In the midst of globalization and the current pro-business anti-regulatory climate, more strategic actions and plans are needed to provide increased worker participation in the political process, better worker education, and recruitment of workers to increase union membership, thereby providing more workers with a united voice to fight for stronger and more effective workplace protections.

Reforming Workers' Compensation

The United States does not have a unified workers' compensation system. Each state has its own standards and practices. The burden of proof that disease is occupationally related lies with workers. They must find physicians who believe that their illnesses are occupationally related. Judges who hear contested cases must be convinced that the illnesses are work related.[37] A national workers' compensation system with uniform benefits should be established. Employers should bear the burden of proof that illnesses are not related to work. Workers' compensation should also not be the "exclusive remedy" for workers seeking to recover damages from employers; pain-and-suffering awards should be allowed.[38]

Promoting the Role of Organized Labor

Workers who can be fired at the whim of their employers cannot be very insistent in demanding safer working conditions. This situation is especially true (a) in workplaces where there is no union, and (b) in jobs where employees can easily be replaced and for which alternative safer jobs at marginally lower wage rates are not available. In addition, the costs associated with switching jobs—such as loss of health care benefits, pension rights, and seniority; the necessity of becoming familiar with a new employer; and the expense and personal disruption of relocation—may be too high a risk for many workers.[11] Labor unions have been a powerful market force to protect workers' rights and to assist workers in confronting employer market power. Starting in the 1980s, however, the power of many labor unions diminished to the point where workers in many industries were forced to accept wage concessions. In other industries, prominent companies replaced unionized workers with nonunion workers and the overall percentage of the U.S. workforce declined considerably, from 22 percent in 1982 to 14 percent in 2004.

Union organizing has become the principal rallying cry for unions in the AFL-CIO. Unions at every level are being asked to shift resources to help workers organize. Unions are recruiting and training new organizers whose diversity reflects that of workers in the United States.[39] Forming a labor organization in the workplace is still a fundamental right. Now, more than ever, workers need a strong and countervailing voice to corporate power, to speak out against the social injustice of an unhealthy work environment. Due to liberalized trade practices, free market economic policies, and the elimination or weakening of protective labor legislation, the risks and costs to workers attempting to organize have increased. Still, however, the possibility remains that unions can win organizing drives—even in hostile organizing climates—if they implement more comprehensive and multifaceted organizing strategies. Humility, class unity, persistence, and determination—combined with the commitment for better wages, better workplace health and safety protection, and fair contracts—form a strong foundation for organizing workers.[12]

Conclusion

Work profoundly defines the well-being of individuals and populations. The structure of the workplace is a reflection of both general social conditions in the society at large and the specific organization within the workplace.

The frightening acceleration of economic disparities, even in the context of boom economies, stands as a major barrier to achieving social justice in the United States. The workplace remains the crucible where social justice must be established. Disparities in working conditions must be addressed if occupational injuries and diseases are to be prevented. To achieve health and safety goals, a large, militant, and principled labor movement is needed—the major tool to achieving democracy in the workplace. Upon that foundation, we believe, rest all measures to expand democracy in general, and to eliminate racial, ethnic, and gender discrimination.

References

1. Levenstein C, Wooding J, Rosenberg B. Occupational health: a social perspective. In: Levy BS, Wegman DH, eds. Occupational health: recognizing and preventing work-related disease and injury. 4th ed. Philadelphia: Lippincott Williams & Wilkins, 2000:27–50.
2. Davis A. Women, race, and class. New York: Vintage Books, 1981.
3. Staples R. The black woman in American history. Chicago: Nelson-Hall Publishers, 1983:14.
4. Haywood H. Negro liberation. Chicago: Liberator Press, 1976.
5. Gindin S. Social justice and globalization: are they compatible? Toronto, Ontario: Monthly Review Press, 2002:1–11.
6. Evans G, Kantrowitz E. Social status and health: the potential role of environmental risk exposure. Annu Rev Public Health 2002;23:303–31.
7. Taylor A, Murray L. Minority workers. In: Levy BS, Wegman DH, eds. Occupational health: recognizing and preventing work-related disease and injury. 4th ed. Philadelphia: Lippincott Williams & Wilkins, 2000:679–87.
8. Green J. The world of the worker: labor in twentieth century America. New York: Hill and Wang, 1980.
9. Morris R, ed. A history of the American worker. Princeton, N.J.: Princeton University Press, 1983.
10. Berman D. Why work kills: a brief history of occupational safety and health in the United States. Int J Health Serv 1977;7:63–88.
11. McGarity T, Shapiro S. Workers at risk: the failed promise of the occupational safety and health administration. Westport, Conn.: Greenwood Publishing Group, 1993.
12. Taylor A. Organizing marginalized workers. Occup Med State Art Rev 1999;14:687–95.
13. Subramanian SV, Kawachi I. Wage poverty, earned income inequality, and health. In: Heyman J, ed. Global inequalities at work: work's impact on the health of individuals, families, and societies. Oxford, England: Oxford University Press, 2003.
14. Wallerstein N. Empowerment to reduce health disparities. Scand J Public Health 2002;30(suppl 59):72–7.
15. Theorell T, Lind E, Floderus B. The relationship of disturbing life changes and emotions to the early development of myocardial infarctions and other serious illness. Int J Epidemiol 1975;4:281–93.
16. Leeflang RLI, Klein-Hesselink DJ, Spruit IP. Health effects of unemployment. II. Men and women. Soc Sci Med 1992;34:351–63.
17. Brackbill R, Siegel P, Ackermann S. Self reported hypertension among unemployed people in the United States. Br Med J 1995;310:568.
18. Levenstein S, Smith MW, Kaplan GA. Psychosocial predictors of hypertension in men and women. Arch Intern Med 2001;161:1341–6.
19. Frumkin H, Walker ED, Friedman-Jiminez G. Minority workers and communities. Occup Med State Art Rev 1999;14:495–517.
20. Murray L. Sick and tired of being sick and tired: scientific evidence, methods, and research implications for racial and ethnic disparities in occupational health. Am J Public Health 2003;93:221–6.
21. O'Connor-Marer P, Schenker MB. Pesticides, adverse effects. In BS Levy, GR Wagner, KM Rest, JL Weeks, eds. Preventing occupational disease and injury. 2nd ed. Washington, D.C.: American Public Health Association, 2005:396.

22. Richardson S, Ruser J, Suarez P. Hispanic workers in the United States: an analysis of employment distributions, fatal occupational injuries, and non-fatal occupational injuries and illnesses. Safety is seguridad: a workshop summary. Washington, D.C.: National Research Council, National Academy Press, 2003.

23. Institute of Medicine. Protecting youth at work: health, safety, and development of working children and adolescents in the United States. Washington, D.C.: National Academy Press, 1998.

24. Ashford N. The economic and social context of special populations. Occup Med State Art Rev 1999;14:485–93.

25. U.S. Chemical Safety and Hazard Investigation Board. Investigation report: refinery fire incident—Tosco Avon Refinery. Washington, D.C.: U.S. Chemical Safety and Hazard Investigation Board (report no. 99-014-I-CA), March 2001.

26. U.S. Chemical Safety and Hazard Investigation Board. Safety bulletin: management of change. Washington, D.C.: U.S. Chemical Safety and Hazard Investigation Board (report no. 2001-05-SB), August 2001.

27. Labor Force Statistics for the Current Population. The employment situation: March 2004. U.S. Department of Labor, U.S. Bureau of Labor Statistics. Released April 2, 2004.

28. Mishel L, Bernstein J, Boushey H. The state of working America 2002/2003. Ithaca, N.Y.: Economic Policy Institute, Cornell University Press, 2003.

29. Burchell B. The effects of labour market position, job insecurity, and unemployment on psychological health. In: Gallie D, et al., eds. Social change and the experience of unemployment. Oxford, England: Oxford University Press, 1994.

30. Bethune A. Unemployment and mortality. In: Drever F, Whitehead M, eds. Health inequalities. London, England: H.M. Stationery Office, 1997.

31. U.S. Census Bureau. U.S. Census: educational attainment of civilians 16 years and over, by labor force statistics. Washington, D.C.: U.S. Census Bureau, 2000.

32. Robinson J. Trends in racial inequality and exposure to work-related hazards, 1968–1986. AAOHN J 1989;37:56–63.

33. Friedman-Jimenez G. Occupational disease among minority workers. AAOHN J 1989;37:64–70.

34. Abell H. Endangering women's health for profit: health and safety in Mexico's maquiladoras. Dev Pract 1999;9:595–600.

35. Frumkin H. Across the water and down the ladder: occupational health in the global economy. Occup Med State Art Rev 1999;14:637–63.

36. U.S. Department of Labor. OSHA citations statistics, 2002. Washington, D.C.: OSHA, 2003.

37. Boden L. Workers' compensation. In: Levy BS, Wegman DH, eds. Occupational health: recognizing and preventing work-related disease and injury. 4th ed. Philadelphia: Lippincott Williams & Wilkins, 2000:237–56.

38. Morris L. Minorities, jobs, and health: an unmet promise. AAOHN J 1989;37:53–5.

39. Sweeney J. Public addresses: building a labor movement strategy for the new century. Georgetown J Poverty Law Policy 2000;VII:163–72.

20

ORAL HEALTH

Myron Allukian, Jr., and Alice M. Horowitz

Introduction

Oral diseases, including dental disorders, represent a neglected or silent epidemic,[1-7] largely due to social injustice. Although they affect almost everyone, the prevention of oral diseases has not received high priority. In fact, the United States in recent years has moved backward, with the elimination or limiting of adult dental services in most state dental Medicaid programs.[8] The most vulnerable people have become even more vulnerable.

A healthy mouth and smile, free from pain and infection, is a valued necessity for those who live and work in the public eye, as witnessed by the large sums of money many people spend to achieve this ideal image and state of health. However, what about the rest of the population?

Health Care versus Medical and Dental Care

A major reason why oral health is such a low priority in the United States is that it is not viewed as an integral component of overall health. Since the first dental school was established in 1840, dentistry developed as a separate profession. Most medical schools teach very little, if anything, about oral health. Because medicine has played a dominant role in the development of health policy and practice in our country, oral health is usually excluded or not considered part of primary health care. This perception is held by many policymakers, and it is reflected in the public financing of health care. Only 4 percent of dental care is financed with public funds, compared with 32 percent for medical care.[6]

Defining Oral Health

Good oral health is being able to eat, chew, talk, smile, kiss, sleep, read, think, study, or work without oral pain, discomfort, or embarrassment. Oral health is having a smile that helps you feel good about yourself and gives others a healthy and positive image of you. Good oral health is essential and integral to overall health and well-being. Poor oral health is associated with diabetes, premature birth and low birth weight,[9–11] heart disease, and stroke.[12–14] As Dr. C. Everett Koop, a former U.S. Surgeon General, has said, "You're not healthy without good oral health." The maintenance of oral health is important for freedom from pain, infection, and suffering; the ability to eat and chew, as well as proper digestion and nutrition; the ability to speak properly; social mobility; employability; self-image and self-esteem; and a higher quality of life.

A Neglected Epidemic

Oral diseases are life-long for most Americans. There has been a marked improvement in our nation's oral health since the 1970s due to community water fluoridation, fluorides, dental sealants, technological advances, dental insurance, and better education of the public and the health professions. But oral diseases remain a neglected epidemic in the United States:

- Seventy-eight percent of 17-year-olds have had tooth decay, with an average of seven tooth surfaces affected.[15]
- Ninety-eight percent of 40- to 44-year-olds have had tooth decay, with an average of 45 affected tooth surfaces.[15]
- Thirty percent of Americans older than 65 have no teeth.[16]
- Twenty-two percent of 35- to 44-year-olds have destructive periodontal disease.[16]
- More Americans die each year from oral and pharyngeal cancer than from cervical cancer or malignant melanoma.[17]

There are great disparities in oral health between the "haves" and "have-nots." For those people who are sophisticated and have the financial resources, personal preventive procedures are used and dental services are obtained on a regular and periodic basis. For everyone else, dental services are crisis oriented. In addition, increasingly less money is being spent on oral health in the United

States. In 2003, the total cost for dental care, about $74.3 billion, represented 4.4 percent of health care expenditures compared with 6.4 percent in 1970—a 31 percent relative decrease.[18]

The Relationship Between Social Injustice and Oral Health

Laws, regulations, policies, customs, and practices can serve as barriers to social justice in oral health. Social injustice especially affects the oral health of vulnerable populations, including children, older people, low-income individuals, poorly-educated people, the developmentally disabled, medically compromised people, the homebound and the homeless, people infected with HIV, migrants, immigrants, uninsured people, institutionalized individuals, residents of rural areas, and members of racial, ethnic, and linguistic minorities.

Vulnerable populations have greater oral health needs and less access to resources to respond to these needs. In the United States:

- Oral diseases represent the most prevalent unmet health need of children.[19]
- The rate of untreated dental disease among low-income children aged 2 to 5 years is almost five times that of high-income children.[20]
- Low-income children have 10 times more unmet dental needs than do higher-income children.[21]
- Low-income children have almost 12 times more days missed from school than do higher-income children.[22]
- The oral cancer mortality rate of African-American males is almost double that of white males.[23]
- Among 14-year-olds, the use of preventive dental sealants is almost four times greater for whites than for African-Americans of the same age.[16]
- The rate of untreated dental disease for American Indian and Alaska Native children aged 2 to 4 years is six times greater than that in white children.[16]
- People without health insurance have four times the rate of unmet dental needs as do those with private insurance.[24]
- Among those aged 18 and older, Asian-Americans and native Hawaiians or other Pacific Islanders have never been to a dentist at a rate about 10 times that of white Americans.[25]
- Only 15.7 percent of adults—and only 2.5 percent of poor adults—aged 65 and over living in rural areas have private dental insurance.[26]

There are strong relationships between both low dental care use and poor oral health status and (a) low education, (b) low income, (c) nonwhite racial status, and (d) lack of health insurance coverage (tables 20-1 and 20-2). (See also box 20-1.) For example, only about 35 percent of people over age 25

TABLE 20-1   Percentage of Persons Aged 25 or Older Who Had a Dental Visit Within the Last Year by Education, Income, and Race, 1993

	Persons Who Had a Dental Visit (%)
Education	
<12 Years	35.1
12 Years	54.8
>12 Years	70.9
Income	
Below poverty	30.4
At or above poverty	55.8
Race and Hispanic Origin	
White, non-Hispanic	56.6
Black, non-Hispanic	39.1
Hispanic	42.1
Education, Race, and Hispanic Origin	
<12 Years	
White, non-Hispanic	41.0
Black, non-Hispanic	33.1
Hispanic	33.0
12 Years	
White, non-Hispanic	60.4
Black, non-Hispanic	48.2
Hispanic	54.6
>12 Years	
White, non-Hispanic	75.8
Black, non-Hispanic	61.3
Hispanic	61.8

From U.S. Department of Health and Human Services. Oral health in America: a report of the Surgeon General. Rockville, Md.: National Institute of Dental and Craniofacial Research, National Institutes of Health, 2000.

with less than 12 years of education have been to a dentist in the past year, compared with about 71 percent of those with more than 12 years of education. Over 20 percent of people over age 2 with a family income less than $10,000 have not been to a dentist for 5 years or more, compared with 5.5 percent for these with a family income of more than $35,000. Over 13 percent of Mexican-Americans have never been to a dentist, compared with 4.4 percent of whites (table 20-2). A national study showed that Mexican-American children and adults had greater unmet dental needs, less dental insurance, and fewer dental visits than other Hispanics or Latinos, as well as Puerto Ricans, Cubans, and Central or South Americans.[26a]

TABLE 20-2 Percentage of Persons, 2 Years or Older, by Time Since Last Dental Visit, by Education, Income, Race, and Insurance, United States, 1989

	5 Years or Longer (%)	Never (%)
Education		
<9 Years	30.6	5.9
9–11 Years	23.5	1.3
12 Years	14.4	0.5
>13 Years	6.9	0.2
Family Income		
<$10,000	20.1	7.0
$10,000–19,999	16.1	6.6
$20,000–34,999	10.4	4.6
>$35,000	5.5	2.9
Race		
White	10.5	4.4
Black	15.1	5.9
Other	10.8	6.7
Hispanic Origin		
Non-Hispanic	10.8	4.1
Hispanic	13.0	9.7
Mexican-American	15.8	13.1
Other Hispanic	9.0	5.1
Dental Insurance Coverage		
With private dental insurance	6.6	3.3
Without private dental insurance	14.2	6.0

From U.S. Department of Health and Human Services. Oral health in America: a report of the Surgeon General. Rockville, Md.: National Institute of Dental and Craniofacial Research, National Institutes of Health, 2000.

Health Literacy and Social Inequality

Higher levels of education are generally associated with better overall health status. Health literacy is recognized as an essential skill not only for managing disease but also for preventing it and for navigating the health care system to facilitate access.[27] Nearly half the U.S. population has low or limited literacy skills[28]—they cannot read and understand directions on prescriptions and over-the-counter medicines; interpret bus schedules, which may preclude getting to health appointments; complete Medicaid forms to determine if their children are eligible for oral health care; and understand what their health care providers tell them.[27] Concomitantly, most health care providers have not been trained to communicate with patients so that patients or their caregivers,

Most oral diseases can be prevented or controlled, yet they often are rampant, especially in developing countries. In many ways, social injustice in oral health in developing countries mirrors that among lower socioeconomic groups in the United States. For example, many poor people in developing countries cannot afford to purchase toothbrushes and fluoride toothpaste, and many do not understand the value of either; many can barely afford to feed themselves, let alone go to a dentist. All too often oral health is not considered important, or even part of overall health. In many developing countries, inadequate education perpetuates myths concerning health. In addition, in many developing countries there are few, if any, sources of dental care. The dentist-to-population ratio in these countries often ranges from 1:36,000 to 1:119,000, compared with 1:1,700 in the United States.[1]

In developing countries, central water supplies often are few and much of the water is not potable. Thus, community water fluoridation is not feasible. However, fluoridated salt, a proven method of ensuring adequate levels of systemic fluoride, could be used in countries where central water supplies are sparse.[2] This method of dental caries prevention is an effective and equitable approach because virtually all people buy and use salt. In Central and South America, the Pan American Health Organization (PAHO) has promoted fluoridated salt, which is usually the same price as nonfluoridated salt. Fluoride toothpaste and other sources of fluoride usually are not available in these countries or they are too expensive. Even toothbrushes are often not available.

U.S. industries export huge quantities of sugar-laden products, especially soft drinks. These products contribute to tooth decay and obesity. Despite efforts by the World Health Organization (WHO) to address the obesity problem by developing a strategic plan for all countries to adopt, the United States has attempted to derail the plan because of the influence of the food and sugar industries that want to continue to sell their products in these countries.[3]

In many developing countries, young children with malnutrition and poor oral hygiene develop noma or cancrum oris, a gangrenous condition that starts in the mouth and destroys the mouth and face. Ninety percent of the children with this condition die without having been treated. This disease is preventable, but the WHO budget for preventing it and other oral health disorders is severely limited.[4]

Worldwide, 4.9 million people died in 2000 as a result of tobacco use. Although tobacco use is decreasing in more affluent countries, its use is rapidly rising in low- and middle-income countries, where most people live.[5] Tobacco-induced oral diseases include periodontitis and oral and pharyngeal cancers, which rank among the three most common cancers in South Central Asia.[4–5]

Use of tobacco also is associated with congenital defects, such as cleft lip and palate, in children whose mothers have smoked during pregnancy. In 2003, the World Health Assembly agreed on a groundbreaking public health

(continued)

treaty to control tobacco supply and consumption.[5] Because the United States has curtailed to a certain extent who can use tobacco products and where they can be used, multinational tobacco industries have turned their attention to other countries where there are few restrictions. Their advertising efforts have worked because they have gained access to Eastern Europe, Asia, and Africa, where markets previously were restricted. In most Asian countries, there is easy access to cigarette machines by children and youth and little effort to educate the public about the dangers of tobacco use. About 25 percent of teenagers in other countries have been offered free cigarettes by company representatives.[6]

The following recommendations would improve the oral health and general health of people in developing countries:

1. The United States must be more responsive to the health and human needs of other countries and should not support the export of U.S. products deleterious to health or safety.
2. Developing countries should place a higher priority on the oral health of their populations and implement community-based primary prevention programs, such as community water fluoridation or salt fluoridation, and school-based dental programs.
3. WHO and PAHO must make oral health a much higher priority, especially in developing countries.

References

1. FDI World Dental Federation. Global dentistry information. Available at: http://www.fdiworldental.org/resources/3_Ofacts.html. Accessed February 22, 2005.
2. Pan American Health Organization. Final report to the W. K. Kellogg Foundation, project no. 43225. Multi-year plan for salt fluoridation programs in the region of the Americas. Washington, D.C.: Pan American Health Organization, World Health Organization, 2000.
3. Stein R. U.S. says it will contest WHO plan to fight obesity. *Washington Post,* 2004, p A3.
4. Petersen PE. The World Oral Health Report 2003: continuous improvement of oral health in the 21st century—the approach of the WHO Global Oral Health Program. Community Dent Oral Epidemiol 2003;31(suppl 1):3–24.
5. Petersen PE. Tobacco and oral health—the role of the World Health Organization. Oral Health Prev Dent 2003;1:309–15.
6. Warren C, Riley L, Asma S, et al. Tobacco use by youth: a surveillance report from the Global Youth Tobacco Survey Project. Bull WHO 2000;78:868–76.

in the case of children or older people, understand. Moreover, if decision-makers are not aware of the importance of health literacy, their health programs will likely be less effective and more expensive.

Overall, adults are not very knowledgeable about many aspects of oral health.[6] Often people with the greatest oral health burdens have the least access to health information and the fewest skills to navigate the health care system.[27] However, most oral diseases can be prevented or controlled.[29] Inadequate government policies at the national, state, and local levels adversely affect the oral health of the public, especially of vulnerable populations.

National Priorities

In the absence of a national oral health program, the United States has created many "ad hoc" or "Band-Aid" programs to respond to the oral health needs that are inadequate, as follows:

- Medicare does not include dental services, except for trauma or cancer.
- Medicaid dental programs nationally serve only about 20 percent of eligible children.[30]
- Dental care is an optional service in Medicaid for adults, and most state Medicaid programs do not provide dental care to adults.[8]
- Until recently, less than half of the federally funded community and migrant health centers did not include dental services.
- There are 2,112 dental health professional shortage areas (DHPSAs) with more than 41 million residents.[31]
- Head Start programs no longer have a meaningful oral health component even though access to dental services is their number-one issue.[32]
- Job Corps dental programs have become a low priority.
- Indian Health Service dental programs have become more fragmented and less effective.

Executive branch federal agencies and the Congress have not made oral health services for the underserved a sufficient priority. U.S. federal agencies have done a good job in documenting the oral health needs of our country, with such initiatives as *Healthy People 2010* and the *U.S. Surgeon's Report on Oral Health*, and in funding some research. However, such reports and research have yet to be translated into effective national programs.

Local and State Priorities

Oral health is a low priority in most states.

- Most states have eliminated or dramatically cut back their adult dental Medicaid programs.[8]
- Only 35 states have a permanent full-time state dental director with a dental education, and most of them are inadequately funded and understaffed.[33]

- Many states have restrictive state practice acts that limit who may practice dentistry in their states and what scope of services may be provided by dental hygienists and dental assistants.
- Most state and local boards of health do not include a dentist or dental hygienist.
- Many local boards of health in nonfluoridated communities have not attempted to achieve fluoridation for their communities, even though it is the most cost-effective preventive measure for better oral health and was designated by the Centers for Disease Control and Prevention as one the of 10 great public health achievements of the twentieth century.[34]
- Most school-based health care centers do not include oral health.
- Only a small minority of local health departments have a dental program.
- Access to dental care is one of the leading cause of discrimination for persons with HIV/AIDS.

School Programs

Many school-age children and youth in the United States do not have access to basic preventive and primary oral and medical care, even though many of them are poor enough to qualify for free school lunches and breakfasts. Because most children and youth in the United States are enrolled in schools, they would benefit from school-based health clinics that include oral health services.[35] This approach to providing health services to children and adolescents is very practical and cost-effective. Less time is lost from classes going to and from a dental care facility located in the school, and parents do not have to miss work to take their children to obtain health services. There are more than 1,500 health centers in schools in the United States, of which few provide oral health preventive and treatment services.[36]

Comprehensive, school-based oral health education and preventive regimens, especially in schools with a high prevalence of youngsters on free-lunch programs, provide an equal opportunity for good oral health.[35] New Zealand, Australia, Denmark, and other countries maintain such school-based oral health programs. Not to provide these services in the richest country in the world is social injustice.

Dental Public Health Infrastructure

Most of the more than 2,800 local health departments in the United States do not employ dentists or dental hygienists who are trained in public health. Although a majority of state health departments employ full-time dentists or hygienists, they generally have very limited funding and small-sized staffs. Of the approximately 150,000 dentists in the United States, only 152 are certified by the American Board of Dental Public Health.[37] Public health dentists are trained to improve and protect the oral health of communities and population groups at the community, town, region, state, or national level. Almost always, the population groups served include vulnerable populations, such as children, low-income people, the homeless, or the elderly.

Although dentists trained in public health, compared with dental clinicians or private practitioners, make a greater impact on improving the oral health of a population, they are not valued by our society. Dentists trained in public health have more education and training than most dental clinicians, but their income is much less because they do not treat individual patients.

Dental Workforce

The dental workforce does not mirror our population. Although 12 percent of the U.S. population is composed of African-Americans, they represent only 2.2 percent of practicing dentists[38]—and the future does not look promising. In 2001–2002, 13 of the 55 dental schools in the United States did not have *any* entering African-American students and 10 schools had only one entering African-American.[39] Hispanic and Native-American dentists also are sorely needed.

Practices of the Food Industry

The food industry in the United States, a $709 billion enterprise in 2002, adversely affects the health of most Americans,[40] including oral health. Nearly 98 percent of adults have had tooth decay[16] and about 60 percent of adults are overweight or obese.[41] The average American consumes about 154 pounds of sugar, most of which is added to processed foods, drinks, and sweets[42]—a 34-pound or 28-percent increase in added sugar or sweeteners since 1982. In 1997, the average American consumed 53 teaspoons of added sugar a day.[42]

The consumption of high-sugared drinks by U.S. children and youth has escalated. Soft-drink consumption among school-aged youth (6 to 17 years of age) increased from a prevalence of 37 percent in 1977–1978 to 56 percent in 1994–1998. During this period, the average daily intake increased from 5 to 12 fluid ounces.[43] At least 56 percent of school-age children drink at least one soft drink daily.

Adolescent males are the highest consumers of soft drinks; 20 percent of them drink four or more servings each day.[44] Each 12-ounce serving of a sweetened soft drink contains 10 teaspoons of sugar. The odds of children becoming obese increase 1.6 times for each additional can or glass of sugar-sweetened soda consumed daily.[45] This increase in consumption of soft drinks has resulted from an aggressive marketing campaign that spends billions of dollars a year to target children and youth.[46]

About 60 percent of middle and high schools sell soft drinks on campus.[47] Recently, there has been an outcry among parents, educators, and health care providers regarding the practice by the soft drink industry of "buying schools"—such as a soft drink company giving money to a school in exchange for exclusive rights to sell high-sugar drinks in the school. Approximately 16 percent of school districts in the United States have made such an arrangement. Because most schools are experiencing severe budget cuts, this approach to supplementing their income has had a huge impact on what students drink on school premises.[47] These contracts have provided schools with more than $20 million in revenue.[48]

Candy sales on school grounds also are a common practice to earn money for team uniforms, recreational equipment, and computers. These sugar-laden products cause tooth decay in children and youth and establish poor health practices that contribute to obesity. Marketing high-fat and high-sugar products to children and youth has resulted in our country having the highest percentage of overweight school-age children in the world, 15 percent.[49] Enticing school-age children and youth to eat high-fat and high-sugar products is a social injustice because many of them are not knowledgeable enough to make appropriate decisions about healthy food choices. In addition, the amount of money the food industry puts into advertising for this vulnerable age group far outweighs attempts to educate children about healthy lifestyles. Also, high-fat and high-sugar products are usually less expensive to purchase than healthy foods, which makes it all the more inequitable for families of low socioeconomic status.

Practices of the Tobacco Industry

In the United States, over 440,000 people die each year from tobacco-related diseases, including cancer,[50] and 4,000 U.S. children and youth begin smoking each day[51]—most between the ages of 10 and 18. The tobacco industry promotes smoking by annually spending billions of dollars on advertising and marketing—since 1999, it has spent more than $101 million to lobby the U.S Congress.[52] The federal government is investing heavily in reducing tobacco use among our youth, but it simply is no match for the tobacco industry.[53] The tobacco industry spent over $11.2 billion in 2001 on marketing—much of which was directed at reaching children and youth, including high-visibility, store-shelf display sales that are more affordable to this age group and "giveaways," such as hats and lighters.[54] Although the tobacco industry does not now invade U.S. school premises as it once did, some schools still allow the tobacco industry to support sporting events and some school districts continue to allow the use of tobacco on school grounds.

Many coaches and teachers are users and the industry continues to advertise directly to youth. In addition, some tobacco companies have increased advertising in youth-directed magazines.[55] Among 12th-grade students, approximately 27 percent reported that they smoke.[51] Because many youth do not graduate from high school, there may be an even higher percentage of youth of this age group who smoke. Directing advertising practices to vulnerable youth is an extreme social inequality because the use of tobacco is addictive and it is very difficult to quit. Frequently, children and youth who are attracted to the use of tobacco are those who already have other disadvantages, which make the inequality all the more burdensome. The use of tobacco products essentially ensures a lifetime of addiction, poor general and oral health, and an early death. In 2000, 32 percent of Americans below the poverty level smoked compared with 23 percent of those at or above poverty level.[55]

What Needs to Be Done

National initiatives could help sensitize policymakers and the general public about the need for better oral health. *Healthy People 2010,* the Surgeon General's report on oral health, and the Surgeon General's National Call to Action[56] have been steps in the right direction, but they have limitations.

Healthy People 2010

This report on the nation's health objectives for the year 2010 includes oral health as one of 28 priority areas. Previous reports focused on national health objectives for the years 1990 and 2000. Oral health has always been included in these objectives, although, in its first draft, the 1990 objectives did not include oral health. The *Healthy People 2000* objectives emphasized disparities. *Healthy People 2010* has two overarching goals: to increase longevity and quality of life and to eliminate disparities. *Healthy People 2010* includes objectives on prevention in a variety of content areas, access, and infrastructure. These national objectives provide a strategic management tool for local, state, and national government agencies and organizations to develop their own health plans with objectives specific to their needs. These national objectives have been helpful in providing guidance to interested parties concerning national needs and priorities. Unfortunately, there have been too few interested parties or any significant funding to achieve these objectives at the national, state, or local level.

Oral Health in America: A Report of the Surgeon General

The first U.S. Surgeon General's report on oral health, published in 2000,[6] raised the visibility of the "silent epidemic of oral diseases" (p. vii) and documented the importance of oral health as essential to overall health and well-being. The report also documented great disparities between the "haves" and "have-nots," and stressed the importance of effective community-based prevention programs and the need for a strong dental public health infrastructure. Its major findings were as follows:

- Oral diseases and disorders affect health and well-being throughout life.
- Safe and effective measures exist to prevent the most common dental diseases: dental caries and periodontal diseases.
- Lifestyle behaviors that affect general health, such as tobacco use, excessive alcohol use, and poor dietary choices, adversely affect oral and craniofacial health as well.
- There are profound and consequential oral health disparities within the U.S. population.
- More information is needed to improve oral health and eliminate health disparities.
- The mouth reflects general health and well-being. Oral diseases and conditions are associated with other health problems.
- Scientific research is key to further reduction in the burden of diseases and disorders that affect the face, mouth, and teeth.

Although this report clearly demonstrated the extent of the dental crisis in the United States and the epidemic of oral diseases, it was not accompanied by any legislation, executive orders, or funding to respond to these great unmet dental needs.

A National Call to Action to Promote Oral Health

In 2003, U.S. Surgeon General Richard Carmona released *A National Call to Action to Promote Oral Health*,[56] as recommended in the Surgeon General's report on oral health. The vision of the Call to Action was to "advance the general health and well-being of all Americans by creating partnerships at all levels of society to engage in programs to promote oral health and prevent disease" (p. 9). Its three goals mirror those of *Healthy People 2010*: to promote oral health, to promote quality of life, and to eliminate oral health disparities. The Call to Action contains five recommended actions to achieve these goals:

1. Change perceptions of oral health.
2. Overcome barriers by replicating effective programs and proven efforts.
3. Build a science base and accelerate science transfer.
4. Increase oral health workforce diversity, capacity, and flexibility.
5. Increase collaborations.

The Surgeon General has recommended that action plans throughout the United States be written, each by a consortium of stakeholders at the local, regional, and state level, using the *Healthy People 2010* objectives to establish goals and to guide needs assessments and outcome measures. Although the Call to Action is an essential step in the right direction, it consists primarily of guidance with no substantive funding or legislation for programs that can make a difference in people's lives, especially for vulnerable populations.

Recommendations

When there is a problem that affects the entire community, the entire community needs to be involved in some way to respond to the problem. Just as it takes a village to raise a child, it will take a village to resolve the neglected epidemic of oral diseases, especially for vulnerable populations. Clinical dentistry alone cannot resolve this epidemic of oral diseases. There are approximately 1,700 people for every dentist in the United States.[39] The average dentist treats about 800 to 900 people a year.[57]

Oral diseases should be a national priority with appropriate leadership, policies, funding, and programs to have a meaningful impact. The following recommendations would dramatically improve the oral health of the U.S. population, especially for those who are most vulnerable.

1. *A national health program.* We need a national health program for all U.S. residents with a comprehensive oral health component that stresses prevention and primary dental care. It must also include targeted initiatives for schoolchildren and other vulnerable populations, as well as population-based preventive measures, such as community water fluoridation, school-based sealant programs, and tobacco prevention and control programs. The obstacles are enormous, including the insurance industry, drug companies, many other major corporations, and much of organized medicine.[58]

2. *Oral health as a national priority.* Oral health must be made a much higher national priority by the federal government and national organizations, agencies, and institutions in all of their health policies and programs. Oral health must be an integral component of all health

programs for all stages of life and for all vulnerable populations. In addition, the federal government must provide appropriate funding for community-based preventive measures, such as water fluoridation and school-based prevention programs. Charity and volunteerism by dental care providers are helpful but not sufficient.

The federal government also must provide the leadership, expertise, and technical assistance to states and local communities to improve oral health through its regional offices. This action would necessitate a significant increase in the recruitment and staffing of dentists with public health expertise in the U.S. Public Health Service and all federal agencies involved in health services. In 1988, a congressional report documented the inadequacy of the federal government's lack of resources and focus to improve oral health, and in 2003, Congress again expressed its concerns about the oral health programs of the Health Resources and Services Administration.[59,60] Although a few improvements were made in oral health as a result of this report, much more needs to be done:

- Targeted initiatives should be implemented to strengthen and dramatically improve oral health programs for high-risk populations served by programs like Head Start, Community Health Centers, National Health Service Corps, Job Corps, Maternal and Child Health, and the Indian Health Service.
- Medicare should include dental services. Medicaid should include dental services for adults, and both Medicaid and the Child Health Improvement Program (CHIP) should upgrade and improve their dental programs for children.
- Nondental professional associations and national organizations, such as the National Governors Association, the National Conference of Mayors, the National Education Association, and the American Association of Retired People (AARP), should include oral health in their policies and programs. The dental profession should work with these organizations so that oral health is part of general health, as it is considered to be by the American Public Health Association.

3. *Health in schools.* All public schools should provide comprehensive health education, with a meaningful oral health component for all children in grades K through 12. Children need to learn to make healthy choices for healthy lifestyles and healthy lives. We recommend the following:
- All schools should be tobacco free.
- No public school should provide "junk" foods or high-sugared drinks.
- Schools with high-risk, low-income, and minority children should have school-based health programs with an oral health component that provides preventive services and dental care onsite.

- Schools of education and teacher training should include health education with oral health in their curricula.
- Medical, nursing, social work, and public health schools should include oral health in their curricula.
- Accreditation standards for schools in the health professions should include oral health.
- National board examinations for medical, nursing, and other health professional students should include oral health.

4. *State and local priorities.* State and local government should make oral health a much higher priority:
   - State and local health departments should integrate oral health into all health policies and programs.
   - State Medicaid programs should upgrade and improve their dental programs and include dental services in their services for adults and in their CHIPs.
   - State and large local health departments should have full-time dental directors who are board certified or board eligible in dental public health, with sufficient resources and staff members to make a meaningful impact.
   - State dental licensing boards should be part of state health departments, with more public health dentists, dental hygienists, and consumers as full voting members.
   - State dental practice acts should be permissive for licensees to be responsive to access issues in their state, by allowing national reciprocity, limited licensure for foreign-trained dentists for public programs and educational institutions, and a broad scope of duties and supervision for dental hygienists and dental assistants.
   - State and local departments of education should integrate health education with a meaningful oral health component into the school curricula for all children in grades K to 12.
   - State and local departments of education should allow only nutritious foods and snacks in the schools and should not allow "junk" food and high-sugared drinks into schools.
   - State and local boards of health and health departments should actively promote community water fluoridation until all communities with a central supply are fluoridated. (For communities without central water supplies, school-based fluoride programs should be implemented.)
   - State and local health departments should implement school-based sealant programs for all schools with high-risk children.

5. *Prevention.* Effective prevention programs, initiatives, and services must be the foundation for all dental programs at the local, state, and

national levels. Effective population-based prevention programs, such as community water fluoridation, tobacco prevention and control programs, and school fluoride and sealant programs, should be the cornerstones of these prevention programs and have targeted funding. Preventive services for children and vulnerable people, such as brushing with fluoride toothpaste, applying sealants, and using topical fluoride, should be promoted. Oral cancer screening, especially for high-risk groups, should also be promoted.

6. *Workforce development.* The oral health workforce needs greater diversity, flexibility, sensitivity, and expertise in population-based oral health prevention programs and services for vulnerable populations. The workforce should reflect the population it serves. Initiatives should be established to enable and support inner-city, rural, minority, and low-income students in middle schools, high schools, and colleges for a future in dentistry, dental hygiene, dental assisting, and public health. These initiatives should focus on African-Americans, Hispanics, Native Americans, and other underrepresented minorities.

Initiatives also should be established to dramatically increase and support the number of dentists trained in population-based oral health and dental public health, especially on community-based prevention and resolution of disparities in oral health. Scholarship and loan repayment programs need to be developed to encourage graduate dental residents to practice in dentally underserved communities.

A national board clinical examination or a national reciprocity program needs to be developed, implemented, and accepted by state licensing boards, so that dentists and hygienists can practice in any state. Training programs for dental hygienists and dental assistants should begin teaching their students to their maximum competency, including expanded duties, so that they can function most effectively and efficiently. Dental schools should again teach their students how to be more productive through a team approach, such as four-handed dentistry using dental assistants and multiple chairs, using auxiliaries more effectively and efficiently.

Conclusion

The neglected epidemic of oral disease is a social injustice for many Americans, especially vulnerable populations. Our country has the money, expertise, and resources, but we continue to ration dental services. Millions of U.S. residents have unnecessary oral diseases and infections because proven cost-effective, population-based preventive measures, such as community water fluoridation, have not been implemented.

Oral health is an integral part of total health. Institutions, agencies, and organizations must understand and promote this concept. The greatest disparities in oral health are between the "haves" and "have-nots." People are much more likely to have poor oral health if they are low-income, uninsured, developmentally disabled, homebound, homeless, medically compromised, and/or members of minority groups or other high-risk populations who do not have access to oral health services. Although the U.S. government has documented well the disparities in oral health with *Healthy People 2010* and the Surgeon General's report on oral health, without funding or legislation, these initiatives will not have much of a national impact.

To make a difference, we recommend the following:

- A national health program should be available for all U.S. residents, with a meaningful comprehensive oral component that stresses prevention and primary dental care.
- A much higher priority should be given to oral health by federal, state, and local government agencies and by nongovernmental organizations and institutions.
- Provision by all public schools of (a) comprehensive health education, with an oral health component, for all children in grades K through 12; and (b) dental care services in all school health clinics and centers for high-risk children.
- Effective prevention programs, initiatives, and services, such as water fluoridation, which must be the foundation for all dental programs at the local, state, and national levels.
- Promoting in the oral health workforce greater diversity, flexibility, sensitivity, and expertise in population-based, oral health prevention programs and services for vulnerable populations.

Once these recommendations are implemented and monitored in a meaningful manner, the United States will have social justice for better oral health.

References

1. Allukian M. The neglected American epidemic. Nation's Health 1990;May–June:2.
2. Allukian M Jr. Oral diseases: the neglected epidemic. In: Scutchfield FD, Keck CW, eds. Principles of Public Health Practice (2nd Edition). Albany, NY: Delmar Publishers, 2003, pp. 387–408, chapter 21.
3. The Dental Health Foundation. The oral health of California's children: a neglected epidemic. San Rafael, Calif.: Dental Health Foundation, 1997.

4. Gotsch AR. The neglected epidemic. The Nation's Health 1999:2.

5. Allukian M Jr. The neglected epidemic and the Surgeon General's Report: a call to action for better oral health (editorial). Am J Public Health 2000;90:843–5.

6. U.S. Department of Health and Human Services. Oral health in America: a report of the Surgeon General. Rockville, Md.: National Institute of Dental and Craniofacial Research, National Institutes of Health, 2000.

7. Krisberg K. Call to action issued on oral health diseases. Nation's Health 2003:2, 19.

8. Schneider D. Adult dental benefits in Medicaid: FY 2000, 2002, and 2003, Personal communication, September 25, 2003.

9. Dasanayake AP. Poor periodontal health of the pregnant woman as a risk factor for low birth weight. Ann Periodontol 1998;3:206–11.

10. Offenbacher S, Katz V, Fertik G, et al. Periodontal infection as a possible factor for preterm low birth weight. Ann Periodontol 1995;67(suppl 10):1103–13.

11. Davenport ES, Willias CE, Sterne JA, et al. The East London Study of Maternal Chronic Periodontal Disease and Preterm Low Birth Weight Infants: study design and prevalence data. Ann Periodontol 1998;3:213–21.

12. Beck JD, Offenbacher S, William R, et al. Periodontitis: a risk factor for coronary heart disease? Ann Periodontol 1998;3:127–41.

13. Genco RJ. Periodontol disease and risk for myocardial infarction and cardiovascular disease. Cardiovasc. Rev. Rep. 1998;19:34–40.

14. Slavkin HC. Does the mouth put the heart at risk? J Am Dent Assoc 1998;19:34–40.

15. Vargas CM. Unpublished estimates, Third National Health and Nutrition Examination Survey, 2000. Personal communication.

16. U.S. Department of Health and Human Services. Healthy people 2010. 2nd ed. With understanding and improving health and objectives for improving health. 2 vols. Washington, D.C.: U.S. Government Printing Office, 2000.

17. Greenlee RT, Murray T, Bolden S, et al. Cancer statistics, 2000. CA Cancer J Clin 2000;50:7–33.

18. Centers for Medicare and Medicaid Services, Office of the Actuary, National Health Statistics Group. Health accounts, table 3: national health expenditures, by source of funds and type of expenditure: selected calendar years 1998–2003. Available at: http://www.cms.hhs.gov/statistics/nhe/historical/t3.asp. Accessed February 23, 2005.

19. Newacheck PW, Hughes DC, Hung YY, et al. The unmet health needs of America's children. Pediatrics 2000;105:989–97.

20. Vargas CM, Crall J, Schneider D. Sociodemographic distribution of pediatric dental caries: NHANES III, 1999–1994. J Am Dent Assoc 1998;129:1229–38.

21. Simpson G, Bloom B, Cohen RA, et al. Access to health care, part I. Vital Health Stat 1997;197:1–47.

22. Adams PF, Marano MA. Current estimates from the National Health Survey, 1994. Vital and health statistics. Hyattsville, Md.: U.S. Department of Health and Human Services, National Center for Health Statistics (series 10, no. 193, 1995).

23. Healthy People 2000 progress review for oral health. Washington, D.C.: National Institute of Dental and Craniofacial Research, U.S. Department of Health and Human Services, 1999.

24. Mueller CD, Schur CL, Paramore C. Access to dental care in the U.S. J Am Dent Assoc 1998;129:429–37.

25. Qiu Y, Ni H. Utilization of dental care services by Asians and native Hawaiian or other Pacific Islanders: U.S., 1997–2000. Hyattsville, Md.: National Center for Health Statistics, 2003 (advance data from Vital and Health Statistics; no. 336).

26. Vargas CM, Yellowitz JA, Hayes KL. Oral health statistics of older rural adults in the U.S. J Am Dent Assoc 2003;134:479–86.

26a. Scott G, Simile C. Access to dental care among Hispanic or Latino subgroups: United States 2000–03. Advance data from vital and health statistics. Hyattsville, Md.: National Center for Health Statistics, 354, May 12, 2005.

27. Rudd RE, Moeykens BA, Colton TC: Health and literacy: a review of medical and public health literature, National Center for the Study of Adult Learning and Literacy annual review of adult learning and literacy, vol. 1. New York: Jossey-Bass, 2000.

28. Kirsch IS, Jungeblut A, Jenkins L Kolstad A. Adult literacy in America. Washington, D.C.: U.S. Department of Education, 1993.

29. Horowitz AM: The public's oral health: the gaps between what we know and what we do. Adv Dent Sci 1995;9:91–5.

30. Children's dental services under Medicaid: access and utilization. San Francisco, Calif.: Office of the Inspector General, 1996 (DHHS publication OEI-09-93-00240).

31. Shortage Designation Branch, National Center for Health Workforce Analysis, Rockville, Md., BHP, HRSA. Dental Health Professional Shortage Areas. June 2003.

32. Brocato R. Head Start and partners forum on oral health. Washington, D.C.: Head Start Bureau, 2001. Head Start Bull 71:1–43, 2001.

33. Perkins D. Personal communication. Jefferson City, Mo.: Association of State and Territorial Dental Directors, January 26, 2004.

34. Ten great public health achievements—United States, 1990–1999. MMWR Morb Mortal Wkly Rep 1999;48:241–3.

35. Horowitz AM, Harris NO. Creating effective, school-based oral health programs. In: Harris NO, Garcia-Godoy F eds. Primary preventive dentistry. 6th ed. Upper Saddle River, N.J.: Pearson Prentice-Hall, 2004:521–53.

36. The Center for Health and Health Care in Schools. Dental and mental health services. Available at: http://www.healthinschools.org. Accessed January 25, 2005.

37. Council on Dental Education and Licensure. Report of national certifying boards for special areas of dental practice. Chicago, Ill.: American Dental Association. April 2004.

38. Brown LJ, Lazar V. Closing the gap. Minority dentists: why do we need them? Washington, D.C.: Office of Minority Health: U.S. Department of Health and Human Services, 1999.

39. Noonan AS, Evans CA. The need for diversity in the health professions. J Dent Educ 2003;67:1030–3.

40. AmberWaves USDA's Economic Research Services. Available at: http://www.ers.usda.gov/AmberWaves/February04/Indicators/behinddata.htm. Accessed January 25, 2005.

41. U.S. Department of Health and Human Services. The Surgeon General's call to action to prevent and decrease overweight and obesity. Rockville, Md.: U.S. Department of Health and Human Services, Public Health Service, Office of the Surgeon General, 2001.

42. Putnam JJ, Allshouse JE. Food consumption, prices, and expenditures, 1970–1997. Washington, D.C.: U.S. Department of Agriculture, 1999 (an economic research and service report, statistical bulletin no. 965).

43. French SA, Lin BH, Guthrie JF. National trends in soft drink consumption among children and adolescents age 6 to 17 years: prevalence, amounts, and sources. J Am Diet Assoc 2003;103:1326–31.

44. Gleason P, Suitor C. Children's diets in the mid-1990s: dietary intake and its relationship with school meal participation. Alexandria, Va.: U.S. Department of Agriculture, Food and Nutrition Service, Office of Analysis, Nutrition and Evaluation, 2001.

45. Ludwig DS, Peterson KE, Gortmaker SL. Relation between consumption of sugar sweetened drinks and childhood obesity: a prospective, observational analysis. Lancet 2001:357:505–8.

46. Advertising Age's leading national advertisers' report 2002, 47th annual report. Advertising Age 2003;24:1–77.

47. Nestle M. Soft drink pouring rights. Public Health Rep 2000;115:308–19.

48. American Academy of Pediatrics. Policy statement. Soft drinks in schools. Pediatrics 2004;113:152–4.

49. National Center for Health Statistics. Health, United States, 2002 with chart book on trends in health of Americans. Overweight children and adolescents 6–19 years of age, according to sex, age, race and Hispanic origin; U.S., selected years 1963–65 through 1999–2000. Hyattsville, Md.: National Center for Health Statistics, 2002.

50. Centers for Disease Control and Prevention, Annual smoking-attributable mortality, years of potential life lost, and economic costs U.S., 1995–1999, MMWR Morb Mortal Wkly Rep 2002;51:300–3. Available at: http://www.cdc.gov/tobacco/sgr/sgr4kids/6facts.htm. Accessed January 25, 2005.

51. Brandt AM, Richmond JB. Tobacco pandemic. The Washington Post, 2004, p A21.

52. Buying influence, selling death. Available at: http://www.tobaccofreekids.org. Accessed January 25, 2005.

53. Tobacco use and public health. Available at: http://www.gao.gov/cgi-bin/getrpt?-GAO-04-41. Accessed January 25, 2005.

54. Federal Trade Commission cigarette report for 2001. Available at: http://www.ftc.gov/os/2003//06/2001cigreport.pdf. Accessed January 25, 2005.

55. Healton C. Nelson K. Reversal of misfortune: viewing tobacco as a social justice issue. Am J Public Health 2004;94:186–91.

56. U.S. Department of Health and Human Services. A national call to action to promote oral health. Rockville, Md.: U.S. Department of Health and Human Services, Public Health Service, Centers for Disease Control and Prevention and the National Institutes of Health, National Institute of Dental and Craniofacial Research (NIH publication no. 03-5303), May 2003.

57. American Dental Association. The 1999 survey of dental practice: characteristics of dentists in private practice and their patients. Chicago, Ill.: ADA, February 2001.

58. Kuttner R. Face it: we're rationing health. Boston Globe, September 14, 2003.

59. HRSA, Interim Study Group on Dental Activities. Improving the oral health of the American people: opportunity for action, a study of the oral health activities of DHHS. Rockville, Md.: HRSA, March 1989.

60. American Dental Association. American Dental Association Federal Dental News, Fall/Winter, 2003.

21

INTERNATIONAL HEALTH

Barry S. Levy and Victor W. Sidel

Introduction

Widespread social injustice leads to profoundly increased rates of illness and premature death in developing countries. This social injustice and resultant morbidity and mortality are related to inadequate public health services and medical care, as well as other factors, both internal and external.

Internal factors include (a) extreme poverty; (b) rampant discrimination against women, indigenous peoples, racial and ethnic minorities, the physically and mentally disabled, and other vulnerable groups; (c) unrepresentative, unaccountable governments and often widespread corruption; and (d) failure to protect human rights.

External factors—many of which result from the policies of developed countries, multinational corporations, and international financial institutions—include (a) high external debt; (b) "structural adjustment," which has reduced health and other human services; (c) trade barriers, which have limited exports to developing countries; (d) export of hazardous substances from developed to developing countries; (e) inadequate financial and technical assistance from developed countries; (f) the "brain drain" of educated people from developing to developed countries; (g) arms trade; and (h) high cost of drugs and vaccines needed to treat and prevent serious and widespread diseases. Several of these factors are discussed in more detail below.

Of the 192 countries in the world, 132 are categorized as "developing (or less-developed) countries," the better-off of which are sometimes considered "industrializing countries" or "countries in transition." The World Health Organization (WHO) classifies 72 of these countries as high-mortality developing countries (46 of them in Africa) and 60 of them as low-mortality developing countries.[1] WHO classifies the other 60 countries as "developed countries," which includes the United States, Canada, Japan, Australia, New Zealand, and all nations in Europe.[1]

Extreme Poverty

Developing countries are characterized by profoundly low levels of income, along with high population density and high fertility[2,3] (table 21-1). There are wide gaps between the very few who are rich and the multitudes who are poor.[4] Approximately 1.1 billion people live on less than the equivalent of US$1.15 per day—almost all in developing countries.[5] Most people in developing countries cannot meet their basic needs for food, clothing, shelter, and health care. Such extreme poverty—often due to multiple forms of social injustice—has a huge impact on health as a result of poor nutrition, limited access to therapeutic and preventive health services, and increased exposure

TABLE 21-1   Characteristics of Selected Developing Countries and, for Comparison, the United States

Country	Total Population (2002)	Gross National Income per Capita (2001) (U.S. dollars)	Population Density (per square kilometer) (2002)	Total Fertility Rate (births per woman) (2002)
Afghanistan	22.9	NA	43	6.8
Guatemala	12.0	1,680	111	4.3
Haiti	8.2	480	301	4.2
Iraq	24.0	NA	55	4.1
Kenya	31.5	350	55	4.2
Pakistan	149.5	420	188	4.5
Peru	26.8	1,980	21	2.6
Sierra Leone	4.8	140	73	5.6
South Africa	44.8	2,820	37	2.8
Vietnam	80.3	410	247	1.9
United States	291.0	34,280	31	2.1

From The World Bank. 2004 World development indicators. Washington, D.C.: The World Bank, 2004:14–16, 96–98.

TABLE 21-2   Annual Per-Capita Expenditures on Health, Total and
Government (in U.S. Dollars, Using Average Exchange Rates, 2001),
Selected Developing Countries and, for Comparison, the United States

Country	Total Per-Capita Expenditures on Health (U.S. dollars)	Government Per-Capita Expenditures on Health (U.S. dollars)
Afghanistan	8	4
Guatemala	86	41
Haiti	22	12
Iraq	225	72
Kenya	29	6
Pakistan	16	4
Peru	97	53
Sierra Leone	7	4
South Africa	222	92
Vietnam	21	6
United States	4,887	2,168

From World Health Organization. World Health Report 2003: shaping the future.
Geneva, Switzerland: World Health Organization, 2003:178–181.

to health and safety hazards. Individuals and governments spend far less
money capita on health than in developed countries[6] (table 21-2).

Education and employment opportunities are extremely limited in developing countries. Primary school completion rates are much lower and adult
literacy rates are much higher than in developed countries[7] (table 21-3).
Inadequate industrial development restricts economic opportunities for individuals and entire countries. As a result, highly educated individuals, including many physicians, nurses, and other health professionals, often leave
their home countries to seek better educational and employment opportunities
in developed countries.[8] As one example of this "brain drain," in 2002 there
were 5,334 nonfederal physicians trained in African medical schools who
were licensed to practice medicine in the United States; other data suggest
that there are even more Africa-trained physicians in the United States.[9]

Failure to Protect Human Rights

In developing countries, protection of human rights is often limited or nonexistent. Threats to human rights include (a) large-scale abuses, such as
genocide[10] and ethnic cleansing (see box 17-2 on p. 306), torture, and forced
migration; and (b) chronic, systemic problems that deny people their basic
rights, including access to safe food and water, health care, security, and a

TABLE 21-3   Primary School Completion Rate (1995–2001) and
Adult Illiteracy Rate for Men and Women (2002), Selected Developing
Countries

Country	Primary School Completion Rate (%)	Adult Illiteracy Rate (%)	
		Men	Women
Afghanistan	8	NA	NA
Guatemala	52	23	38
Haiti	70	46	50
Iraq	55	NA	NA
Kenya	63	10	21
Pakistan	59	47	71
Peru	98	9	20
Sierra Leone	32	NA	NA
South Africa	98	13	15
Vietnam	101*	6	13

*Artifact of calculation.

From The World Bank. 2003 World development indicators. Washington, D.C.: The World Bank, 2003:84–86; and The World Bank. 2004 development indicators. Washington, D.C.: The World Bank, 2004:84–86.

healthy working and living environment; freedom of religion, speech, and assembly; and protection against arbitrary use of governmental power. Human rights problems also include the following:

- Discrimination based on gender, age, racial and ethnic status, political opinion, sexual orientation, health, and disability status
- Child labor, with more than 250 million children between the ages of 5 and 14 working—approximately half of them working full-time
- Trafficking in human beings (box 21-1)
- Design and implementation of health policies that adversely affect health
- Civil wars and international conflicts.[11]

Although women provide 70 to 80 percent of all health care in developing countries, are the heads of the households in at least 20 percent of all households in Africa and Latin America, and grow 80 percent of the food consumed domestically in parts of Africa and at least 50 percent of export crops, they face widespread and serious discrimination in many developing countries.[12] One-third to one-half of women become mothers before reaching the age of 20. Forty percent of all women of reproductive age are anemic. And many girls (about 6,000 worldwide) are subject to genital mutilation each day. In sub-Saharan Africa, 1 in 22 women dies from pregnancy-related complications.[12]

BOX 21-1 Trafficking in Persons

"Trafficking in persons," or human trafficking, is the "recruitment, transportation, transfer, harboring or receipt of persons," by threat or use of force or other coercion, abduction, fraud, deception, abuse of power or position of vulnerability, or giving or receiving of payments or benefits in order to achieve the consent of a person having control over another person for the purpose of exploitation.[1]

From Himalayan villages to Eastern European cities, people—especially women and girls—are attracted by the prospect of a well-paid job as a domestic servant, waitress, or factory worker. Traffickers recruit victims through false advertisements, mail-order bride catalogs, and casual acquaintances.

Upon arrival at their destination, victims are placed in conditions controlled by traffickers, while they are exploited to earn illicit revenues. Many are physically confined, their travel or identify documents are taken away, and they or their families are threatened if they do not cooperate. Women and girls who have been forced to work as prostitutes are blackmailed by the threat that traffickers will tell their families. Trafficked children are dependent on the traffickers for food, shelter, and other basic necessities. Traffickers also play on victims' fear that authorities in a strange country will prosecute or deport them if they ask for help.

Trafficking in human beings is a crime in which victims are moved from poor environments to more affluent ones, with the profits flowing in the opposite direction, a pattern often repeated at the domestic, regional, and global levels. It is a crime believed to be growing the fastest in Central and Eastern Europe and the former Soviet Union. In Asia, girls from villages in Nepal and Bangladesh, most of whom are under age 18, are sold to brothels in India for $1,000. Trafficked women from Thailand and the Philippines are increasingly being joined by women from other countries in Southeast Asia. It is estimated that the industry is now worth several billion dollars a year.

Trafficking in human beings is not confined to the sex industry. Children are trafficked to work in sweatshops as laborers and men work illegally at jobs that are dirty, difficult, and dangerous. An estimated 45,000 to 50,000 women and children are brought to the United States every year under false pretenses and are forced to work as prostitutes, abused laborers, or servants. Many of them come from developing countries. More than 200,000 children are enslaved by cross-border smuggling in West and Central Africa. The children are often "sold" by unsuspecting parents who believe their children are going to be looked after, learn a trade, or be educated. Trafficking is fostered, in part, by social and economic disparities that create a supply of victims seeking to migrate and the demand for sexual and other services that provide the economic impetus for trafficking.

(continued)

Addressing the Problem

Deterrence and criminal punishments are important elements, but addressing the underlying conditions that drive both supply and demand are also necessary. Another important preventive measure is public information to mobilize support for effective laws, raise the awareness of key law-enforcement and other officials, and inform socially marginalized groups from which victims are often recruited about trafficking so they will be less likely to be deceived when approached by traffickers.

The United Nations Global Program Against Trafficking in Human Beings aims to shed light on the involvement of organized criminal groups in human trafficking and to promote the development of effective criminal justice–related responses. At the country level, this program raises awareness; trains law enforcement officers, prosecutors, and judges; advises on drafting relevant legislation; advises on and assists in strengthening anti-trafficking programs; and improves victim and witness support. At the international level, the program assists agencies, institutions, and governments in designing effective programs and measures against trafficking in human beings.

Reference

1. United Nations Office on Drugs and Crime. The protocol to prevent, suppress and punish trafficking in persons. Available at: http://www.unodc.org/unodc/en/trafficking_protocol.html. Accessed March 8, 2005.

Adapted from Office on Drugs and Crime, United Nations. Trafficking in human beings. Available at: http://www.unodc.org/unodc/en/trafficking_human_beings.html. Accessed March 8, 2005.

Inadequate Foreign Assistance

Many developed countries are providing less financial aid and technical assistance to developing countries than they did 20 years ago. This has occurred for a variety of reasons, including the end of Cold War competition in foreign assistance between the United States and the Soviet Union. The United Nations has recommended that developed countries contribute 0.7 percent or more of their gross domestic product (GDP) for official development assistance. In 1999, Denmark, Norway, the Netherlands, and Sweden met this standard. Although the United States contributed more than 0.7 percent of its GDP for foreign assistance in the early 1960s, this percentage has substantially declined; in 2002, the United States contributed only 0.13 percent of its gross national income (GNI) for foreign assistance[13] (fig. 21-1).

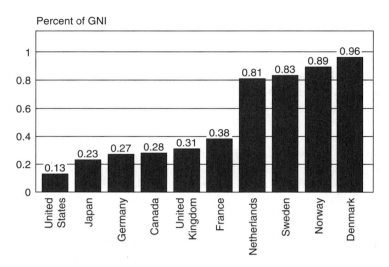

Percent of GNI

Figure 21-1 Official development assistance as a percent of gross national income (GNI), 2002. (From United Nations Development Program. Human development report, 2004. New York, N.Y.: Oxford University Press, 2004.)

External Debt Burdens and Structural Adjustment Policies

Developing countries suffer the effects of huge external debt. By the late 1990s, 41 of the most heavily indebted poor countries (mostly in Africa) had a total debt of approximately $200 billion. This debt developed largely during the 1970s and 1980s as a result of high interest rates and recessions in developed countries, weak commodity prices, the high price of oil, and domestic factors within these countries, including high trade and budget deficits, low savings rates, poor public sector management, weak economic policies, and protracted civil wars.[14]

Structural adjustment policies (SAPs) are economic policies that nations must adopt to qualify for new loans from the World Bank and the International Monetary Fund and to receive assistance in repaying previous debts to the World Bank, other governments, and commercial banks. These SAPs often require debtor nations to devalue their currencies against the dollar, lift import and export restrictions, balance their budgets, and remove price controls and state subsidies. This devaluation leads to these countries' goods becoming cheaper for other countries to buy and makes imported goods from other countries more expensive. The International Monetary Fund encourages affected nations to balance their budgets by reducing government spending, which often leads to sharp reductions in health and other human services that hurt the poor the most.[15,16]

Unrepresentative Governments and Corruption

In many developing countries, the general population has only a limited role in political and economic decisions. In addition, because civil society is disorganized in many developing countries, there are relatively few nongovernmental organizations (NGOs), and those that do exist have less influence on government decisions. Corruption and mismanagement of resources are widespread in many developing countries, with those in power often using corrupt policies and practices to stay in power and to siphon off funds for their own personal gain. This corruption goes unchecked in many countries where public participation in decision-making is limited and NGOs are weak.

Major sources of corruption in the health sector include contracting and procurement, petty theft, selling accreditation or positions, disappearance of public funds, absence of physicians and other health professionals from their government jobs, and the need for informal payments by patients or their families to obtain services.[17] In a recent World Bank survey, in 10 of 22 developing countries and countries in transition, health was perceived among the top four most corrupt sectors. In this survey, absence rates among health care workers in several countries was in the range of 30 percent, and the frequency of informal payments by patients or their families for hospital services ranged from 15 to 65 percent.[17]

Some practical elements encountered in the implementation of human rights in developing countries include bad governance and embezzlement of public funds, the absence of law and order in countries confronted with civil war or those where civil peace is extremely disturbed, absence of legitimate governments and nationally autonomous democratic systems based on the protection of human rights, poverty and underdevelopment, and the debt burden.[18]

Economic Globalization

Economic globalization has benefited some individuals in some developing countries but has often undermined governments, social structures, and national cultures. Free-enterprise zones have been established in some developing countries, where low-wage jobs are available, but organization of workers into labor unions is prohibited and many occupational health and safety problems exist. Often very hazardous industries have flourished in these zones. (See box 19-1 on p. 346.)

Impact of Social Injustice on Public Health in Developing Countries

Endemic and Epidemic Diseases

Life expectancy is significantly lower in developing countries[19] (table 21-4). While infectious diseases, such as tuberculosis and other respiratory diseases, HIV/AIDS, diarrheal diseases, and malaria, continue to account for a substantial proportion of deaths in developing countries, cardiovascular diseases and malignant neoplasms, as in developed countries, are the leading causes of death[20] (fig. 21-2). Nevertheless, HIV/AIDS has had, and continues to have, a catastrophic impact on developing countries; for example, by the end of 2003, there were 25 million people living with HIV/AIDS in sub-Saharan Africa, accounting for approximately two-thirds of all people living with HIV/AIDS in the world at that time and representing a prevalence of 7.5 percent of HIV/AIDS among adults there.[21] In addition, during 2003, there were 2.2 million deaths due to AIDS in sub-Saharan Africa, representing more than three fourths of deaths due to AIDS worldwide in that year.[21] Depression and other mental disorders are widespread and people who suffer from them are typically stigmatized. (See also chapters 13, 15, and 16.)

Social injustice has a profoundly negative impact on children's health, leading to much malnutrition, illness, and premature death that could otherwise be prevented. Leading causes of death in children in developing countries are perinatal conditions (23 percent of all childhood deaths), lower respiratory

TABLE 21-4 Life Expectancy at Birth (in years, 2002), Males and Females, Selected Developing Countries and, for Comparison, the United States

Country	Life Expectancy	
	Males	Females
Afghanistan	42	43
Guatemala	63	69
Haiti	49	51
Iraq	59	63
Kenya	50	52
Pakistan	61	62
Peru	68	72
Sierra Leone	32	35
South Africa	49	53
Vietnam	67	72
United States	75	80

From World Health Organization. World health report 2003: shaping the future. Geneva, Switzerland: World Health Organization, 2003:146–153.

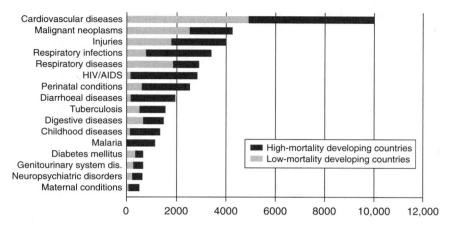

Figure 21-2 Deaths attributable to 16 leading causes in developing countries, 2001. (From the World Health Organization. World health report 2003: shaping the future. Geneva, Switzerland: World Health Organization, 2003:86.)

infections (18 percent), diarrheal diseases (15 percent), and malaria (11 percent).[20] Malnutrition contributes to high rates of childhood mortality, as a result of dietary deficiencies of protein, energy, and micronutrients; it also inhibits children's ability to fight infection and adversely affects physical and mental development[22] (table 21-5 and box 21-2). (See also chapter 14.)

TABLE 21-5   Infant Mortality Rate (IMR, Infant Deaths per 1,000 Live Births, 2002), Under-5 Mortality Rate (U5MR, Deaths per 1,000 Children, 2002), and Percent of Weight-for-Age Malnourished Children Under Age 5 (1996–2002), Selected Developing Countries and, for Comparison, the United States

Country	IMR	U5MR	Percent Malnourished
Afghanistan	165	257	49
Guatemala	36	49	24
Haiti	79	123	17
Iraq	102	125	16
Kenya	78	122	22
Pakistan	76	101	NA
Peru	30	39	7
Sierra Leone	165	284	27
South Africa	52	65	NA
Vietnam	20	26	34
United States	7	8	NA

From The World Bank. 2004 World development indicators. Washington, D.C.: The World Bank, 2004:100–102, 108–110.

BOX 21-2 Hunger and Malnutrition in Developing Countries

The number of people affected by hunger in the world has grown by 4.5 million people a year since 1995, mainly due to drought, war, trade barriers, and AIDS. This increase has been especially severe in the developing countries of sub-Saharan Africa. Between 1991 and 2001, more than 840 million people were affected by hunger, of whom 798 million lived in the developing world. For example, in Ethiopia, between 1995 and 2001, 47 percent of children were malnourished, and in Congo, between 1999 and 2001, 75 percent of the total population was malnourished. War and sanctions accounted for much childhood malnutrition in Iraq in the 1990s. The increase in hunger occurred while the world was producing sufficient amounts of food.[1,2]

The Food and Agriculture Organization of the United Nations has attributed much hunger to a lack of political will. The Hunger Project, a nonprofit independent organization, has attributed much hunger in the world to discrimination against women—which leads to less education, less literacy, less paid employment, lower income, and malnutrition during pregnancy and breastfeeding.

Poor health adds to these problems. For example, HIV/AIDS results in and worsens food security in several ways. Most HIV/AIDS victims die young, during what would otherwise be their most productive years. It is estimated that by 2020 HIV/AIDS will have killed one fifth or more agricultural workers in most of southern Africa. HIV/AIDS victims leave behind survivors who are mainly elderly and young—many of them orphans—who do not have the strength, resources, or know-how to grow commercial and staple crops; they therefore cannot grow enough food to survive. Not only does HIV/AIDS cause more hunger, but hunger increases the spread and hastens the course of the disease. Hungry people often migrate from rural areas to urban slums, where HIV infection rates are increased and where women and children, in order to survive, may have to barter sex for food or money.[1]

References

1. Food and Agriculture Organization. The state of food insecurity in the world 2003. Rome, Italy: FAO, 2003.
2. Sengupta S. Hunger worsens in many lands, U.N. says. New York Times, November 26, 2003, p A3.

Inadequate prenatal and maternity care accounts for poor birth outcomes, including high infant mortality from perinatal conditions and high maternal mortality ratios[23] (table 21-6). Immunization rates, while increasing, are still lower in developing than in developed countries. Measles, pertussis, and tetanus account for almost 10 percent of all childhood deaths in developing countries.[24]

TABLE 21-6 Percentage of Low Birth Weight Infants (1998–2002), Percentage of Births Attended by Skilled Health Staff (1995–2002), and Maternal Mortality Ratio (Maternal Deaths per 100,000 Live Births, Modeled Estimates for 2000), Selected Developing Countries and, for Comparison, the United States

Country	Percent of Low Birth Weight Infants	Percent of Births Attended by Skilled Staff	Maternal Mortality Ratio
Afghanistan	NA	12	1,900
Guatemala	13	41	240
Haiti	21	24	680
Iraq	15	72	250
Kenya	11	44	1,000
Pakistan	19	20	500
Peru	11	59	410
Sierra Leone	NA	42	2,000
South Africa	15	84	230
Vietnam	9	70	130
United States	8	99	17

From The World Bank. 2004 World development indicators. Washington, D.C.: The World Bank, 2004:96–98, 100–102.

Access to Adequate Medical Care and Public Health Services

People in developing countries generally have inadequate access to effective medical care and public health services.[25] Many governments in developing countries spend less than the equivalent of US$5 per capita on health. Facilities, equipment and supplies, and human resources are shamefully inadequate. And the number of physicians, nurses, midwives, dentists, and pharmacists is woefully below standards in most developing countries. For example, in Afghanistan, there are 11 physicians per 100,000 population; in Haiti, 8; in Kenya, 13; and in Yemen, 23, compared with 279 in the United States.[26] In Afghanistan, there are 18 nurses per 100,000 population; in Haiti, 11; in Kenya, 90; and in Yemen, 51, compared with 972 in the United States.[26] (WHO recommends a minimum of 20 physicians and 100 nurses per 100,000 population.)

Greater Impact on the Poor

Throughout developing countries, there are serious inequalities in health status and health care. The poorest women and children face the greatest risks to their health, and they are far less likely to use necessary health services than are those who are better off financially. For example:

- Poorer women have more children and have them earlier in their lives.

- The poorest adolescents aged 15 to 19 are three times more likely to give birth than are the richest in this age group.
- The poorest children are three times more likely to be stunted (low height for age) and twice as likely to die as the wealthiest children.
- The poorest women are twice as likely to be malnourished, one fourth as likely to use contraceptives, and one fifth as likely to have medically trained assistants during labor and delivery.[27]
- In developing countries, poor people generally lack almost all of the factors necessary for good health, such as education, knowledge related to health, nutrition, and utilization of health services. For example, the poorest women are on average one ninth as likely to have a fifth-grade or higher education compared with the richest women.[27]

Environmental Health Issues

Developing countries face a wide range of environmental health issues.[28] Water contamination with microorganisms and chemicals, such as pesticides, occurs frequently in developing countries. Approximately 1.1 billion people worldwide, mainly in developing countries, lack access to what is termed an "improved water supply," such as a household connection to a water supply, a protected deep well or spring, or a rainwater collection system.[29] About 2.4 billion people lack access to what is termed "improved sanitation," such as a connection to a public sewer or septic system or a pour-flush, simple-pit, or ventilated improved-pit latrine.[29] Water contamination with microorganisms contributes to much diarrheal disease and to many of the 5,000 deaths that occur daily due to diarrheal disease, of which 99 percent occur in developing countries.[29] Exposure to heavy metals represents another significant environmental hazard, such as exposure to lead from the exhaust of gasoline engines and industrial sources—an especially important risk to children.[30] Global warming is likely to increase vector-borne disease, food and water shortages, flooding, and extreme weather in developing countries with disastrous effects on health[31] (see chapter 17).

Living Conditions

Relatively few people in developing countries have access to adequate housing.[32] Although most people in developing countries live in rural areas, many people live in urban slums (fig. 21-3). Typically, young men leave their wives and children behind in rural areas as they seek jobs in cities. In urban slums, housing is typically overcrowded and lacks adequate safe water and sanitation.[33] Within developing countries, about 25 million people are internally displaced, most often because of national economic problems and/or civil war; their basic needs are usually not met.[34] In addition, about 12 to 20 million

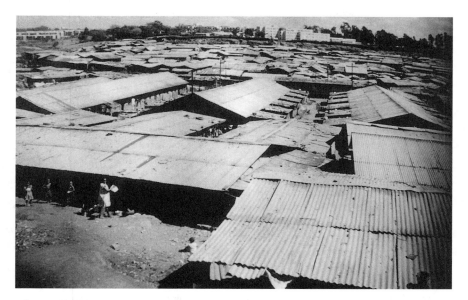

Figure 21-3 Mathare Valley slum area in Nairobi, Kenya, where 100,000 people have lived in crowded housing with no electricity and little running water. (Photograph by Barry S. Levy.)

refugees—86 percent from developing countries—have left their homes seeking political or economic asylum elsewhere[35] (see chapter 11).

Occupational Health and Safety Issues

Many developing countries face serious problems in occupational health and safety[36,37] (see chapter 18). These problems reflect a lesser state of industrial development and the import of hazardous substances from developed countries (box 21-3). Many countries are in such need of economic development and of "hard cash" to pay off their debt burdens that they are willing to establish or import hazardous industries. Similarly, many people in developing countries are so desperate for work that they are willing to take unsafe and hazardous jobs. In addition, there is less infrastructure for diagnosing, treating, and preventing occupational health and safety problems in developing countries and fewer laws and regulations, which are less stringently enforced.[38]

Violence

Many people in developing countries face the consequences of war and other forms of conflict, especially civil wars, which continue to rage in many

BOX 21-3 Import of Hazardous Substances Into
Developing Countries

The import of hazardous substances, waste, and even entire industries is a major challenge facing developing countries. Tobacco and pesticides are among hazardous substances most frequently imported into developing countries.

Tobacco

There are approximately 1.25 billion smokers worldwide, with 800 million living in developing countries. Large multinational tobacco countries based in Great Britain and the United States are largely responsible for increased smoking in developing countries, often leading national tobacco companies to increase their marketing activities in response. Following World War II, the United States began exporting tobacco under the Food for Peace Program. In the first 25 years of this program, the United States exported almost $1 billion of tobacco, exposing developing countries to Western-style cigarettes. By 1994, 220 billion U.S.-manufactured cigarettes were shipped abroad—a 55-percent increase since 1989.[1]

Almost three-quarters of the world's tobacco is grown in developing countries. Multinational tobacco companies exploit developing countries in a number of ways. Although the initial cost of seed, tools, curing barns, and other materials is high, the multinational tobacco companies make loans to small farmers for fertilizers and insecticides, thus trapping them in a cycle of debt. Serious environmental costs are associated with tobacco production, especially deforestation, erosion, and desertification. Multinational tobacco companies often seek to strengthen their presence in developing countries by engaging their economies and communities. Seemingly philanthropic acts of building schools and hospitals allowed the tobacco companies to buy into health and education sectors of society. Poorer developing countries are less likely to resist such financial aid and more likely to look favorably on the tobacco industry.[1]

By 2030, tobacco is expected to be the single largest cause of death worldwide, accounting for about 10 million deaths a year. In Bangladesh, for example, tobacco consumption has a direct impact on the health of poor households, with poor people spending less on food, resulting in malnutrition. The typical poor smoker could add over 500 calories to the diet of one or two children if he or she stopped smoking. Applied to the entire country of Bangladesh, an estimated 10.5 million people currently malnourished could have an adequate diet if money spent on cigarettes was spent on food instead.[1]

An important step toward controlling tobacco worldwide is the World Health Organization Framework Convention on Tobacco Control. This new

(continued)

legal instrument addresses issues of tobacco advertising and promotion, agricultural diversification, smuggling, taxes, and subsidies.[2]

Pesticides

The export of banned and restricted pesticides from the United States and other developed countries to developing countries accounts for much unnecessary illness and death. Between 1997 and 2000, for example, the United States exported 3.2 billion pounds of pesticide products—an average of 45 tons per hour. Nearly 65 million pounds of these exported pesticides were either forbidden or severely restricted in the United States.[3] Over many years, the United States has exported pesticides known to cause adverse effects on the reproductive system,[4] cancer, or birth defects.

International efforts to reduce the trade of hazardous pesticides may be bearing fruit. No banned pesticide export was recorded for the year 2000, 2.2 million pounds of pesticides regulated under a treaty on persistent organic pollutants (POPs)[5] were exported between 1997 and 1999 with no such export in 2000.[3] These findings indicate that progress is possible and that international efforts should be expanded.[3] Nevertheless, the United States continues to export large amounts of pesticides designated "extremely hazardous" by the World Health Organization (89 million pounds), pesticides associated with cancer (170 million pounds), and pesticides associated with endocrine destroying effects (368 million pounds), mostly to developing countries.

References

1. Action on Smoking and Health. Fact sheet no. 21: tobacco in the developing world. Available at: http://www.ash.org.uk/html/factsheets/html/fact21.html. Accessed July 11, 2004.
2. World Health Organization. WHO Framework Convention on Tobacco Control. Available at: http://www.who.int/tobacco/areas/framework/en. Accessed January 25, 2005.
3. Smith C. Pesticide exports from U.S. ports, 1997–2000. Int J Occup Environ Health 2001;7:266–74.
4. Levy BS, Levin JL, Teitelbaum DT, eds. DBCP–induced sterility and reduced fertility among men in developing countries: a case study of the export of a known hazard. Int J Occup Environ Health 1999;5:115–53.
5. POPs treaty in force today. Pesticide Action Network Updates Service, May 17, 2004. Available at: http://www.panna.org/resources/panups/panup_20040517.dv.html. Accessed January 25, 2005.

developing countries in Africa, Asia, and Latin America.[39,40] War not only causes immediate morbidity and mortality but also leads to long-term physical and mental health consequences among survivors and their families. War causes widespread damage to the environment. In addition, war and the preparation for war sap economic, human, and other resources that could otherwise be used for health and human services. Domestic and community violence, often byproducts of war, continue to take a heavy toll among the populations of developing countries. The import of arms, both legally and illegally, into developing countries has been one of a number of factors that have exacerbated these conflicts[41] (see box 17-1 on p. 298).

What Needs to Be Done

The Millennium Development Goals provide a framework for addressing the problems discussed in this chapter (table 21-7). (See chapter 28.) A multisectoral approach to achieving these goals is needed, in which health professionals can play important roles.

1. *Promoting approaches that focus on the poor.* It is important that resources be directed to areas of greatest need. Measures that focus on the poor include the following:

- Adopting policies in education, labor, and primary health care that promote benefits of growth and development flowing to the poor

TABLE 21-7   Millennium Development Goals (1990–2015)

1. Eradicate extreme poverty and hunger
   - Halve the proportion of people with less than $1 a day
   - Halve the proportion of people who suffer from hunger
2. Achieve universal primary education
   - Ensure that boys and girls alike complete primary schooling
3. Promote gender equality and empower women
   - Eliminate gender disparity at all levels of education
4. Reduce child mortality
   - Reduce by two-thirds the under-5 mortality rate
5. Improve maternal health
   - Reduce by three-fourths the maternal mortality ratio
6. Combat HIV/AIDS, malaria, and other diseases
   - Reverse the spread of HIV/AIDS
7. Ensure environmental sustainability
   - Integrate sustainable development into country policies and reverse loss of environmental resources
   - Halve the proportion of people without access to potable water and adequate sanitation
   - Significantly improve the lives of at least 100 million slum dwellers
8. Develop a global partnership for development
   - Raise official development assistance
   - Expand market access
   - Encourage debt sustainability

From http://www.developmentgoals.org. Accessed April 12, 2005.

- Investing in education to decrease health inequalities by enabling people to obtain better and safer jobs, improve health literacy, take preventive measures, avoid risky behaviors, and demand higher quality health services
- Directing programs toward living areas and health problems of poor people
- Providing all people with a basic package of cost-effective health services
- Increasing and improving primary care facilities and services
- Developing partnerships between governments and nongovernmental organizations (NGOs)
- Mobilizing community resources, including training community-based health workers, involving traditional healers, and ensuring that services are provided at the local level
- Establishing prepayment for health care through taxes or insurance, with the amount of these contributions related to a person's ability to pay.[42]

Promoting and providing microcredit programs for the poorest of the poor is also extremely important. Microcredit is the extension of small loans to entrepreneurs too poor to qualify for traditional bank loans; it has been demonstrated to be an effective and popular measure in reducing poverty. For example, the Grameen Bank Project, established in 1976 in Bangladesh, has lent over $4 billion to more than 3 million borrowers, of whom 96 percent are women. The bank, which has over 1,200 branches in almost 45,000 villages, has a loan recovery rate of almost 99 percent. Loans have been made not only for small enterprises but also for housing and for education, enabling many of the poorest of the poor to substantially improve their lives. The Grameen system promotes credit as a human right and is not based on any collateral in contracts—it is based on trust. It provides service at the doorstep of the poor based on the principle that people should not have to go to the bank, the bank should go to the people. The Grameen system believes that poverty is not created by the poor but rather by the institutions and policies that surround poor people and that, to reduce poverty, it is necessary to make appropriate changes in the institutions and policies and to develop new ones.[43]

2. *Promoting and protecting human rights and reducing discrimination and its impact.* Human rights—especially for indigenous people, as well as women, children, older people, and other vulnerable populations—need to be promoted and protected.[11,44] The Universal Declaration of Human Rights (see box 1-2 on p. 14) provides a strong foundation for these initiatives.[45] The United Nations and its component agencies and committees play a vital role in building global partnerships for human rights, preventing human rights violations and responding to emergencies, promoting human rights

along with democracy and development as guiding principles for lasting peace, and coordinating the systemwide strengthening of the United Nations Human Rights Program.[46]

Six core human rights treaties provide for monitoring mechanisms concerning human rights. These include monitoring of the implementation of the International Covenant on Civil and Political Rights; the International Covenant on Economic, Social, and Cultural Rights; and international conventions concerning racial discrimination, discrimination against women, the rights of children, and torture and other cruel, inhumane, or degrading treatment or punishment.[46] The work of the United Nations and individual countries for promoting and protecting human rights depends on a dynamic network of partnerships throughout the world, with NGOs and other representatives of civil society, such as academic institutions and citizens' groups, playing critically important roles. (See also chapter 22.)

A number of specific suggestions have been made to improve respect for human rights in developing countries, including the following:

- Improve democratic institutions and the rule of law.
- Establish massive campaigns to explain human rights to the general public and policymakers.
- Identify areas where rapid progress can be made.
- Establish free legal procedures concerning human rights in the context of elections.
- Increase aid for development and make it more effective.
- Reinforce national and international mechanisms for the protection of human rights.[18]

Much needs to be done to reduce discrimination and its impact. For example, to address discrimination against women and its adverse effect on health, the World Bank recommends a package of essential health services for women, including prevention and management of unwanted pregnancies; safe pregnancy and delivery services; prevention and management of sexually transmitted diseases; promotion of positive health practices, such as public education and individual counseling to encourage delayed childbearing, safe sex, and adequate nutrition; and prevention of practices harmful to health, such as gender discrimination, domestic violence, rape, and female genital mutilation. In addition, it recommends a wider choice of family planning methods, nutrition assistance for women before and beyond reproductive age, cervical and breast cancer screening and treatment, and greater attention to the health problems of women beyond reproductive age.[47]

3. *Improving health care systems.* Health care systems in developing countries are critically important for reducing social injustice and its impact

on health. New facilities need to be developed to widen access to medical care. More professionals need to be trained—not only physicians but also nurses, physician's assistants, nurse-midwives, community health workers, and other health personnel. Incentives need to be strengthened to encourage these health professionals to serve where they are most needed. In addition, policies need to be designed and implemented to encourage health professionals who train abroad to return to their home countries. Discriminatory practices in medical care need to be reduced so that all people have adequate access to medical care. In addition, there needs to be a greater emphasis on prevention—not only clinical preventive services that are designed to detect and treat disease at an early stage but also community-based public health services to improve individual and community health. Finally, capabilities need to be developed within developing regions of the world for the manufacture of essential medicines, including antiretroviral drugs to treat HIV/AIDS.

4. *Improving education and health literacy.* Because literacy and educational status are so closely linked to health status, it is extremely important to improve access and quality of education in developing countries. This improvement will not only enhance employment opportunities but also increase people's understanding of and access to health services. Health literacy has been defined as "the degree to which individuals have the capacity to obtain, process, and understand basic health information and services needed to make appropriate health decisions."[48] Low health literacy is a contributing factor to poor health outcomes. As a result of low health literacy, people lack knowledge about medical care and medical conditions, do not understand or use preventive services, and have poorer health status.[49] Health literacy can be improved by improving readability of health education materials and medical care information, as well as by providing appropriate training of physicians, nurses, and other health care providers.

5. *Increasing foreign assistance.* Increased foreign assistance from developed countries can provide critically important financial and human resources to reduce social injustice and improve health in developing countries. It is important that foreign assistance promote sustainable policies and programs that rely on local resources and policies and programs that are culturally, politically, and socioeconomically appropriate. Health professionals and others need to create the popular and political will in developed countries so that governments and the general public in developed countries recognize that it is in their enlightened self-interest to provide adequate assistance to developing countries.

6. *Reducing the export of hazards from developed to developing countries.* Development and enforcement of international treaties and other agreements can do much to reduce the import of (a) hazardous products and wastes and (b) industries that are hazardous. The recent agreements of the World Health

Assembly on the international tobacco trade[50] and on persistent organic pollutants (POPs), which initially targets for elimination 12 toxic chemicals,[51] provide excellent models for restricting exports of hazardous substances from developed to developing countries. The export of health activism has been proposed as another remedy for the export of hazards.[52]

7. *Preventing war and other forms of violence.* The potential for war and other forms of violence can be minimized by reducing the international arms trade; promoting nonviolent means of conflict resolution; strengthening international treaties and conventions concerning antipersonnel landmines as well as nuclear, chemical, and biologic weapons[53]; and promoting a culture of peace. A reduced potential for war will decrease military expenditures, which drain scarce financial and human resources—a particularly tragic situation in many developing countries (see chapter 17).

8. *Promoting representative government and reducing corruption.* Policies and programs must be developed to promote more representative governments in developing countries that are accountable to the populations they serve. Public participation needs to be improved in many ways. The United Nations Development Program is playing an important role in promoting democratic governance by strengthening parliamentary oversight representation and lawmaking; electoral systems and processes; access to justice and human rights; access to information; decentralization, and local government; and public administration and civil service reform.[54] In addition, NGOs need to be strengthened so they can influence decisions at all levels of government. This will help to reduce corruption among government officials. A variety of remedies have been proposed to reduce corruption in developing countries and its adverse effect on health, including enactment of governmentwide anticorruption policies, promotion of a culture of public service, adoption and enforcement of procurement and contracting rules, adoption of public standards of conduct and oversight, improvement of the public management of health services, and compensation of health care providers at appropriate levels for their work. In addition, improvement of fiscal oversight with enforcement of penalties for unlawful practices is important.[17]

9. *Changing international economic policies.* International lending institutions, including the World Bank, need to continue to reduce the debt burden on developing countries, which plays an increasingly adverse role in restricting their ability to promote sustainable human development.[55] Governments relieved of their external debt burdens will have substantially more money to support delivery of needed health services. In addition, structural adjustment policies by the World Bank and the International Monetary Fund, which decrease health and other human services, need to be altered.

Developed countries need to reduce their import tariffs that make it difficult or impossible for farmers and others in developing countries to sell their crops or other products in the United States and other developed countries. These tariffs have played a disastrous role in many developing countries by preventing farmers and others from these countries from competing in world markets on a level playing field. These measures would help reduce poverty in developing countries and, as a result, improve the health of the population.

10. *Promoting sustainable development.* Reducing social injustice and resultant poor health in developing countries requires, among other things, sustained economic growth to increase productivity and income in these countries. (See chapter 28.) Development involves, however, more than economic growth. Sustainable development also requires attention to environmental and social issues. As stated in the World Development Report 2003 of the World Bank, *Sustainable Development in a Dynamic World: Transforming Institutions, Growth, and Quality of Life*[56]:

> Lack of assets, opportunity and effective voice for large segments of the population blocks the emergence of general welfare-enhancing policies, impedes growth and undermines the potential for positive change. At the national level, it robs us of the talents of those left out in society. And at the international level, it deprives us of the contribution poor countries can make to a more just and sustainable future. A more sustainable development path is more socially inclusive. It enables societies to transform and solve collective problems. The challenge, now and in the future, is to develop the courage and commitment to manage the processes that underpin human life and well-being and to bring about a transformation that improves the quality of the environment, strengthens our social fabric, and enhances the quality of people's lives. The more people heard, the less assets wasted.

Conclusion

There is much to be done to ensure social justice for people in developing countries. Health professionals in both developing and developed countries have important roles to play in education and training, advocacy for improved national and international policies to promote social justice and to protect human rights, and consultation and technical assistance to reduce social injustice in these countries and to minimize its health consequences. Social justice in developed countries cannot be achieved until it is achieved in developing countries.

References

1. World Health Organization. The world health report 2003: shaping the future. Geneva: World Health Organization, 2003:183.
2. World Health Organization. World health report 2003: shaping the future. Geneva: World Health Organization, 2003:146–8.

3. The World Bank. 2003 World development indicators. Washington, D.C.: The World Bank, 2003:14–6.

4. Sarin R. Rich-poor divide growing. In: The Worldwatch Institute. Vital signs 2003: the trends that are shaping our future. New York, N.Y.: W.W. Norton & Company, 2003:88–9.

5. The World Bank. World development indicators 2004. Washington, D.C.: The World Bank, 2004, p. 1.

6. World Health Organization. World health report 2003: shaping the future. Geneva: World Health Organization, 2003:178–81.

7. The World Bank. 2003 World development indicators. Washington, D.C.: The World Bank, 2003:84–6, 88–90.

8. Physicians for Human Rights. An action plan to prevent brain drain: building equitable health systems in Africa (a report by physicians for human rights). Boston, Mass.: Physicians for Human Rights, 2004.

9. Hagopian A, Thompson MJ, Fordycel M, et al. The migration of physicians from sub-Saharan Africa to the United States: measures of the African brain drain. Human Resources for Health 2004;2:17.

10. Power S. "A problem from hell": America and the age of genocide. New York, N.Y.: Basic Books, 2002.

11. Mann JM, Gruskin S, Grodin MA, Annas GJ, eds. Health and human rights: a reader. New York, N.Y.: Routledge, 1999.

12. The World Bank Group. A new agenda for women's health and nutrition. Avilable at: http://www.worldbank.org/html/extdr/hnp/health/newagenda/women.htm. Accessed January 25, 2005.

13. United Nations Development Program. Human development report 2004. New York, N.Y.: Oxford University Press, 2004.

14. International Monetary Fund Staff. The logic of debt relief for the poorest countries. Washington, DC: International Monetary Fund, 2000. Available at: http://www.imf.org/external/np/exr/ib/2000/092300.htm. Accessed January 25, 2005.

15. The Whirled Bank Group. Structural adjustment program. Available at: http://www.whirledbank.org/development/sap.html on August 19, 2004. Accessed January 25, 2005.

16. Shah A. Structural adjustment—a major cause of poverty. Available at: http://www.globalissues.org/TradeRelated/SAP.asp on August 19, 2004. Accessed January 25, 2005.

17. Lewis M. Corruption and health in developing and transition economies. 11th International Anticorruption Conference, Seoul, Republic of Korea, May 25–28, 2003.

18. Kobila JM. Comparative practice on human rights: north-south. In: Coicaud JM, Doyle MW, Gardner AM, eds. The globalization of human rights. Tokyo, Japan: United Nations University Press, 2003:89–115.

19. World Health Organization. World health report 2003: shaping the future. Geneva, Switzerland: World Health Organization, 2003:146–53.

20. World Health Organization. World health report 2003: shaping the future. Geneva, Switzerland: World Health Organization, 2003:86.

21. Steinbrook R. The AIDS epidemic 2004. N Engl J Med 2004;351:115–7.

22. West KP Jr, Caballero B, Black RE. Nutrition. In: Merson MH, Black RE, Mills AJ, eds. International public health: diseases, programs, systems, and policies. Gaithersburg, Md.: Aspen Publishers, 2001:207–91.

23. The World Bank. 2003 World development indicators. Washington, D.C.: The World Bank, 2003:100–2, 104–6.

24. The World Bank. 2003 World development indicators. Washington, D.C.: The World Bank, 2003:96–8.
25. Mills AJ, Ranson MK. The design of health systems. In: Merson MH, Black RE, Mills AJ, eds. International public health: diseases, programs, systems, and policies. Gaithersburg, Md.: Aspen Publishers, 2001:515–57.
26. World Health Organization. WHO estimates of health personnel: physicians, nurses, midwives, dentists and pharmacists (around 1998). Geneva, Switzerland: World Health Organization.
27. Population Reference Bureau. The wealth gap in health: data on women and children in 53 developing countries. Washington, D.C.: Population Reference Bureau, May 2004.
28. Shahi GS, Levy BS, Binger Al, et al, eds. International perspectives on environment, development, and health: toward a sustainable world. New York, N.Y.: Springer Publishing Company, 1997.
29. World Health Organization data. The global water supply and sanitation assessment 2000. Available at: http://www.who.int/docstore/water_sanitation_health/Globassessment/Global1.htm. Accessed March 8, 2005.
30. Silbergeld EK. The international dimensions of lead exposure. Int J Occup Environ Health 1995;1:336–48.
31. McMichael AJ, Campbell–Lendrum DH, Corvalan CF, et al, eds. Climate change and human health: risks and responses. Geneva, Switzerland: World Health Organization, 2003.
32. Merson MH, Black RE, Mills AJ, eds. International public health: diseases, programs, systems, and policies. Gaithersburg, Md.: Aspen Publishers, 2001:404–7.
33. Koop CE, Pearson CE, Schwarz MR, eds. Critical issues in global health. San Francisco, Calif.: Jossey-Bass, 2001.
34. Hampton J, ed. Internally displaced people: a global survey. London, England: Earthscan, Norwegian Refugee Council and Global IDP Survey, 1998.
35. Reed H, Haaga J, Keely C., eds. The demography of forced migration: summary of a workshop. Washington, D.C.: National Academies Press, 1998.
36. Heymann J, ed. Global inequalities at work: work's impact on the health of individuals, families, and societies. New York, N.Y.: Oxford University Press, 2003.
37. Levy BS. Hazards in the international setting: general issues. In: Fleming LE, Herzstein JA, Bunn WB III, eds. Issues in international occupational and environmental medicine. Beverly, Mass.: OEM Press, 1997:105–14.
38. Reich MR, Okubo T, eds. Protecting workers' health in the third world: national and international strategies. New York, N.Y.: Auburn House, 1992.
39. Levy BS, Sidel VW, eds. War and public health (updated edition). Washington, D.C.: American Public Health Association, 2000.
40. Stockholm International Peace Research Institute. SIPRI yearbook 2003: armaments, disarmament and international security. New York, N.Y.: Oxford University Press, 2003.
41. Cukier W, Chapdelaine A. Small arms, explosives, and incendiaries. In: Levy BS, Sidel VW, eds. Terrorism and public health: a balanced approach to strengthening systems and protecting people. New York, N.Y.: Oxford University Press, 2003:155–74.
42. Carr D. Improving the health of the world's poorest people (health bulletin 1). Washington, D.C.: Population Reference Bureau, 2004.
43. Grameen: Banking for the poor. Available at: http://www.grameen-info.org. Accessed January 25, 2005.
44. Kim JY, Millen JV, Irwin A, et al, eds. Dying for growth: global inequality and the health of the poor. Monroe, Me.: Common Courage Press, 2000.

45. General Assembly, United Nations. The universal declaration of human rights. New York, N.Y.: United Nations, December 10, 1948.

46. United Nations. A United Nations priority: human rights in action. New York, N.Y.: United Nations. Available at: http://www.un.org/rights/HRToday/action.htm. Accessed January 25, 2005.

47. The World Bank. A new agenda for women's health and nutrition. Available at: http://www.worldbank.org/html/extdr/hnp/health/newagenda/women.htm. Accessed March 8, 2005.

48. U.S. Department of Health and Human Services. Healthy people 2010. 2nd ed. Washington, D.C.: U.S. Government Printing Office, 2000, Objective 11-2.

49. Andrus MR, Roth MT. Health literacy: a review. Pharmacotherapy 2002;22:282–302.

50. World Health Organization. WHO Framework Convention on Tobacco Control. Available at: http://www.who.int/tobacco/areas/framework/en. Accessed January 25, 2005.

51. POPs treaty in force today. Pesticide Action Network Updates Service, May 17, 2004. Available at: http://www.panna.org/resources/panups/panup_20040517.dv.html. Accessed January 25, 2005.

52. Belmar R, Drucker E, Michaels D, Sidel V. The export of health activism: a remedy for the export of hazardous industry. In: Ives JH, ed. The exportation of hazardous industries, technologies, and products to developing countries (report to the National Institute for Occupational Safety and Health), 1982:88–93. (Available from Department of Family and Social Medicine, Montefiore Medical Center, 111 East 210th Street, Bronx, N.Y. 10467.)

53. Levy BS, Sidel VW, eds. Terrorism and public health: a balanced approach to strengthening systems and protecting people. New York, N.Y.: Oxford University Press, 2003: 168, 180, 202, 226–7.

54. United Nations Development Program. Available at: http://www.undp.org/governance/index.htm. Accessed January 25, 2005.

55. Rich B. Mortgaging the earth: the World Bank, environmental impoverishment, and the crisis of development. Boston, Mass.: Beacon Press, 1994.

56. The World Bank. World development report 2003. Sustainable development in a dynamic world: transforming institutions, growth, and quality of life. New York, N.Y.: Oxford University Press, 2003: 197.

Further Reading

Evans T, Whitehead M, Diderichsen F, et al., eds. Challenging inequities in health: from ethics to action. New York, N.Y.: Oxford University Press, 2001.

Feachem RG, Kjellstrom T, Murray CJ, et al., eds. The health of adults in the developing world. New York, N.Y.: Oxford University Press, 1992.

Kim JY, Millen JV, Irwin A, et al., eds. Dying for growth: global inequality and the health of the poor. Monroe, Me.: Common Courage Press, 2000.

Koop CE, Pearson CE, Schwarz MR, eds. Critical issues in global health. San Francisco, Calif.: Jossey-Bass, 2001.

Leon D, Walt G, eds. Poverty inequality and health: an international perspective. New York, N.Y.: Oxford University Press, 2001.

Merson MH, Black RE, Mills AJ, eds. International public health: diseases, programs, systems, and policies. Gaithersburg, Md.: Aspen Publishers, 2001.

Sachs JD. The end of poverty: economic possibilities for our time. New York, N.Y.: The Penguin Press, 2005.

Part IV

What Needs to Be Done

22

ADDRESSING SOCIAL INJUSTICE IN A HUMAN RIGHTS CONTEXT

Sofia Gruskin and Paula Braveman

Introduction

The violation or neglect of human rights jeopardizes health directly by interfering with physical, mental, and social well-being. In this chapter,* we consider the relevance of human rights to public health in three major spheres: (a) as legal standards and obligations of governments, (b) as a conceptual framework for analysis and advocacy, and (c) as guiding principles for designing and implementing policies and programs.

Core Concepts

Human rights are internationally recognized norms and standards that apply equally to people everywhere and that define obligations of governments toward individuals and groups. International human rights law is based on legal agreements to which governments have agreed with the purpose of

---

*This chapter was adapted from a paper by the authors: Braveman P, Gruskin S. Poverty, equity, human rights and health. Bull WHO 2003;81:539–45.

promoting and protecting these rights. Governments are accountable, as signatories of human rights treaties, to set targets and show good-faith movement toward achievement of the full realization of all human rights. Signatory nations are responsible for reporting periodically to the relevant international monitoring bodies on their compliance with human rights treaties.

International human rights law not only prohibits direct violations of rights but also hold governments responsible for progressively ensuring conditions that enable individuals to realize their rights as fully as possible. Governments are responsible for progressively removing the obstacles to individuals achieving all of their rights, with particular attention to those individuals or groups that have more obstacles to realizing their rights, such as the poor, the marginalized, and the excluded.[1]

The term "human rights" within the United States generally calls to mind civil and political rights, such as freedoms of speech, assembly, and religion and freedom from torture or arbitrary arrest. However, human rights norms and agreements also span entitlements that are economic, social, and cultural in nature. This wide scope of human rights has tremendous implications for those committed to social justice.

While it is possible to identify different categories of rights, it is also critical to rights discourse and action to recognize that all rights are interdependent and interrelated and that individuals rarely suffer neglect or violation of one right in isolation. For historical reasons, the rights described in human rights documents were divided into two categories: (a) civil and political rights including, among others, the rights to liberty, to security of person, to freedom of movement, and to vote; and (b) economic, social, and cultural rights including, among others, the rights to the highest attainable standard of health, to work, to social security, to adequate food, to clothing and housing, to education, and to enjoyment of the benefits of scientific progress and its applications.

Although the Universal Declaration of Human Rights (1948)[2] contains both categories of rights, these rights were artificially split into two treaties due to Cold War politics, with the United States focusing on civil and political rights and the former Soviet Union mainly focusing on economic, social, and cultural rights. Since the end of the Cold War, acknowledgment of the indivisibility and interdependence of rights has, again, become commonplace. The Convention on the Rights of the Child (1989),[3] the first human rights treaty to be opened for signature since the end of the Cold War, includes civil, political, economic, and social rights considerations—not only within the same treaty but within the same right. (The United States and the collapsed nation of Somalia are the only countries not to have ratified the Convention on the Rights of the Child.)

Perhaps the right most relevant to the concerns of this book is the right to health, defined as the right to the highest attainable standard of health.[4] We operationalize the highest attainable standard of health as that experienced by the most privileged social stratum in a society.[5] The right to health reinforces government responsibility for prevention, treatment, and control of disease and for the creation of conditions necessary to ensure access to health care facilities, goods, and services that are essential for health.[6,7]

However, in addition to the right to health and of equal importance in pursuing the right to health, are human rights to a wide range of conditions that are needed for optimal health—such as water, food, shelter, safe working conditions, education, information, participation, and enjoyment of the benefits of scientific progress. Because human rights principles hold that all rights—economic, social, cultural, civil, and political—are interdependent and indivisible, governments are accountable for progressively addressing conditions that may impede not only the realization of the "right to health" but also the realization of related rights.[8] Every country is now party to at least one treaty addressing health-related rights.[9,10]

The principle of nondiscrimination, the overarching principle that cuts across all rights, is of great relevance for social justice. It covers not only explicit or direct discrimination but also structural discrimination—the discrimination inherent in societal structures that subtly, but systematically, keeps some groups at a disadvantage. Governments can be understood to be obligated to remove barriers, such as linguistic or cultural obstacles, that can (a) discourage groups that have historically experienced discrimination from making appropriate use of health care services or from receiving necessary education, or (b) track marginalized groups into health-damaging jobs and neighborhoods.

Human Rights as Legal Standards and Obligations of Governments

Human rights and ethical principles related to health are strongly consonant. In particular, equal opportunities to be healthy (distributive justice) and the human rights obligation to remove barriers so that individuals and groups can realize their right to health seem to be closely related. However, human rights instruments provide a unique and powerful contribution to efforts for social justice in public health by removing the concerns for improving the health of disadvantaged groups from the voluntary realms of ethics, charity, and solidarity to the realms of law and entitlement.

Human rights standards and legal obligations relevant to social justice are unfortunately not being sufficiently fulfilled in many, perhaps most, places in the world today, making it clear that the existence of entitlements and laws is not sufficient to guarantee their reality. However, the enforcement of human rights and the effectiveness of human rights accountability mechanisms could be greatly strengthened if they were used as a matter of course by leaders in public health and other development and social sectors committed to social justice.

Official and unofficial mechanisms now exist to monitor compliance with international and regional human rights norms and standards. At the international level, governments that ratify human rights treaties are obliged to report every several years to the specific body responsible for monitoring government action under a given treaty. They are responsible for demonstrating how they are and are not in compliance with treaty provisions. They must show constant improvement in their efforts to respect, protect, and fulfill the rights in question. Each of the treaty bodies meets several times each year to assess the government reports that have been submitted and to provide concluding comments and observations as to what must be improved in the future. There are seven international human rights treaty monitoring bodies—each corresponding to a major human rights treaty (table 22-1). In addition, existing international political bodies of the United Nations, most notably the General Assembly, are charged with following up on agreements made at major summits, such as the Millennium Development Goals (see table 21-7 on p. 394).

TABLE 22-1   Human Rights Treaties and Their Monitoring Bodies

Treaty	Monitoring Body
International Convention on the Elimination of All Forms of Racial Discrimination	Committee on the Elimination of All Forms of Racial Discrimination
International Covenant on Economic, Social, and Cultural Rights	Committee on Economic, Social, and Cultural Rights
International Covenant on Civil and Political Rights	Human Rights Committee
International Convention on the Elimination of All Forms of Discrimination Against Women	Committee on the Elimination of All Forms of Discrimination Against Women
Convention Against Torture, and Other Cruel, Inhuman or Degrading Treatment or Punishment	Committee Against Torture
Convention on the Rights of the Child	Committee on the Rights of the Child
International Convention on the Protection of the Rights of All Migrant Workers and Members of Their Families	Committee on the Protection of the Rights of All Migrant Workers and Members of Their Families

All of the human rights treaty bodies have expressed a commitment to exploring government obligations under the treaties for health and for specific issues raised by HIV/AIDS, disability, and reproductive and sexual health. Health-oriented United Nations institutions, such as the World Health Organization (WHO), UNAIDS, and the United Nations Children's Fund (UNICEF), are invited to provide information on the state of health and the performance of health systems in the countries under review. Nongovernmental organizations (NGOs) can also submit informal reports—often termed "shadow reports"—providing additional information and stating their views on the situations and issues at stake. NGOs, such as Amnesty International, Oxfam, and Physicians for Human Rights, and the news media, through their public statements, also play major, albeit unofficial, roles in monitoring compliance with human rights norms and agreements.

While these accountability structures exist, use of these formal mechanisms is clearly in need of strengthening. Health leaders committed to social justice could play an important role, for example, by (a) institutionalizing a routine process of review of data on health and health care from a social justice and human rights perspective, using the relevant concluding comments and observations of the monitoring bodies to guide their analysis, and (b) using this review to stimulate public debate and consideration by national-level human rights monitoring bodies of the implications for health and the promotion and protection of human rights.

The recognition of human rights norms as entitlements and legal standards can also be a powerful tool to influence national policies. For example, affirmative action—preferential action in favor of historically disadvantaged or disenfranchised groups, such as racial and ethnic minorities, as well as women—has been a potentially important tool for social justice, with implications for health, such as in ensuring a diverse health workforce to serve disadvantaged populations and in focusing attention and resources on reducing health disparities. However, affirmative action in the United States continues to face many legal and other challenges. Reference to human rights principles may be helpful in building consensus for the legitimacy of affirmative action. Particularly relevant is the crosscutting principle of nondiscrimination, and human rights agreements that call for concerted action by governments to remove obstacles for women and marginalized groups, including indigenous peoples.

Human Rights as a Conceptual Framework for Analysis and Advocacy

Human rights principles can provide a useful, systematic framework for analyzing health and social justice issues and advocating effectively for social justice in public health. This framework focuses attention on how violations or lack of attention to human rights can have serious health consequences and how the design or implementation of health policies, programs, and practices can promote or violate rights. A human rights lens brings attention not only to the technical and operational aspects of health-related interventions but also to the civil, political, economic, social, and cultural factors that surround them.[11] For strategies to achieve social justice in public health, human rights principles and standards provide guidance about (a) who should be considered disadvantaged and (b) the importance of addressing the nonmedical, as well as the medical, determinants of health. Human rights norms also provide a framework—and forums—for institutionalizing a social justice perspective across all ongoing health-sector actions.

Who is disadvantaged? According to human rights norms, the disadvantaged are those with underlying obstacles affecting their ability to realize all of their rights. A human rights perspective can thus provide a universal frame of reference for identifying social justice concerns. For example, whether a given disparity constitutes an injustice may be a matter of dispute. More-privileged groups have at times claimed that health disparities adversely affecting the health of, for example, a disenfranchised ethnic group merely reflect different "cultures" or "lifestyles." Or privileged groups have claimed that the poor have poorer health because they engage in health-damaging behaviors, such as smoking and eating less-nutritious food; implicitly, they view these behaviors as entirely freely chosen rather than as shaped by the conditions in which disadvantaged groups live because of social position. Such a view provides a rationale for not committing more public resources to addressing the conditions in disadvantaged communities that support health-damaging behaviors.

By contrast, human rights norms assert rights to living standards needed for optimal health and expressly prohibit discrimination on the basis of such factors as gender, racial or ethnic group, national origin, religion, and disability. Particularly where certain groups, such as women and disenfranchised racial and ethnic groups, are systematically excluded from decision-making, human rights standards can play a crucial role in agenda setting by strengthening consensus about the existence of inequities in health and the need to reduce them. For example, in some western European countries during the past 15 to 20 years, systematic monitoring and public discussion of socioeconomic inequalities in health have played an important role in building consensus among the more-advantaged segments of society about the need to address those inequalities. As another example, the 2003 California state ballot initiative to ban the collection and analysis of information on race or ethnicity in public data sets (Proposition 54) was defeated, in part, by arguments stressing the need to monitor the size of racial and ethnic disparities in order to determine if they are being reduced. In both of these examples, human rights perspectives were generally not invoked explicitly but were implicit. We believe that such efforts would be strengthened by explicit reference to human rights principles, about which the public should be educated.

Are nonmedical determinants of health, including poverty and lack of education, appropriate concerns for health workers who care about social justice? Both social justice and human rights principles dictate striving for equal opportunity for health for groups who have historically experienced discrimination or social marginalization. Taken seriously, achieving equal opportunities for health entails not only buffering the health-damaging effects of poverty and marginalization by providing health services but also reducing disparities among populations in the underlying conditions necessary to be healthy, such as access to clean water and sanitation, nutritious food, adequate shelter, education, and a clean environment. Addressing these underlying determinants of health and health care requires attention to both social justice and human rights perspectives. Human rights principles provide a particularly compelling argument for government responsibility—not only to provide health services but also to alter the conditions that create, exacerbate, and perpetuate economic poverty, social and economic deprivation, and marginalization or social exclusion.

Few people would contest that economic poverty—with and without its associated social disadvantages—plays a central role in creating, exacerbating, and perpetuating ill health. Even in the absence of absolute deprivation, relative inequalities in economic resources have damaging effects on the health of all members of a society—including the most advantaged.[12–16]

Although poverty is not, in and of itself, a violation of human rights, government action or inaction leading to poverty and government failure to adequately address the conditions that create, exacerbate, and perpetuate poverty and marginalization often reflect, or are closely connected with, violations or denials of human rights.[1] For example, lack of access to education, especially primary education, can be understood as both (a) the denial of a right—in and of itself; and (b) inextricably connected with poverty and ill health. Education, which fosters empowerment and participation in informed decisions about health-related behaviors, is crucial to breaking the poverty–ill health cycle. Health workers can play an important role in advocating for policies to improve education and to eliminate poverty by speaking to the health implications of these policies.

Institutionalizing the Routine Systematic Application of Social Justice and Human Rights Perspectives Within All Health-Sector Actions

Most public health efforts are intended to benefit whole populations and sometimes particularly the disadvantaged, but experience has shown that a strategic approach is necessary to overcome the tendency for the poor or marginalized to benefit too little from even the best-intentioned efforts.[17,18] Work on social justice and human rights must be integrated as an ongoing priority—not as an afterthought—in all programs of health institutions. This approach will require the use of simple, practical tools that health personnel perceive as helpful to their work, as well as training and ongoing support. Presenting social justice principles within a human rights framework could reinforce their importance, in part by showing that they reflect a broad worldwide consensus. Social justice principles and human rights norms should routinely be used to frame discussion of the findings from monitoring efforts to assess social disparties in health. And these results should then be presented in forums for monitoring of human rights.

Monitoring the Social Justice and Human Rights Implications of Policies in All Sectors That Affect Health

Routine assessment, using human rights norms, of potential health implications for people in different social strata should become standard practice in the design, implementation, and evaluation of all development policies that could conceivably affect health, not only policies within the health sector. Social justice and human rights principles suggest that routinely collected population data on health and health care and other health determinants be disaggregated by degree of social advantage. For example, relevant data should be analyzed by gender, race, ethnicity, and other factors that reflect social position. Without monitoring, there is no accountability for the potentially different impact of policies on population groups of different degrees of social disadvantage.[5,19,20] The fact that most societies have far less tolerance for social disparities in health than in wealth or other social privileges provides the health sector a powerful tool for mobilizing public opinion.[21]

Strengthening Arguments and Building Public Consensus for Achieving Equitable Financing of Health Care

Equitable financing means that those with the least resources pay the least, both in absolute terms and as a proportion of their total resources. It also means that lack of personal resources does not restrict an individual from receiving needed services that are recommended on the basis of prevailing norms and scientific knowledge. Equitable financing would increase access to health care, which—if health care services are effective—should improve people's health and, thus, their ability to earn a living, which, in itself, is essential to realizing a range of rights. Equitable financing of health care could also reduce poverty more directly by protecting those who are most vulnerable from impoverishment resulting from health care expenses. Equitable financing is likely to be sustainable with, for example, risk pooling.[22] Implementation of this strategy requires building public consensus regarding commitment to social justice, which can be strengthened by showing the linkages to the human rights obligations of governments.

Human Rights as Guiding Principles for Designing and Implementing Policies and Programs

Designing and Implementing Health Services

Human rights principles require that health institutions systematically consider how the design or implementation of policies and programs may directly or indirectly affect social marginalization, disadvantage, vulnerability, or discrimination. For example, improving the geographic and financial accessibility of preventive health services may not alleviate disparities in their use, without active outreach and support for the groups most likely to be underutilizers despite equal or greater need.[17,23] This requires identifying and addressing the obstacles, including unconscious and de facto discrimination—such as language, cultural beliefs, racism, gender discrimination, and homophobia—that keep disadvantaged groups from receiving the full benefits of health initiatives. Although many policies and programs to reduce poverty and improve the health of the poor routinely consider and address these concerns, many, unfortunately, do not.[24] Explicit adoption of human rights approaches can help bring systematic attention to social disadvantage, vulnerability, and discrimination in health policies and programs.

Human rights principles require that public health institutions ensure that services effectively address the major causes of preventable ill health—and associated impoverishment—among the disadvantaged. This approach requires systematic and sustained efforts to build infrastructure, to overcome the complex barriers to receiving health care that often accompany low social position, and to achieve comprehensive and high-quality universal services. Access and quality are inseparable; perceived low quality is a widespread barrier to use of available services by the disadvantaged.[25]

Particularly among agencies supporting health programs in lower-income countries, resource constraints are at times cited as a rationale for focusing on a limited number of conditions—such as malaria, tuberculosis, HIV/AIDS, or maternal morbidity/mortality—that disproportionately affect the poor. A human rights commitment to "progressive realization" of all rights requires this narrowed focus to be temporary. Targets must be set within a long-range plan to progressively ensure comprehensive, high-quality services relevant to the health needs of the entire population.[26]

Strengthening and Extending Public Health Functions to Address the Social Determinants of Health

The health sector can make a major contribution to addressing social justice and human rights concerns by strengthening and extending those crucial public health functions—beyond health care services—that address the basic conditions needed to achieve health and to escape from the vicious cycle of poverty and ill health. These functions include setting and enforcing standards for water and sanitation, food and drug safety, tobacco control, and working, housing, and environmental conditions. These functions benefit society as a whole, and they particularly benefit the disadvantaged.

The health sector, however, has little or no direct control over most of the underlying conditions necessary for health. Thus, traditional public health functions can be expanded through collaboration with other sectors to develop strategic plans addressing these conditions in light of both social justice and human rights concerns. Reflecting human rights norms, these expanded public health functions could include promoting an adequate food supply; education permitting full economic, social, and political participation; housing and neighborhood environments that promote health; and dignified, safe employment.[4] Such efforts would require collaboration with a range of sectors that have not traditionally been health-sector partners, such as those sectors addressing economic, social, political, educational, environmental, and general development activities. These expanded public health functions would not involve the health sector dictating what other sectors should do but would rather enable the health sector to serve as a key partner, providing evidence on health—within social justice and human rights frameworks—that could shed light on policy directions.

Conclusion

Health workers should be aware that human rights norms, standards, laws, and accountability mechanisms are highly relevant tools that can enhance efforts to achieve social justice in health, both globally and within countries. Human rights treaties and other agreements can provide important mechanisms to strengthen accountability of governments for moving toward greater social justice in health. Although these accountability mechanisms need to be strengthened, their increased use—for example, by the health sector—could be a major step toward this goal. Furthermore, human rights principles and norms can strengthen advocacy efforts for social justice in health, in part by emphasizing a broad international consensus on (a) key issues, such as the need to eliminate gender, racial, and ethnic discrimination; and (b) the right to health and related rights to water, food, shelter, information, education, and the benefits of scientific progress. Human rights perspectives and instruments can also strengthen the analytic frameworks that we use to develop strategies to achieve social justice, particularly with respect to the importance of addressing the nonmedical determinants of health. Finally, human rights norms can provide guidance on how to shape the design of health programs to reduce obstacles to realization of the right to health and related rights and with explicit attention to the human rights principle of nondiscrimination. This principle provides a crucial framework for efforts toward greater social justice in public health.

One of the most valuable contributions of human rights principles and standards to struggles for greater social justice in public health may be the obligation of governments not only to not directly violate human rights but also to promote them, ensuring the realization of the conditions needed to enable individuals and groups to achieve all of their rights. This approach justifies and strengthens advocacy for the need to address underlying unjust societal conditions and structures, moving beyond attempts only to buffer their health-damaging effects by providing health services. And in so doing, this approach provides a framework that can guide strategies within the health sector to achieve greater social justice in health.

Acknowledgments The authors wish to acknowledge Eva Wallstam and Eugenio Villar Montesinos of the World Health Organization (WHO), whose idea it was initially to address the linkages between human rights and social justice in relation to health. The authors are solely responsible for the opinions and perspectives expressed in this chapter.

References

1. Gruskin S, Tarantola D. Health and human rights. In: Detels R, Beaglehole R, eds. Oxford textbook on public health. New York, N.Y.: Oxford University Press, 2002, pp. 311–35.
2. Universal Declaration of Human Rights, G.A. res. 217A (III), U.N. Doc A/810 at 71 (1948).
3. United Nations. Convention on the Rights of the Child (1989). UN General Assembly Document A/RES/44/25.
4. Constitution of the World Health Organization as adopted by the International Health Conference, New York, 19–22 June, 1946, signed on 22 July 1946 by the representatives of 61 States (official records of the World Health Organization no. 2,

p. 100); International Covenant on Economic, Social and Cultural Rights (ICESCR), G.A. Res. 2200 (XXI), UN GAOR, 21st session, supp. no. 16, at 49, UN Doc. A/6316 (1966) and entered into force, 3 January 1; United Nations Committee on Economic, Social and Cultural Rights. The right to the highest attainable standard of health: E/C.12/2000/4. CESCR general comment 14. Geneva, Switzerland: United Nations, 2000.

5. Braveman P, Gruskin S. Defining equity in health. J Epidemiol Commun Health 2003;57:254–8.

6. Kirby M. The right to health fifty years on: still skeptical? Health Human Rights 1999;4:7–24.

7. Leary V. The right to health in international human rights law. Health Human Rights 1994;1:24–56.

8. Eide A. Economic, social and cultural rights as human rights. In: Eide A, Krause C, Rosas A, eds. Economic, social and cultural rights: a textbook. Dordrecht, the Netherlands: Martinus Nijhoff, 1995.

9. Tomasevski, K. Health rights. In: Eide A, Krause C, Rosas A, eds. Economic, social and cultural rights: a textbook. Dordrecht, the Netherlands: Martinus Nijhoff, 1995.

10. United Nations. Manual on human rights reporting. Geneva, Switzerland: United Nations Center for Human Rights, 1996 (UN document no. HR/PUB/96/1).

11. Gruskin S, Tarantola D. HIV/AIDS and human rights revisited. Canadian HIV/AIDS Policy Law Rev 6(1/2), 2001.

12. Wilkinson RG. Socioeconomic determinants of health. Health inequalities: relative or absolute material standards? BMJ 1997;314:591–5.

13. Wilkinson RG. Unhealthy societies: the afflictions of inequality. New York, N.Y.: Rutledge, 1996.

14. Lynch JW, Kaplan GA. Understanding how inequality in the distribution of income affects health. J Health Psychol 1997;2:297–314.

15. Kawachi, I, Kennedy BP, Lochner K, Prothrow-Stith D. Social capital, income inequality, and mortality. Am J Public Health 1997;87:1491–8.

16. Deaton A. Inequalities in income and inequalities in health. NBER (National Bureau of Economic Research) working paper W7141, May 1999. Available at: http://www.nber.org/papers/w7141. Accessed May 21, 2005.

17. Hart JT. The inverse care law. Lancet 1971;1:405–12.

18. Braveman P, Tarimo E. Screening in primary health care. Geneva, Switzerland: World Health Organization, 1994.

19. Braveman P. Monitoring equity in health and health care: a policy-oriented approach in low- and middle-income countries. Geneva, Switzerland: World Health Organization, 1998 (WHO/CHS/HSS/98.1, equity initiative document no. 3).

20. Braveman P, Tarimo E, Creese A. Equity in health and health care: a WHO initiative. Geneva, Switzerland: World Health Organization, October 1996.

21. Birdsall N, Hecht R. Swimming against the tide: strategies for improving equity in health. Human resources development and operations policy (HROWP 55). Washington, D.C.: World Bank, 1995.

22. Davies P, Carrin G. Risk-pooling—necessary but not sufficient. Bull WHO 2001; 79:587.

23. Aday LA, Andersen RM. Equity of access to medical care: a conceptual and empirical overview. Med Care 1981;19:4–27.

24. Feinstein O, Picciotto R, eds. Evaluation and poverty reduction: proceedings from a World Bank Conference. Washington, D.C.: World Bank, 2000.

25. Haddad S, Fournier P, Machouf N, Fassinet Y. What does quality mean to lay people? Community perceptions of primary health care services in Guinea. Soc Sci Med 1998;47:381–94.
26. Gruskin S, Loff B. Do human rights have a role in public health work? Lancet 2002; 360:1880.

23

PROMOTING SOCIAL JUSTICE THROUGH PUBLIC HEALTH POLICIES, PROGRAMS, AND SERVICES

Alonzo Plough

Introduction

Public health policies, programs, and services—collectively termed public health practice—in the United States have been the subject of a series of reports by the Institute of Medicine (IOM)[1,2] and considerable commentary by the federal government, professional associations, and academic institutions.[3–5] However, social injustice as a focus of practice is rarely discussed.

Most assessments of the state of public health practice have dealt with such issues as organizational structure, funding shortfalls, and capacity limitation. They have typically focused on defining functional capacity (to provide the 10 essential public health services*) and the growing gaps

*The ten essential public health services are: (1) monitor health status to identify community problems; (2) diagnose and investigate health problems and health hazards in the community; (3) inform, educate, and empower people about health issues; (4) mobilize community partnerships and action to identify and solve health problems; (5) develop policies and plans that support individual and community health efforts; (6) enforce laws and regulations that protect health and ensure safety; (7) link people to needed personal health services and assure the provision of health care when otherwise unavailable; (8) assure a competent public health and personal health care workforce; (9) evaluate effectiveness, accessibility, and quality of personal and population-based health services; and (10) research for new insights and innovative solutions to health problems.

between population health challenges and resources invested in the public health system.[6]

Broad assessments of a system in "disarray," particularly at the local level, abound. Federal- and state-level attempts to bring coherence to public health practice through standards and performance measures are presented as remedies for the diagnosis of systemic dysfunction. Current strategic planning at the Centers for Disease Control and Prevention (CDC) looks to the private sector and individual health care providers as an underused component of public health practice.[7]

These analyses also mention, one way or another, the imperative of public health to improve the social conditions in specific communities that largely determine health and well-being. Social determinants of health, community-based public health, community-based participatory research, and the social/ecological model* all appear as descriptors of a component of public health practice. However, this domain of practice is not considered essential. No national standards or performance measures explicitly deal with the promotion of social justice as a public health practice core capacity.

To better understand how social justice can and does become an object of public health practice, there must be (a) a recognition that public health practice is overwhelmingly a government activity—in organizational delivery and in financing, and (b) a debunking of much of the conventional judgment that public health practice is in disarray. Because the performance of activities and interventions to promote social justice challenges the broader political economy and explicitly identifies social injustice as a causal element in the poor health status of a particular community, government public health practice is placed in a difficult context. How health departments approach this problem will depend on (a) the level of government—federal, state, or local—in which the agency is located, (b) the political ideology of elected officials who oversee the agency, (c) the capacity and commitment of public health officials, (d) the ability of agency staff members to meaningfully engage community residents in collaborative endeavors, and (e) the competing demands of public health challenges, such as SARS, bioterrorism preparedness, routine outbreaks of disease, inspections of various facilities, and service delivery mandates. An operational focus on root causes of poor health, such as poverty, income and wealth inequality, and racism—all factors related to social injustice—requires a public health capacity not often discussed. This is the

---

*The social/ecological model describes how social, physical, and genetic factors influence health status. This includes contextual and relational influences on health, such as social and community networks, living and working conditions, institutional influences, and political and economic policies, all of which interact to shape population and individual health.

capacity to effectively manage the urgent demands of public health practice while simultaneously and explicitly understanding the social context and root causes of the poor health of populations. Importantly, this understanding of social context and root causes must inform both current practice and future strategic planning.

Public Health Agencies and Social Justice

Federal Agencies

The capacity to address social injustice in public health practice, or the ability to develop it, varies with the level of government in which a health agency operates. Federal agencies such as CDC and the Health Resources and Services Administration (HRSA) have a national scope, extensive grants and contracts, and multiple delivery and research programs that could focus on social injustice as a core problem in public health practice. Although there are some isolated examples of social justice as a key component of federal agency policy, these do not represent a central tendency. Too often, such promising policy directions like HRSA's 100 Percent Access and Zero Disparities initiative during the Clinton administration or the environmental justice focus of CDC's National Center for Environmental Health during the same period have had marginal funding and program development. The administration of each U.S. president has a different capacity to envision social injustice as an operational policy and program direction. As a result, there has been little sustained effort to address this fundamental problem at the federal level.

State Health Departments

State-level public health practice faces similar challenges, with frequent changes in governors, high turnover of public health officials, and widespread inability to gain sustained political support for explicit public heath activities to address social injustice. As is the case with federal-level public health practice, state health departments are often not directly connected with community-based public health practice. The default mode of public health practice at the state level is the pass-through of federal funds to local agencies, very general and aggregated statewide policy development, and regulatory activities. Advocacy and activism of health officials—which are essential ingredients for successful policy interventions to reduce social injustice—are very constrained at this level.

The average tenure of state public health directors is only 2.9 years.[8] As a result, directors are usually just starting or about to leave positions, making it quite difficult to provide the sustained and visible leadership needed to address social injustice as an essential function of public health practice. A review of the websites of the 50 state health departments found only one department with an extensive and explicit incorporation of social justice as a standard of practice.[9] The Association of State and Territorial Heath Officials (ASTHO) website contains no reports on or any references to addressing social justice as a core public health practice strategy.

Clearly, federal- and state-level public health agencies could influence critical policy areas that are shaped at the state level of government, such as education, taxation, housing, and economic development. The scale of federal- and state-level bureaucracy and the siloed nature of agency behavior make such direct action and collaboration difficult, especially on politically charged topics.

Federal and state public health agencies, however, can facilitate social justice interventions at the local level through funding that is sufficiently flexible to allow for community-driven approaches to prevention that can address social determinants of health. Funding approaches, such as the Racial and Ethnic Approaches to Community Health (REACH) program that has funded local coalitions to address health disparities in AIDS/HIV, diabetes, and infant mortality, have resulted in effective community-level interventions that address root causes of ill health and represent a social justice framework. The Steps to a Healthier United States (STEPS) grants program holds similar promise, although this program has been implemented too recently to evaluate its impact.

Local Health Departments

The local level of government public health practice is best situated to explicitly address social injustice. Local health departments represent the backbone of the government public health system, but they have been poorly represented in studies and reports on the current and projected status of public health practice.[10] Both of the influential IOM reports indicate that the public health system—from the perspective of conventional standards and technical capacity—is in disarray. Local health departments in particular are cited as having limited public health capacity.

There are a number of flaws, however, in the conventional analysis of local public health capacity.[11] In the United States, 70 percent of the population and almost all highly populous urban areas—where health disparities based on race, ethnicity, and poverty abound—are served by metropolitan health departments that are highly functional and have developed many effective policies, programs, and services. These health departments are also the most community-embedded components of the government public health structure and are beginning to develop public health practice models that explicitly consider addressing social injustice as a core organizational competency.

The best examples of a commitment to social justice as a part of public practice are associated with the policy commitment of the National Association of County and City Health Officials (NACCHO) to social justice. There are numerous references to social justice on the NACCHO website, which operates as a technical resource to local public health practitioners.[12] In 2001, NACCHO formed the Health and Social Justice Partnership together with three other organizations:

- The Center for the Advancement of Health, a private organization that focuses on accelerating the application of new research on prevention to improve health policy
- America's Health Together, a university-based entity that coordinates research and service activities to eliminate racial and ethnic disparities in health
- The Center for Minority Health at the University of Pittsburgh, an advisory organization dedicated to raising awareness of the relationship of social inequality to health.

The goal of this partnership is to

> eliminate inequalities in health status by raising awareness about their relationship to social and economic inequality, and what can be done to act on the conditions that produce them.... The partnership seeks to create a national dialogue and propose public policy agendas directed towards eliminating the root causes and consequences of inequalities (through) op-eds, magazine articles and other media related strategies. (p. 2)[13]

Its board has adopted a resolution that has, in part, urged "support for ideas, activities, social movements, and policies that advance action to build health equity through social justice" (p. 1).[14] In 2002, NACCHO revised its strategic plan to define as a core strategic action of local public health practice the capacity "to address issues of health equity and social justice, oppose racism, and support diversity and cultural competence" (p. 3).

In the world of public health practice, this dramatic difference in a professional association's explicit support for incorporating social justice as a core competency and providing tools, training, workshops, and other technical assistance to local practitioners to implement strategies and specific actions is profound. This support has provided grants and other resources that build strategic action in many local communities across the nation. Importantly, such a professional practice framework provides a much-needed legitimacy for advocacy work at the local level. When a local board of health member or city official questions why a health department is involved in land use or environmental justice as a policy and program area, the ability to point to a national organization's strategic plans and practice guidelines often provides the evidence for these actions being seen as "standard" public health practice.

Local public health practice is grounded in specific communities and is part of a local network of community-based organizations and public and private institutions with a shared local governmental context. The broad range of social conditions that adversely influence health outcomes—such as unemployment rates, poverty, disinvestments in public education, unsafe neighborhoods, and suburban sprawl (as a deterrent to community cohesion)—have a daily immediacy at this level of public health practice. The definition of public health as a "social enterprise" with a mandate to align the technical tools of epidemiology and assessment with effective community partnerships and advocacy can become operational in local health departments with the leadership and commitment to engage with their communities in challenging social injustice. The much longer tenure of local public health officials, compared with their state counterparts, increases the possibilities for catalytic leadership and sustained practice efforts grounded in a social justice framework. Staff members of local health departments are also members of the community, helping to increase linkages between communities that experience health problems related to social injustice and local public health programs and services that should be accountable to these communities.

Clearly, all government public health agencies—including local health departments—are challenged in creating authentic community partnerships. To be effective in a community-linked approach to addressing social injustice requires public health agencies to incorporate new approaches to collaboration that go far beyond the traditional expert-driven approach to professional public health practice.[15] Roz Lasker and Elisa Weiss[16] present a very thoughtful approach to the essential principles of collaboration required to facilitate activities that address the root causes of health disparities and other social and economic conditions that decrease the well-being of communities. The key components of their community health governance model suggest that effective collaboration requires empowerment, community building (the bridging of social ties), and community engagement. All of these are essential activities of public health practice, without which public health agencies would probably revert to the rhetoric of community engagement without the impact from true power sharing with community members. Too often, public health agencies use the language of the social determinants of health and the need to reduce health disparities but do not internally transform in ways that would allow for the nontraditional actions required to address social injustice as a risk to the public's health. Using the language of social justice while applying the traditional top-down tools of public health practice has a limited impact.

The major challenge of public health practice is to move theoretical knowledge about the relationship of social injustice to increased health risks and poor health outcomes into broad and sustainable changes in agency policies and practices. These changes include (a) providing support and training to staff members in partnership development, and (b) creating the capacity to extend public health practice beyond the agency walls to dynamic partnerships with other disciplines, such as economic development, land use planning, housing, transportation, and education.

Local public health practitioners are particularly effective when local data are generated and communicated through accessible reports that highlight the impact of specific social and economic factors on health outcomes. Effective use of local media is an essential tool of public health practice in broadening the public's awareness of the impacts of social injustice on community health. Careful, data-driven presentations to local elected officials and health board members are essential components of public health practices that address social injustice. However, this type of political advocacy is not always the most significant form of community and political mobilization activities.

Effective local public health practice depends largely on capabilities to (a) build on a general base of community-driven partnerships (some of which are not explicitly health focused), (b) identify root causes and leverage points for change, and (c) select the most effective set of tools and strategies that match specific manifestations of social injustice. Root causes of social injustice are often best addressed by focusing on policies concerning labor and employment, taxation, environmental conditions, housing, land use, and child development and support. The critical responsibility of public health practice that is oriented to social justice is to recognize the broader context of causation and to not constrict programs and interventions to those that are based on individual behaviors or a specific disease.

Public Health Practice Oriented to Social Justice

Two Case Studies

This section examines two examples of how public health policies, programs, and practices can highlight the relationship between social injustice and the public's health. Each example provides some practical insights into how community partnerships can be used to deepen knowledge of root causes of poor health, mobilize and activate political and community leadership, and make initial efforts sustainable. The case studies are drawn from local public health agencies in San Francisco and Seattle. Each case study focuses on a health-related problem with significant social determinants, with each public health agency and its community partners deploying different strategies to link the broader social justice problem with a specific approach to health improvement at the community level. The scale of impact and the possible sustainability of the efforts in each of these case studies are different. They highlight the complexities of addressing social injustice through public health practices and policies that are primarily governmental.

Case Study 1

The San Francisco Department of Public Health is a city and county health department serving a diverse metropolitan population. Its practice framework is linked to the strategies to promote social justice in local public health practice at a national level. For example, its environmental health section supports the Program on Health, Equity, and Sustainability, the goal of which is "to make San Francisco a livable city for all residents and to foster environmental, community, and economic conditions that allow residents to achieve their human potential."[17]

In 2002, the department facilitated a process to address environmental health disparities in asthma, particularly in relation to indoor-air exposure to poor children. Recognizing that some neighborhoods have a high concentration of substandard housing and drawing on published studies relating poor indoor-air quality to the presence of mites, cockroaches, and mold, the department raised the level of community awareness through data presentation and community mobilization. Setting the context with an estimate of 54,000 residents diagnosed with asthma, the department pointed out the disproportionately more severe outcomes among communities of color and placed this risk in a broader community context by stating, "The health and well-being of San Francisco's residents, families, and community are at stake."[17]

An important community-mobilizing strategy was the development of the San Francisco Asthma Task Force. Chaired by a local nongovernment social-service provider, the composition of the group reflected the diversity of the community, including representatives of nonprofit organizations and community-advocacy organizations and community members, many of whom had experienced asthma in their own families. The task force developed focused working groups that had a diversity of members. These working groups gained information from tenants with asthma, property owners, managers, builders, and contractors to develop a community-based definition of the problem. Then teams from the Department of Public Health and the task force applied the interdisciplinary tools of environmental health, environmental epidemiology, building and housing code enforcement, and tenant organizing to further define intervention and policy approaches. Through an open community process, including retreats, the task force developed recommendations that focused on improving indoor-air quality for lower-income tenants. The final report of the task force highlighted the structural deficiencies of buildings that exacerbate asthma by exposure to molds, fumes, and other hazards. These factors, which represent significant forms of housing injustice, were presented by the group as root causes of asthma. There was explicit recognition, based on the findings of the work groups, that low-income people have few housing options and are disproportionately exposed to these factors.[18]

Recommendations resulting from this locally driven public health partnership reflect insights gained and action strategies developed when public health workers and community partners create dynamic collaborations to address social injustice. The major action strategies that it developed to address environmental determinants of asthma included the following:

1. *Establishing a cross-agency group to inspect public-housing properties and to create accountability mechanisms that rapidly brought conditions into compliance with the housing code.* This strategy involved creating interagency collaborations among the health department, the housing agency, and agencies involved with code enforcement, the police, and the legal and judicial systems, all of which focused on improving the underlying social conditions that account for income-based disparities in asthma.
2. *Establishing standards and guidelines for comprehensive healthy housing, including roles for property owners—requiring government entities to strengthen the relationship between building codes and landlords' legal obligation to tenants to reduce housing-related health risks.*
3. *Instituting a legal housing-advocacy program for poor patients identified with asthma.* This intervention implemented a monitoring and engagement strategy that raised awareness about environmental determinants of asthma and linked poor asthma patients using hospital emergency departments with information and housing advocates.

This case study demonstrates how many of the elements of a social justice-oriented public health practice are developed and implemented. While the overall project recognized the clinical and disease control issues, its thrust addressed the root causes of asthma in housing and economic policies. The health department was a key participant, but the project was broadly based in the community and led by community organizations. Finally, recommendations addressed the social context of risk and incorporated nontraditional approaches for providing public health programs and services.

Case Study 2

Public Health–Seattle and King County is a large metropolitan local health department serving nearly 2 million people. The department has long recognized the critical importance of social justice in public health practice, as reflected in its mission and value statements and its organizational structure. A specific interdisciplinary unit—Community-Based Public Health Practice (CBPHP)—was established in 1998 to develop community-driven activities grounded in a deep understanding of the social determinants of health.[19] A major focus of CBPHP was eliminating disproportionately poor health status in communities of color.

To develop an approach to this problem that was oriented to social justice, the department initiated a series of surveys and studies that documented growing disparities among economically marginalized King County racial and ethnic groups. Specific examination of disparities in infant mortality, teen pregnancy, diabetes, and other poor health outcomes set the stage for a more contextual examination of root causes of these problems.[20] The results of these studies were published in an easily accessible form and were made widely available on the Internet and through other communication channels. Health department staff members worked closely with advocates to increase community awareness of these problems and to engage community members in strategies to improve the underlying social and economic bases of the poor health outcomes. This work involved specific community-driven assessment of health and examination of the critical social contexts in specific communities, including American Indians and Alaska Natives, African-Americans, members of specific Asian and Pacific Island groups, and Hispanics.

The King County Ethnicity and Health Survey revealed that discrimination influenced all health disparities. For example, 32 percent of African-Americans thought that they had been discriminated against when receiving health care services at some time.[21] Lower percentages of members of ethnic groups also reported experiencing discrimination. Because discrimination is a potent cause of social injustice, a broader strategy was required for effective advocacy and change. Community partners and health department staff members recognized that racism was the root cause and that how racism influenced health status and health-seeking behavior of specific ethnic populations had to be addressed. In the health care setting, perceptions of discrimination can powerfully impact health-seeking behavior and, potentially, health status. Giving voice to individuals who had experienced racism in health care settings provided a more grounded presentation of the problem. By presenting the issues in human terms, the report presented a dramatic and compelling sense of the problem—much more than could have been achieved with a presentation of statistical data. As a result, the information was more likely to improve staff behavior in institutions where discrimination had occurred.

The health department contracted with a community-based organization to develop and conduct the Racial Discrimination in Health Care Interview Project.[22] The results were reported in a community report and a public health report that was broadly distributed among health care practitioners and their institutions, as well as political and community leaders.[23] The reports high-lighted the extensive range and frequency of perceived discrimination among those interviewed. The discrimination events, which had taken place at nearly 30 different public and private health care facilities throughout King County, included racial slurs and blatant examples of rude behaviors and differential treatment. As the report stated, most interviewees reported changing their behaviors as a result of discrimination they had experienced. Some reported delaying treatment due to their negative experiences and not knowing where else to seek care.

These descriptive and experience-based examples from the survey were presented in numerous public settings, including press conferences with the county executive, community meetings, conferences of health professional associations, and board of health meetings. They generated much media at-tention. The results of the series of studies on race, ethnicity, and health were presented to the chief executives of the major hospitals and health plans in the region. A call to action was delivered in all of those settings, seeking a broad community consensus to adopt the recommendations of the reports, including training health care providers, establishing uniform institutional policies to enforce nondiscrimination, and collecting data and performing monitoring by including questions regarding discrimination on patient satisfaction surveys. Many of the recommendations were implemented by local institutions. The work to eliminate discrimination continues.

Additional Examples of Public Health Practice That Address Social Injustice

These two case studies provide good examples of how public health practice can incorporate a social justice framework that influences policy and service. There are many other ways that government public health, especially at the local level, can address injustice. One example is using public health sur-veillance data to identify the adverse health effects of social injustice. Pub-lic health agencies can closely monitor a set of social indicators—such as measures of poverty, income inequality, housing costs, parents who read to young children, and unemployment—that are highly related to health and human development. It is increasingly important to link these types of social indicators to the more traditional vital statistics and health status measures and to use census tracts and ZIP codes as units of analysis. By this approach, public health departments can develop, with their community partners, neighborhood-focused assessments that can assist communities in advocating to improve social and economic conditions that underlie health disparities. Sometimes the advocacy might be focused on ensuring access to preventive services, such as prenatal care for poor women through community and public health clinics. Increasingly, such assessments find that addressing factors such as inadequate housing, lack of jobs with a livable wage, unsafe workplaces, and community exposures to environmental hazards are even more important than providing traditional, client-focused public health services. Given recent budget cuts for public health services in most jurisdictions, it is unlikely that public health agencies can directly ensure that all appropriate services are available and accessible. However, public health practice can align funded services to populations with the greatest needs and aggressively present the political and social context for the critical gaps in access to preventive services.

An Action Agenda for a Social Justice Core Competency in Public Health Practice

For public health practice to better address social injustice, there will need to be a fundamental shift in what is currently viewed as core or essential public health activities. Evolving local, state, and federal standards for public health in the United States clearly prioritize the traditional role of disease prevention and health promotion, although this is greatly complicated by the even higher prioritization of bioterrorism preparedness. Although community involvement, even community engagement, is seen as a core public health activity, its goals are articulated and its outcomes are measured primarily as changes in individual behavior that reduce conventional disease risk factors. For example, it may be stated that more people eat a healthy diet or perform physical exercise or that more young people understand the risk factors associated with drug use due to community assessment and partnership activities.

A public health practice competency addressing the impact of social injustice on health goes beyond affecting individual behavior change and improving the effectiveness of practices within the traditional boundaries of health services. It focuses on enabling more accountable public and private decisions concerning the basic needs of groups of people who have poor health because of discrimination based on race, income, language, ethnicity, or sexual orientation. Its outcomes can be measured by sustainable reductions in the social determinants of this discrimination.

What Are Some of the Barriers to Wider Acceptance of a Core Public Health Competency Demonstrating Ability to Reduce Social Injustice?

First, as reflected in curricular and other requirements of schools of public health and public health programs, academic public health faculty members are just beginning to develop courses that train students in methods and skills relevant to reducing the impact of social injustice on health. Research and courses on health disparities, minority health, and social determinants of health are more prevalent than ever before in this country, but these courses focus on description of problems and policy issues—generally not on methods of engaging communities to develop sustainable actions to address the root causes of health disparities. Courses on community-based public health practice should go beyond community-based assessment of conventional health risk factors and should focus on community-organizing and empowered collaborative practices that can address root causes of social injustice. These courses could link to public health practice settings, where people who have suffered poor health due to social injustice could serve as adjunct faculty members.

A second and closely related barrier to wider acceptance of this core public health competency is the lack of federal funding to support the development of public health practice approaches to address social injustice. This inadequacy includes limited funding for campus/practice/community partnerships to develop and disseminate best practices. More extensive federal funding to local health departments is required to enable their staff members to understand how to develop effective community partnerships and to develop expertise in nontraditional areas of practice. Clear but flexible mandates for authentic community partnerships in policy and program development are needed.

State health departments need to recognize that the community-driven nature of the social determinants of health requires a decentralized focus on local leadership and community development. This requires a shift in focus away from aggregated state plans for reducing disparities to legislative and regulatory policy approaches to reduce the impact of social injustice on the public's health. It requires legislators and policymakers at all levels of government to understand, for example, that housing and land-use/zoning decisions have a major influence on the public's health.

The third and final barrier to wider acceptance of this core public health competency involves raising money to support its promotion during a period of budgetary constraints. Public health practitioners at all levels will need to creatively use data on the social determinants of health to inform and influence the decisions of elected officials. The greatest challenge may be the perception that social injustice is rarely eliminated by public health services alone—although services can reduce the impact of social injustice on individuals who receive these services. A public health practice commitment to incorporating social justice as a core capacity means going far beyond providing services—it means being a catalyst for sustainable structural change to reduce social injustice.

References

1. Institute of Medicine. The future of public health. Washington, D.C.: Academy Press, 1988.
2. Institute of Medicine. The future of the public's health in the 21st century. Washington, D.C.: National Academy Press, 2003.
3. Fraser M. State and local health department structures implications for systems change. transformations for public health. Turning Point Newsletter 1998;1(4).
4. National Association of County and City Health Officials. Local public health agency infrastructure: a chartbook. October. Available at: http://www.naccho.org/pubs/detail. Accessed January 28, 2005.
5. Freund CG, Liu Z. Local health department capacity and performance in New Jersey. J Public Health Manage Pract 2000;6:42–50.
6. Mays GP, Miller CA, Halverson PK (eds.). Local public health practice: trends and models. Washington, D.C.: American Public Health Association, 2000.
7. Centers for Disease Control and Prevention. The futures initiative: creating the future of CDC for the 21st century. Available at: http://www.cdc.gov/futures/update.htm. Accessed January 28, 2005.
8. Meit MB. I'm OK, but I'm not too sure about you: public health at the state and local levels. J Public Health Manage Pract 2001;7:vii–viii.
9. Minnesota Department of Health. Benefits of community engagement. Available at: http://www.health.state.mn.us/communityeng/index.html. Accessed January 28, 2005.
10. Barry MA, Centra L, Pratt E, Brown CK, Giordano L. Where do the dollars go? Measuring local public health expenditures. 1998. Submitted to the Office of Disease Prevention and Health Promotion, Department of Health and Human Services, by National Association of City and County Health Officials, National Association of Local Boards of Health, and Public Health Foundation. Available at: http://www.phf.org. Accessed January 28, 2005.
11. Plough AL. Understanding the financing and functions of metropolitan health departments: a key to improved public health response. J Public Health Manage Pract 2004;10:421–427.
12. National Association of County and City Health Officials. Creating health equity through social justice. Washington, D.C.: NACCHO, September 2002.
13. National Association of County and City Health Officials. Health and social justice partnership 2001. Available at: http://www.naccho.org/general577.cfm. Accessed January 28, 2005.
14. National Association of County and City Health Officials. Resolution to promote health equity. July 2002. Available at: http://www.naccho.org/resolution94.cfm. Accessed January 28, 2005.
15. Plough AL. Common discourse but divergent actions–bridging the promise of community health governance and public health practice. J Urban Health 2003;80:53–7.
16. Lasker RD, Weiss ES. Broadening participation in community problem-solving: a multidisciplinary model to support collaborative practice and research. J Urban Health 2003;80:14–47.
17. San Francisco Department of Public Health. Program on Health, Equity and Sustainability 2004. Available at: http://www.dph.sf.ca.us/ehs. Accessed January 28, 2005.
18. The San Francisco Asthma Task Force. Strategic plan on asthma for the city and county of San Francisco. San Francisco, Calif.: San Francisco Board of Supervisors, June 2003, p 3.

19. Public Health–Seattle and King County. Strategic direction: a guide to public health programs over the next 5 years. September 1999.

20. Public Health–Seattle and King County. Data watch: racial disparities in infant mortality 1990–1998. August 2000.

21. Public Health–Seattle and King County. The King County Ethnicity and Health Survey for King County. October 1998. Available at: http://www.metrokc.gov/health/reports/ethnicity/index.htm. Accessed January 28, 2005.

22. Public Health–Seattle and King County. Racial Discrimination in Health Care Interview Project. January 2001.

23. Public Health–Seattle and King County. Public health special report: racial and ethnic discrimination in health care settings. January 2001.

24

STRENGTHENING COMMUNITIES AND THE ROLES OF INDIVIDUALS IN COMMUNITY LIFE

**Robert E. Aronson, Kay Lovelace,
John W. Hatch, and Tony L. Whitehead**

Introduction

Strengthening communities and the roles of individuals in community life can help prevent disease and disability and expand resources for promoting social justice. Among the potential strengths of communities are social networks, social support, social capital, and the capacity of communities to identify and solve their own problems. Social networks refer to the set of social connections between people, and these networks can be characterized as to their size, the qualities of the ties between members, and the characteristics of the members. Social support refers to the emotional and instrumental assistance provided through social network ties. Social capital most often refers to the level of cohesiveness, trust, and reciprocity within communities and societies. These concepts are not new, but recently they have been the subject of much research and discussion, especially concerning disparities in health.[1–5]

Community health professionals recognize that the community is an important source of both protective factors and potentially harmful factors such as oppressive social controls or limited connections to social resources in the wider society.[6–8] Researchers have investigated community-level protective factors, such as social integration, social connection, social networks,[9,10] and social capital,[11] and their relationship to health.

We contend that hope plays an important role in protecting individuals and their communities from the effects of chronic stressors. We also contend that mediating structures in society provide a means for oppressed communities to meet some of their needs, beyond the resources provided through either government or market forces.

Social networks have been linked to health outcomes through behavioral, psychological, and physiological pathways.[4] Lisa Berkman and colleagues[4] highlight five mechanisms through which social networks may influence health:

1. Networks provide social support. Although emotional support may affect health through the love and caring that people experience, informational, instrumental, and appraisal support may help individuals' health by improving access to resources and goods.
2. Networks are a source of social influence—through both one-on-one influence and shared norms concerning health.
3. Networks promote social participation and social engagement, and thus define and reinforce societal roles as well as provide opportunities for companionship.
4. Networks affect health by providing or preventing exposure to infectious disease.
5. Networks provide access to material goods, resources, and services.

In addition to affecting health directly, networks, through their patterns of associations, may afford opportunities for individuals to work in concert, to problem solve, and to take action. Thus, social networks may be the mechanism through which much community capacity is achieved.

Social capital comprises aspects of a social structure that facilitate action[12] or norms of reciprocity and civic engagement, social trust, and networks of social relations that can be mobilized for civic action.[13] Research linking social capital to health is only beginning but may explain some differences in health outcomes.[11,14,15] However, a major problem in drawing conclusions from current research in this area is the lack of consensus on an operational definition of "social capital," including the level at which it should be measured and the actual measures used in studies.[2] Further, the emphasis given to social cohesion—one aspect of social capital—and its relationship to health outcomes has been criticized for diverting attention from such structural determinants of health as income inequality, discrimination, and institutional racism.[3,5] Another critique is that social capital, when defined as social cohesion, can have both negative and positive social effects.[16] For example, social capital can be quite strong within antisocial groups, such as white supremacy organizations, the militia movement, and neighborhood gangs.

Community capacity comprises the characteristics of a community that enable it to mobilize, identify, and solve community problems.[17] Researchers have identified numerous dimensions of community capacity; some of these dimensions have been linked to improved program implementation and health outcomes, both theoretically and empirically.[18,19] Community-level traits, resources, and patterns of association can be identified and called on to solve community problems and contribute to community health improvement.[20] Mobilizing community capacity to identify and solve problems is a fundamental ingredient of changing oppressive social structures and patterns of meanings. Transformative changes cannot be sustained without an engaged and mobilized citizenry.

Hope and optimism, at the individual level, are thought to positively influence health and protect against the effects of stress.[21,22] In contrast, a lack of hope is thought to diminish health.[23] In his essay "Nihilism in Black America," Cornell West discusses the problem of hopelessness in black America and its deep-grained effects on culture and society.[24] Hope has not been investigated as a community-level construct, but it is a critical component of individual—and possibly community—transformation.

The protective aspects of community life are not only beneficial to community health but also amenable to change through community-organizing and community-building strategies.[25] Health and community development workers, working alongside communities, have tackled issues such as infant mortality, crime, violence, teenage pregnancy, and gang-related activities. These community-building participatory approaches aim to strengthen the capacity of communities to deal with both these issues and any other issues that come their way.[25] Many community health experts believe that identifying and strengthening community resources—as opposed to focusing solely on community risks—is essential to bringing about the kind of community-based change needed to improve health outcomes.[25–27]

Addressing Social Injustice Through Community Transformation

In considering strategies to address social injustice and its effects on the health of communities and population groups, one should keep in mind three key precepts:

1. Understand the local context when working with communities.
2. In doing so, look upstream to understand the social production of health disparities—the root causes.
3. Encourage strategies that lead to social change.

Multiple, multilevel strategies are needed to repair the fallout from social inequalities and social injustice and to stop the societal perpetuation of these problems. As public health workers, we need strategies to assist individuals and communities in their own transformation as they address health disparities and their root causes. We need strategies to improve access to, and the quality of, facilities and services—including public health programming—and we need strategies to stimulate macroeconomic, political, and cultural change.[28]

The emphasis in public health over the past two decades has been to develop and implement effective approaches to reduce the burden of disease in populations, especially by primary prevention—which aims to prevent the occurrence of illness or injury before it occurs. Primary prevention strategies, however, have focused almost exclusively on influencing the behavioral risk factors of individuals, using a variety of strategies with individuals, communities, and even policies. As we examine the social production of health disparities, we must ask, "How can we achieve social change to stop this injustice?" We believe the answer lies in primary prevention.

Building on the understanding of the relationship between individuals and societies proposed by Anthony Giddens,[29] we believe society is transformed when individuals and communities change the routinized patterns of social organization and meaning. To eliminate health disparities, individuals and communities must come together to change these patterns in ways that alter the power structures that hold social inequalities in place. This approach is not new; it has been part of the professional practice in the fields of community development, community organizing for health, and even some forms of comprehensive community-oriented primary health care. Examples appear in the literature of approaches that were viewed as real threats to the status quo, the political elite, and international interests.[30,31]

To effectively address health disparities, we need to use both ameliorative and fundamental approaches to public health practice.[32] Ameliorative approaches do not directly alter underlying inequalities that contribute to health disparities; rather, they target specific risk factors that are associated with health outcomes, in a given community context, and facilitate development of protective factors to enhance the health of individuals, communities, and populations.[32] In contrast, fundamental approaches seek to transform the elements of society that give rise to inequalities and health disparities.

We need to use these approaches at the individual, community, and societal levels. It should not be assumed that societal-level approaches will necessarily be addressing root causes.[32]

Principles to Guide the Work of Community Transformation

Working with communities to effectively strengthen community capacity and the role of individuals in community life requires certain skills and orientations. We propose the following set of principles, based on the work of one of us (J.W.H.) over almost five decades in the Mississippi Delta, Boston, and North Carolina. Building on his mentorship, the other three of us have applied these principles to our work in Baltimore, Washington, D.C., and North Carolina.

1. *Health worker/organizer, know thyself.* Working with poor communities to eliminate social injustice requires that public health workers are able to think reflectively about their own views of the community, their own privilege, and their own comfort level with different roles in promoting health. Nowhere is this more critical than when organizing or working with communities that are different than that of oneself. Personally mediated racism has both unintentional and intentional aspects.[33] For example, devaluation of individuals based on race, which is one form of personally mediated racism, may be evidenced by either an expression of surprise at someone's competence or an effort to stifle someone's aspirations. It occurs when organizers have a view of a community as "half-empty" rather than "half-full." Organizers might do more for the community than necessary and thus increase—rather than decrease—dependency. Organizers might not challenge their own views of what the community has to offer and might believe that their own way of doing things is more informed and more effective. All of these actions devalue what community members might be able to do.

   Public health workers must also know their ability to conduct—and their comfort level with—a structural analysis of the conditions holding disparities in place. Powerful persons and institutions may be challenged by such an analysis. Without a structural analysis, health workers may not see the ways in which they have privilege not held by the community members with whom they work. This will affect the ability of health workers to be in partnership with the communities in which they work.

2. *Build on a foundation of hope.* Efforts to improve the health of individuals and communities within the context of social injustice must begin with a foundation of hope. The erosion of dignity, self-worth, and a useful role in society have given rise to far too many people who have little hope that things will ever improve for themselves or their communities. This lack of hope can also be seen when some people in

groups in the community believe that other people or groups are beyond being helped. The loss of hope can be threatening to the survival of a sense of morality and community among African-Americans.[24,25]

Paulo Freire described the dehumanization that occurs as a result of oppression and social injustice and the impact of this dehumanization on self-esteem:

> Self-depreciation is another characteristic of the oppressed, which derives from their internalization of the opinion the oppressors hold of them. So often do they hear that they are good for nothing, know nothing and are incapable of learning anything— that they are sick, lazy, unproductive—that in the end they become convinced of their own unfitness.[34]

According to Freire, the first step in surmounting oppression is critically recognizing its causes. In doing so, the oppressed can begin to see themselves and their humanity more fully. Public health strategies to restore dignity, self-respect, and regard for others are needed to repair the damage caused by societal oppression. Only when individuals see themselves as fully human can they act to end their oppression.

3. *Recognize the resources that exist within communities.* Communities are built on strengths and assets—not on problems.[35] Understanding the community context in which health problems arise should include an assessment of community assets and ways they have helped to solve previous problems. In African-American communities, institutions parallel to those of the wider society have served as bases of belonging, self-esteem, leadership development, and social activism.[36] Because blacks were often not able to gain access to broader societal institutions or were not treated equally to whites when such access was gained, they were left to develop and nurture parallel institutions.[37] These institutions have included fraternal organizations; clubs; secret societies; economic and educational institutions, such as historically black colleges and universities; and, of great importance, black churches. These parallel institutions have facilitated the survival of African-Americans, led the civil rights movement, and nurtured community capacity.

Lay health advisor programs are one type of program that builds on the strengths of African-American churches to reduce health disparities.[38,39] Among the projects conducted with these churches with an aim to reduce health disparities are those that have focused on nutrition,[40,41] breast health,[42] prostate cancer,[43] diabetes,[44] and physical activity.[45]

4. *Start where the people are.* Public health practice can address social injustice and health problems by joining with communities to address their concerns. Health educators in communities need to start "where the

people are."[46] This principle is important from the perspectives of both ethics and practicality.[47] From an ethics perspective, starting "where the people are" acknowledges a community's right to self-determination, liberty, and actions based on the values of the community members. From a practical perspective, problems and solutions defined by outside consultants or health workers have a long history of failure and mismatch with community motivations and concerns. Although health workers may be responding from a population perspective to critical health issues, such as cardiovascular disease, diabetes, or infant mortality, these concerns are rarely the same as those of community members. Thus, when health workers focus solely on their concerns or the concerns raised by data, they may have difficulty getting the community involved. In contrast, when health workers join with communities in addressing their concerns, it is often possible to address not only community concerns but eventually also the concerns of the health workers or funding agencies.

5. *Strengthen and expand social networks in communities and beyond communities.* Social networks influence the health of individuals in many ways.[4] They can produce adverse effects related to social control and reduced behavioral options that may encourage risk behaviors harmful to health. Social networks may provide redundant types of social support that offer less linkage to the goods and services of society if the members of the network are relatively homogeneous in terms of education, occupation, and social class.[48] We do not recommend an approach that simply tries to encourage community members to interact with one another, thereby expanding social networks in communities. Rather, we encourage strategies that build networks of support for community and societal change and for greater access to the goods and services of society.

In a 13-county area in eastern North Carolina, two of us (R.E.A. and J.W.H.) worked with a network of 105 churches in a major African-American denomination. To develop the churches' role in promoting health among their members, the existing networks within churches needed to expand outside these churches' walls and into their communities. The training of lay health educators involved a combination of (a) dialogue/problem-posing workshops on the nature of community health problems, and (b) lectures led by local representatives of public health departments, health associations, and other community agencies. The involvement of professionals from outside these churches helped to create links between these churches and these professionals. This expanded the network of the churches to include service providers with access to goods and services not routinely available in the churches' networks. These links were mutually beneficial: church networks developed larger pools of resources for assistance on important community issues, and the network of service providers (including county health departments as well as nonprofit organizations, such as the American Heart Association and the American Red Cross) had greater access to the populations that they were seeking to serve.

6. *Strengthen the capacity of local institutions, networks, and community groups.* Efforts to address health issues through local institutions, networks, and community groups are important strategies to help people to live healthfully in their communities. According to the 2002 Institute of Medicine report, "The Future of the Public's Health in the 21st Century":

> Government public health agencies, as the backbone of the public health system, are clearly in need of support and resources, but they cannot work alone. They must build and maintain partnerships with other organizations and sectors of society, working closely with communities and community based organizations, the health care delivery system, academia, business, and the media.[49]

Although formal public health institutions are in need of resources and support, community-based institutions with which they partner may have even greater needs. As public health professionals work with community-based institutions, they must bring some of these resources to these institutions to meet their needs. Their needs for capacity building may include the development of (a) basic technical skills, such as budgeting and proposal writing; (b) leadership; and (c) financial and human resources. Strengthening of local institutions, networks, and community groups makes it more likely that efforts to address health disparities will be sustainable.

7. *Maintain a long-term perspective on foundational issues.* By maintaining a long-term vision, while addressing immediate needs, all of the above principles can contribute to reducing the social injustices that contribute to poor health. By using local efforts in a way that will create leadership, activated social networks, and problem-solving mechanisms, communities may be better able to advocate and demand change. One of us (J.W.H.), reflecting on his work in the Mississippi Delta, described how a perspective on long-term social change was always a part of his framework, even when addressing immediate needs in ways that were nonconfrontational:

> Focus of much of the action was on practical concerns, such as digging wells, building outdoor sanitary toilets, and reducing health risk conditions in the local environment. Small successes nurtured the belief that change was possible through collective action. Many who doubted the possibility of positive change began to attend meetings

related to the Health Council and the Farm Cooperative. For many, this was a political awakening. People involved with these organizations were recruited by civil rights groups, such as Delta Ministry and the Mississippi Democratic Freedom Party, to lead voter-registration campaigns. Organizing strategies used to educate, recruit, and involve people in the farm cooperative developed skills similar to those required for political action.

8. *Be aware of the dangers of organizing among the oppressed.* Because community and social transformation leading to the elimination of health disparities involves upsetting and transforming routinized patterns of power, it is usually accompanied by conflict. Root causes of health disparities, such as income and wealth inequalities, racism, and sexism, are held in place by powerful interests, which must lose some power if meaningful change is to occur. Health workers and organizers face a number of dilemmas. Such organizing is often dangerous, leading to backlash, exploitation, and oppression. Historically, in the civil rights movement, local leaders were beaten, jailed, or forced to leave after outside organizers moved on. At other times, organizers and leaders were killed.

   There are differing views about how the danger of organizing should be handled. One approach would be to temper social activism by having the community decide how far to take confrontation-based tactics—which is especially important because the community is often left to deal with the fallout from such an approach. Building on an analysis of the root causes of injustice and of the powers that sustain it can enable organizers to enter situations with their eyes open and to anticipate potential backlash.

9. *Continue to exert pressure from outside the community.* The production of social injustice and health disparities is global. Efforts to address this injustice and these disparities therefore require worldwide coordination. Global health issues include environmental global degradation, greenhouse gas emissions, biodiversity loss, water shortages, declines in fisheries, increasing poverty, financial instability, taxation, food insecurity, trade in health-damaging products (such as tobacco, arms, and toxic waste), war and conflict, and governance.[50] What happens in our backyard affects what happens worldwide. For example, World Trade Organization policies result in disinvestment in small, family-based sustainable agriculture, which, in turn, reduces food security.[51] Addressing these issues effectively will take joint action from within and outside communities, from members of community-based organizations, academic and scientific institutions, and government agencies.

An Agenda for Action

What can we do at the community level to address social injustice and its effects on health?

First, we must recognize that community-level strategies must be part of a larger concerted effort leading to social change. Individuals, organizations, and institutions within society each must play their roles in contributing to a movement for change in our society and change in the nature of global economic and social relations. The task is daunting—perhaps even unachievable. Yet the ethic of public health as social justice compels us to push on.

The following represents a suggested agenda for action to address social injustice and its effect on the health of populations. While not exhaustive, it represents general strategies and specific measures that will strengthen communities and the roles of individuals in communities to be able to address health disparities and the social injustice that contributes to their development.

1. *Understand the local context, listen to the community.* To understand the role that the local context plays in the lives and health of community members, we must look beyond numbers and rates to the stories and experiences of community members. If disenfranchised populations are not having their concerns heard and addressed, it may be because no one is listening. How can we listen if we do not interact in meaningful ways with the populations we serve? Public health researchers and practitioners must hear the voices of the people we serve to better understand the social issues that most significantly affect their lives and their health. For example, one of us (R.E.A.) explored, through focus groups, community concerns and notions of what makes a community a good place in which to live for women and children. Figure 24-1 depicts the contrasts between the broad set of concerns voiced by community residents and the narrow focus taken by typical infant mortality prevention programs. The items in this list of residents' concerns should take a prominent role on our agenda for action.

2. *While addressing these important issues, build race, class, and international bridges.* William Julius Wilson, a noted Harvard sociologist, contends that the political muscle needed to address some of the social problems facing our country cannot be achieved without a broad-based multiracial coalition—one that focuses on issues that are important to most Americans and emphasizes their interdependence.[52] These issues include congressional policies for vulnerable families, trade policies that reduce employment opportunities and displace workers, monetary

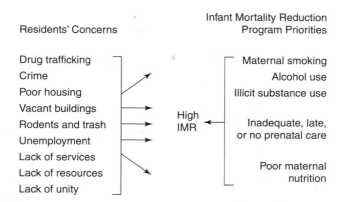

Figure 24-1 Contrasting community and program priorities (IMR = infant mortality rate).

policies that promote full employment, livable-wage policies, and policies to restore American cities.

Many economic forces that have disproportionately affected African-Americans have arisen from global economic forces that are nonracial in origin. These forces include trade policies, such as those of the North American Free Trade Agreement (NAFTA), that have resulted in a decline in lower-skilled, low-wage jobs in the United States. Among less-educated blacks, nearly half of recent job losses have resulted from the loss of manufacturing jobs.

The importance of building bridges between citizens of the United States and other nations is particularly relevant for environmental issues and trade agreements. Free-trade/investment agreements have undermined public health by increasing social inequalities, depleting natural resources, and increasing environmental pollution.[51] The importance of building bridges with activists from other countries in the tobacco control movement is also clear.[53] Tougher tobacco control legislation in the United States has resulted in more aggressive marketing of tobacco control products internationally. Partnerships among countries help groups to frame tobacco issues in an international context and provide information, advice, and resources across borders. In addition, sometimes examples of egregious behavior exhibited by tobacco companies in other countries can be used to deal with their behavior in the United States.

3. *Support efforts that build participatory democracy and an engaged citizenry.* Community-based strategies to address public health problems are most effective when the population is mobilized and engaged in the identification of problems and the development of solutions. The development of broad-based coalitions or collaborative groups of existing

community-based organizations, agencies, associations, and concerned citizens can be a powerful way to mobilize and engage the population. Building broad-based coalitions that address issues facing most Americans will take an engaged citizenry, which is not currently present in the United States. U.S. democracy is threatened by corporations and persons of wealth purchasing access to government decision-makers. Approaches to working with disenfranchised communities on issues of health disparities should use participatory strategies that maximize the potential for individual and community learning and empowerment. Lessons learned and power gained through such strategies, multiplied across communities, can help to strengthen our democracy and address social injustices. Eugenia Eng and colleagues[19] have found that communities with higher rates of participation in addressing health issues are more likely to address other issues in the community.

4. *Work with other organizations to address "the public's health."* Now that we are gaining an increased awareness of the power that context wields in the health of populations, public health professionals should embrace comprehensive approaches to improving the context of people's lives. This may mean that we become involved in issues not typically seen as part of the public health domain. It may mean that we have to expand our set of partners to include those sectors of government and the community that also seek to improve the context of people's lives.

Many of the upstream causes of health disparities are addressed by organizations in the community beyond the local public health agency and thus require action by all agencies concerned with the public's health.[54] As one example, public organizations, private organizations, and government entities could develop fruitful collaborative partnerships to address health disparities due to the built environment. Together, societal sectors of environmental health, community planning, economic development, housing, transportation, social services, public health, justice, and community health could collaboratively tackle issues associated with low-income neighborhoods. Private partners might include local architects, developers, and organizations such as Habitat for Humanity. Built-environment features that emphasize physical activity, such as parks and sidewalks, also strengthen community life by making social connections easier. Parks provide contact with other people and with nature—features of our environment that promote health.[55]

5. *Funding for community-based research and practice should emphasize community building.* With the increased attention given to the impor-

tance of context to population health, funding for research and public health practice should contribute to the process of improving people's lives. Greater emphasis should be placed on participatory research strategies that seek to engage communities in the process of defining research priorities and developing research strategies. The community brings an understanding of the context, including issues of concern and knowledge of how the community "gets things done." Participation by community members helps to restore trust in the public health system and builds skills and community capacity that are important for an engaged citizenry. Funding for public health programs, likewise, should emphasize comprehensive and community-building strategies to improving the context in which people live. State and national funding agencies should consider requiring research staff members and project personnel to complete an orientation to ethics of community-based research and practice—similar to the online training required for research involving human subjects.

Conclusion

Health disparities suffered by poor and minority populations are socially produced; they result largely from current and historical social injustice. Efforts to address these health disparities require approaches that are both ameliorative and fundamental, addressing both current problems and root causes. Furthermore, comprehensive approaches are needed that work across the broad social ecology—individuals, families, communities, organizations, institutions, and the broader society. Communities possess strengths and assets that can be used to address the health problems that they face. In addition, communities can be strengthened in their capacity to address their current health problems and the root causes of these health problems. Public health research and interventions in communities should be designed and implemented in ways that build community capacity and the skills of individuals to contribute to community problem solving. An engaged and critically conscious citizenry is needed to sustain efforts for social change.

Public health professionals need new skill sets and intervention strategies to assist communities in meeting the challenges they face. Understanding of the effects of context on health must include an understanding of how health problems are experienced by people living within these contexts. This understanding should lead us to consider broader approaches to improving the context of people's lives by working collaboratively with communities as well as with government and other sectors.

References

1. Cohen D, Farley TA, Mason K. Why is poverty unhealthy? Social and physical mediators. Soc Sci Med 2003;57:1631–41.
2. Macinko J, Starfield B. The utility of social capital in research on health determinants. Milbank Q 2001;79:387–427.
3. Lynch J. Income inequality and health: expanding the debate. Soc Sci Med 2000; 51:1001–5.
4. Berkman L, Glass T, Brissette I, et al. From social integration to health: Durkheim in the new millennium. Soc Sci Med 2000;51:843–57.
5. Muntaner C, Lynch JW. Income inequality and social cohesion versus class relations: a critique of Wilkinson's neo-Durkheimian research program. Int J Health Serv 1999; 29:59–81.
6. Brodsky A, O'Campo PJ, Aronson RE. PSOC in community context: multi-level correlates of a measure of psychological sense of community in low-income, urban neighborhoods. J Commun Psychol 1999;27:659–79.
7. Roberts E. Neighborhood social environments and the distribution of low birthweight in Chicago. Am J Public Health 1997;87:597–603.
8. Brooks-Gunn J, Duncan GJ, Klebanov PK, et al. Do neighborhoods influence child and adolescent development? Am J Sociol 1993;99:353–95.
9. Berkman L. The role of social relations in health promotion. Psychosomat Med 1995;57:245–54.
10. House J, Landis KR, Umberson D. Social relationships and health. Science 1988; 84:541–5.
11. Kawachi I, Kennedy BP, Lochner K, et al. Social capital, income inequality, and mortality. Am J Public Health 1997;87:1491–8.
12. Coleman J. Social capital in the creation of human capital. Am J Sociol 1988;94: S95–120.
13. Putnam R. The strange disappearance of civic America. Am Prospect 1996;24: 34–48.
14. Kreuter M, Lezin N, Baker B. Social capital: when best practices aren't enough. Indianapolis, Ind.: 48th Annual Meeting of the Society of Public Health Education, 1997.
15. Sampson R, Raudenbush S, Earls F. Neighborhoods and violent crime: a multilevel study of collective efficacy. Science 1997;277:918–24.
16. Kreuter M, Lezin N. Social capital theory. In: DiClemente R, Crosby RA, Kegler MC, eds. Emerging theories in health promotion practice and research. San Francisco, Calif.: Jossey-Bass, 2002.
17. McLeroy K. Community capacity: What is it? How do we measure it? What is the role of the prevention centers and CDC? Atlanta, Ga.: Sixth Annual Prevention Centers Conference, Centers for Disease Control and Prevention, National Center for Chronic Disease Prevention and Health Promotion, 1996.
18. Goodman R, Speers M, McLeroy K, et al. An initial attempt at identifying and defining the dimensions of community capacity to provide a basis for measurement. Health Educ Behav 1998;25:258–78.
19. Eng E, Briscoe J, Cunningham A. Participation effect from water projects on EPI. Soc Sci Med 1990;30:1349–58.
20. Norton B, McLeory KR, Burdine JN, et al. Community capacity: concept, theory, and methods. In: DiClemente R, Crosby RA, Kegler MC, eds. Emerging theories in health promotion practice and research. San Francisco, Calif.: Jossey-Bass, 2002.

21. Scheier M, Carver CS. Optimism, coping, and health: assessment and implications of generalized outcome expectancies. Health Psychol 1985;4:219–47.
22. Snyder C, Harris C, Anderson JR, et al. The will and the ways: development and validation of an individual-differences measure of hope. J Personality Soc Psychol 1991;60:570–85.
23. Scheier M, Carver CS. Effects of optimism on psychological and physical well-being: theoretical overview and empirical update. Cogn Therapy Res 1992;16:201–28.
24. West C. Race matters. New York, N.Y.: Vintage Books, Random House, 2001.
25. Minkler M, Wallerstein N. Improving health through community organization and community building: a health education perspective. In: Minkler M, ed. Community organizing and community building for health. New Brunswick, N.J.: Rutgers University, 1997.
26. McKnight J. Two tools for well-being: health systems. In: Minkler M, ed. Community organizing and community building for health. New Brunswick, N.J.: Rutgers University, 1997.
27. Walter C. Community building practice. In: Minkler M, ed. Community organizing and community building for health. New Brunswick, N.J.: Rutgers University, 1997.
28. Benezeval M, Judge K, Whitehead M. Tackling inequalities in health: an agenda for action. London, England: King's Fund, 1995.
29. Giddens A. The constitution of society. Los Angeles: The University of California Press, 1984.
30. Heggenhougen H. Will primary health care efforts be allowed to succeed? Soc Sci Med 1984;19:217–24.
31. Morgan L. International politics and primary health care in Costa Rica. Soc Sci Med 1990;30:211–9.
32. Geronimus A. To mitigate, resist, or undo: addressing structural influences on the health of urban populations. Am J Public Health 2000;90:867–72.
33. Jones C. Levels of racism: a theoretic framework and a gardener's tale. Am J Public Health 2000;90:1212–5.
34. Friere P. Pedagogy of the oppressed: new revised 20th-anniversary edition. New York, N.Y.: The Continuum Publishing Company, 1993.
35. McKnight J. The careless society: community and its counterfeits. New York, N.Y.: Basic Books, HarperCollins Publishers, 1995.
36. Hatch J, Lovelace K. Involving the southern rural church and students of the health professions in health education. Public Health Rep 1980;95:23–6.
37. Whitehead TL. Health disparities among African Americans: a history of social injustice and processes of environmental stress and adaptation. Working Document of the Cultural Systems Analysis Group, University of Maryland, College Park, Md., 2003.
38. Campbell MK, Demark-Wahnefried W, Symons M, et al. Fruit and vegetable consumption and prevention of cancer: the black churches united for better health project. Am J Public Health 1999;89:1390–6.
39. Eng E, Hatch J, Callan A. Institutionalizing social support through the church and into the community. Health Educ Q 1985;12:81–92.
40. Ammerman A, Washington C, Jackson B, et al. The PRAISE! project: a church-based nutrition intervention designed for cultural appropriateness, sustainability, and diffusion. Health Promotion Practice 2002;3:286–301.
41. Resnicow K, Jackson A, Wang T, et al. A motivational interviewing intervention to increase fruit and vegetable intake through black churches: results of the Eat for Life Trial. Am J Public Health 2001;91:1686–93.

42. Derose KP, Fox SA, Reigadas E, et al. Church-based telephone mammography counseling with peer counselors. J Health Communication 2000;5:175–88.
43. Weinrich S, Holdford D, Boyd M, et al. Prostate cancer education in African American churches. Public Health Nursing 1998;15:188–95.
44. McNabb W. The PATHWAYS church-based weight loss program for urban African-American women at risk for diabetes. Diabetes Care 1997;20:1518–23.
45. Hatch J, Cunningham A, Woods W, et al. The fitness through churches project: description of a community-based cardiovascular health promotion intervention. Hygiene 1986;5:9–12.
46. Nyswander, D. Education for health: some principles and their applications. Health Educ Monogr 1956;14: 65–70.
47. Minkler M, Pies C. Ethical issues in community organization and community participation. In: Minkler M, ed. Community organizing and community building for health. New Brunswick, N.J.: Rutgers University, 1997.
48. Granovetter M. The strength of weak ties. Am J Sociol 1973;78:1360–79.
49. Institute of Medicine. The future of the public's health in the 21st century. Washington, D.C.: National Academies Press, 2003.
50. Labonte R, Spiegel J. Setting global health research priorities: burden of disease and inherently global health issues should both be considered. BMJ 2003;326:722–3.
51. Labonte R. International governance and World Trade Organization (WTO) reform. Critical Public Health 2002;12:65–86.
52. Wilson WJ. The bridge over the racial divide: rising inequalities and coalition politics. Berkeley, Calif.: University of California Press, 1999.
53. White A. Global partnerships for tobacco control. Boston, Mass.: 2003 National Conference on Tobacco and Health, 2003.
54. Halverson PK. Embracing the strength of the public health system: why strong government public health agencies are vitally necessary but insufficient. J Public Health Manage Pract 2002;8:98–100.
55. Frumkin H. Healthy places: exploring the evidence. Am J Public Health 2003; 93:1451–6.

25

PROMOTING SOCIAL JUSTICE THROUGH EDUCATION IN PUBLIC HEALTH

Robert S. Lawrence

Introduction

This chapter examines the opportunity to promote social justice through education programs for students in schools of public health, medical school departments of community and preventive medicine, and elsewhere and, through that education, to equip public health practitioners and researchers with a social justice lens that will guide their future work.

Two major developments of the past half-century provide crucial information and values for developing and implementing social justice curricula. First, the evolution of human rights law since the end of World War II and the emergence of the health and human rights movement have provided new ways of thinking about the right to health and the ethical framework for considering the health of populations. Second, great progress has occurred in the quantitative and qualitative analyses of the social determinants of health and how inequalities and inequities are among the most potent determinants of premature morbidity and mortality. Together, richer and deeper reflections on the right to health and the social determinants of health provide the material for placing education to promote social justice at the heart of the public health curriculum.

Principles of Social Justice and Education in Public Health

By framing the issue of social justice in the context of risk factors for premature morbidity and mortality caused by unjust treatment of subgroups within the population, public health practitioners can apply the core population health tools of epidemiology, biostatistics, social and behavioral sciences, environmental and occupational health, and policy analysis to identify key determinants of risk, prioritize policies or interventions to lower risk, and evaluate and communicate the results. Analysis of health status by population groups identified by race, ethnicity, gender, sexual orientation, religious beliefs and practices, country of origin, insurance and employment status, social status, or class often reveals profound differences. These differences, in turn, usually reflect the inequitable distribution of society's resources—whether in the form of material benefits of better housing or safer worksites or in the amount of control one has over one's life and the opportunities for social engagement, tolerance, and respect.

John Rawls, considered by many to be the most important political philosopher of the second half of the 20th century, further developed, in his theory of justice as fairness, the traditional idea of the social contract to introduce the concept of distributive justice.[1] Distributive justice emerges when, behind a "veil of ignorance" about what status we might have in a theoretical society, we establish as the "original position" (p. 136) the circumstances we would be willing to accept if we were among the least favored members of the society. As science advances our understanding of the social determinants of health, the necessary elements of the "original position," from a population health perspective, emerge more clearly, reinforcing with detail the more general statements rooted in the language of the right to health found in the United Nations Charter, the Universal Declaration of Human Rights, and the International Covenant of Economic, Social and Cultural Rights.[2]

On April 23, 1992, at a ceremony celebrating the seventy-fifth anniversary of the founding of the Johns Hopkins School of Hygiene and Public Health (now the Bloomberg School of Public Health), faculty and students at the school embodied these concepts of social justice and the right to health in the "International Declaration of Health Rights"[3] (see box 1-3 on p. 20). James Grant, Executive Director of the United Nations Children's Fund (UNICEF); Hiroshi Nakajima, Director General of the World Health Organization (WHO); Alfred Sommer, Dean; and hundreds of others in attendance signed the declaration, which is read each year by a graduating student at the school's commencement exercises.

Several other schools of public health have adopted the International Declaration of Health Rights for use in their commencement exercises,[4] and similar pledges to uphold the right to health are included in mission statements of many schools of public health. These encouraging developments are among the predisposing conditions for including social justice issues in educational programs for public health. The moral development of students in the professions occurs when they move beyond the stage of basing their behavior on the values and norms of those around them to a "more principled stage where they identify and attempt to live by personal moral values" (p. 504).[5] Public health educators have a duty to assist in this transformation by being examples in action and word of the centrality of social justice to the ideals of public health.

Logic of Science Added to Moral and Ethical Reasons for Social Justice

Recent contributions from epidemiology, social and behavioral sciences, economics, and human rights studies have strengthened and clarified the scientific basis for the relationship between health and well-being. Advocacy for social justice in the past was often predicated on the link between the elimination of discrimination and prejudice and the fulfillment of civil and political rights. Public health professionals were among the first to connect the realization of human rights to the ability to shape the social and economic forces that create the conditions for improved health. Now a growing body of empirical data adds the logic of science to the moral and ethical reasons for demanding greater social justice.[6–9] Integration of these two fields provides the essential elements for transforming the education of public health professionals. Values clarification and commitment to the principle of the right to health and the knowledge of the social gradient will equip graduates to help them fulfill their professional obligation to address root causes of ill health, including social injustices that determine so much of the burden of preventable morbidity and premature mortality among marginalized groups in society.

Historical Context

The epidemiology of scrotal cancer among London chimney sweeps was one of the earliest observations in the West of the association between socioeconomic status, occupational exposure, and health. Percival Pott, a London physician, described in 1776 the incidence of scrotal cancer in young chimney sweeps, who were usually orphans or abandoned children prized for their small size and in desperate need for employment of any kind. The House of Lords finally approved an Act of Parliament in 1864, after many years of campaigning by child advocates, to outlaw the use of children for climbing chimneys.[10] The delay of almost nine decades between the scientific observation of the problem and the implementation of a policy to protect children established what became a familiar pattern of delay in building political will to correct an injustice. The Industrial Age did bring a growing awareness of the link between health and conditions of work and living subject to public sector regulation. In 1848, Parliament passed the Public Health Act to address poor labor conditions, and over the next half-century, it adopted additional laws to protect the public from risks in the workplace.

In the first half of the twentieth century, progress was slow in developing a coherent view of the social determinants of health. Most regulations protecting the health of the public in the United States focused on safety in the workplace, control of infection by vaccines and quarantine, and protecting the purity of food and water supplies. The increasing definition of health as a public as well as a personal matter led to the establishment of the Pan American Health Organization in 1902, the Office International d'Hygiène Publique in 1907, the International Labor Organization in 1919, and WHO in 1946.[11] WHO developed the idea of health as "a state of complete physical, mental and social well-being and not merely the absence of disease or infirmity."[12] The broadened definition of health included the concept of well-being, which depends on a physical and social environment that creates the conditions necessary to achieve health.

WHO is one of several United Nations agencies rooted in the post–World War II renunciation of war and violence as a means to settling disputes. The Preamble of the Charter of the United Nations includes among the purposes for establishing the UN in 1945[13]:

> to reaffirm faith in fundamental human rights, in the dignity and worth of the human person, in the equal rights of men and women and of nations large and small, and to establish conditions under which justice and respect for the obligations arising from treaties and other sources of international law can be maintained, and to promote social progress and better standards of life in larger freedom. (p. 1)

On December 10, 1948, the Universal Declaration of Human Rights declared, in Article 25,[14]

> Everyone has the right to a standard of living adequate for the health and well-being of himself and of his family, including food, clothing, housing and medical care and necessary social services, and the right to security in the event of unemployment, sickness, disability, widowhood, old age or other lack of livelihood in circumstances beyond his control. (p. 2)

Similar language later appeared in the International Covenant on Economic, Social and Cultural Rights, which entered into force January 3, 1976—sadly, without the ratification of the United States.[15] The right to health—and the other economic, social, and cultural rights—falls within the category of positive, aspirational, and nonjusticiable rights, in contrast to those articulated in the International Covenant on Civil and Political Rights. States are urged to respect, protect, and fulfill these economic and social rights to the "maximum of its available resources, with a view to achieving progressively the full realization of the rights" (p. 1).[15] Some have argued that these rights have no real meaning without the power of legal recourse and that closer attention to civil and political rights would be more likely to ensure conditions of social justice and thus improve well-being. But the declarations of the right to health had struck responsive chords in many countries, leading to the widespread endorsement of the 1978 Declaration of Alma-Ata on Primary Health Care, which laid down the challenge of health for all by the year 2000.[16]

"Good health is the bedrock on which social progress is built. A nation of healthy people can do those things that make life worthwhile, and as the level of health increases so does the potential for happiness" (p. 2).[17] These opening words of *A New Perspective on the Health of Canadians,* often called "The Lalonde Report," speak to the close links between social justice and health. Thirty years ago, Canadian Prime Minister Pierre Trudeau identified health disparities among different racial and ethnic groups as one of the important problems to address as part of his new administration's commitment to promoting social justice. He appointed Marc Lalonde, Minister of National Health and Welfare Canada, as chair of a commission to review the determinants of health and prepare recommendations for actions and policies to improve health and reduce disparities.

The commission grouped the determinants of health in four "fields"—human biology, environment, lifestyle, and health care organization. Contrary to their initial assumptions, the members of the commission concluded that health care organization contributed only a modest amount to the health status of Canadians and that much more attention needed to be given to environmental and lifestyle factors to reduce health disparities. Lack of education, substandard housing, inadequate environmental protections, food insecurity, and poverty emerged as the critical factors leading to premature morbidity and mortality among indigenous people and other marginalized groups in Canada. The idea of using social policy as an explicit tool to improve health status became part of Health Canada's strategy to reduce disparities.

Sir Douglas Black, Chief Scientist to the United Kingdom Department of Health from 1973 to 1977, described the concept of disparities in health status and their relationship to the above demographic variables in 1980 in a report commissioned by the Labor government of the United Kingdom in 1977 and suppressed by the government of Margaret Thatcher that had just come to power.[18] Only several hundred photocopies were distributed, but the report had a great impact on political thought. Both WHO and the Office for Economic Co-Operation and Development (OECD) used it to examine health inequalities in 13 countries (not including the United Kingdom). The report provided robust data showing that the poorest in the United Kingdom had the highest rates of poor health and premature death. Black argued that income, education, and lifestyle alone could not explain the disparities. He asserted that the disparities were also the result of a lack of a coordinated policy that would provide for more equitable provision of services, health goals, increased benefits, and restrictions on tobacco.

Eight years later, the U.S. Institute of Medicine (IOM) released a report, entitled *The Future of Public Health*, which stated that the mission of public health is to "fulfill society's interest in assuring conditions in which people can be healthy" (p. 1).[19] The report also described the three functions of public health—assessment, policy formulation, and assurance—that have become an important organizing principle for education in public health.

Fifteen years later, the IOM published *The Future of the Public's Health in the 21st Century*, revisiting many of the themes in the earlier report.[20] New language had appeared, however, influenced by the discourse on the right to health. The report called for government and a broad spectrum of society to "work effectively together as a public health system and individually to create the conditions that allow people in the United States to be as healthy as they can be. Such a commitment will require political will that has yet to be mobilized" (p. 41).

Education of the future public health workforce to advocate for social justice is one important part of generating that political and social will.

Using Education in Public Health to Promote Social Justice

Although recent trends include increasing numbers of undergraduate public health programs or majors, this discussion will focus on graduate education. Education in public health in the United States occurs mainly at the graduate school level in the 34 schools of public health, which are members of the Association of Schools of Public Health (ASPH), and in the 39 medical schools with departments offering the Master of Public Health (MPH) degree accredited by the Council on Education for Public Health (CEPH).[21] An additional eight schools of public health are associate members of ASPH and will become full members when accredited by CEPH. Graduate programs in community health education are accredited by CEPH at 16 universities.[22] In the 2002–2003 academic year, 17,933 students were enrolled in the 32 schools of public health then accredited. In 2002, 5,664 students were graduated.[22] Of the U.S. students enrolled, 4,864 (33 percent) belonged to minority groups: Asian, 11.9 percent; black, 11.1 percent; Hispanic, 9.4 percent; and Native American/Alaskan Native, 0.8 percent.

In the past decade, minority applications to schools of public health increased by 104 percent compared with an increase in overall U.S. citizen applications of 44 percent. Blacks and Asians were the groups with the greatest increase. A study of 45,000 students matriculating at U.S. universities from the early 1970s to the early 1990s revealed that race-sensitive admissions created a learning environment that improved the capacity of both minority and majority students to live and work with persons of different races and to have more successful careers.[23] Diversity among students in public health is one of the essential components of an educational environment that prepares students to be effective in working for social justice.

Courses in the core disciplines of public health—epidemiology, biostatistics, environmental health sciences, behavioral sciences/health education, and health services administration—are required for a school of public health or an MPH program housed in a school of medicine to meet CEPH standards for accreditation. These core courses should be enriched to include case studies and problem sets with a social justice perspective to demonstrate the important contribution to health disparities related to inequities and inequalities in social and economic status. For example, Public Health Problem Solving is a core course at the Bloomberg School of Public Health that is required of all MPH students, in which case studies are used to stimulate analysis of key determinants of health—biologic, socioeconomic, environmental, behavioral, and health services—from the perspective of the social gradient in health. Concepts of quintile spread, the Gini coefficient,* and fairness and justice in the distribution of goods and services are introduced. Students work in small groups to examine an important public health problem using a stepwise methodology—problem definition, magnitude of problem, key determinants, policy and intervention options, priority setting, implementation, evaluation, and communication—to prepare a written report and make a presentation in the form of a briefing to a legislative body. The written report includes an analysis of the human rights impact of the policy or program being implemented, using the methodology developed by Lawrence Gostin and Jonathan Mann.[24] Use of this analysis provides an excellent pedagogic method to educate public health students about the linkage between "least restrictive policies" from a human rights perspective and the promotion of social justice and protection against unintended policy consequences that might exacerbate inequalities.

---

*A measure of inequality or dispersion in a set of values, such as income levels—the larger the Gini coefficient, the larger is the spread of values.

In a seminar on health and human rights, we have used readings, discussions, and case studies to explore topics such as structural violence, the health impacts of conflict, human rights violations—both civil and political as well as social, economic, and cultural—and their health effects, complex humanitarian emergencies, refugee health, environmental justice, the human poverty index, and the role of advocacy in promoting health for marginalized populations. The seminar is part of the requirement for the Certificate in Health and Human Rights offered at the Bloomberg School of Public Health since 1996. During the 2003–2004 academic year, a new concentration in Humanitarian Assistance, Health and Human Rights was introduced. The capstone projects at the end of the year included a broad range of topics addressing social justice and human rights challenges, ranging from sexual violence among Sudanese refugees in Uganda to the development of a new index of social inequalities to be used in Baltimore.

The CEPH requirement for capstone or practicum experiences has stimulated links with organizations working to promote social justice through service to vulnerable groups. The Albert Schweitzer Fellowship provides service-learning opportunities for graduate students in the health professions and law in six cities or regions of the United States. The Baltimore Albert Schweitzer fellows work with safety-net organizations in the poorest neighborhoods of Baltimore, learning firsthand the lessons of the close relationship between social injustice and poor health. Many of the 200 hours of service during the fellowship year consist of a transforming experience, reinforcing their commitment to use their professional training to advocate for social justice.

Participation in research provides students the opportunity to acquire skills and methods to expand knowledge about the social gradient, to design and implement programs to reduce health risk among vulnerable populations, and to influence policy. Doctoral students conducting dissertation research on health disparities are found in most schools of public health.

Students can participate in advocacy for social change at the local or regional level through groups such as the student chapters of Physicians for Human Rights (PHR). The Juvenile Justice Project and the Ban Landmines Campaign are two PHR projects that have attracted widespread student engagement. Physicians for Social Responsibility, Physicians for a National Health Program, and other local or national advocacy groups provide excellent training in social justice advocacy.

An Agenda for Action

The ultimate goal is to make education and training for public health careers, all of which focus to some degree on social justice, central to the educational mission of public health. The strategy most likely to succeed is to influence the accreditation criteria used by CEPH. An explicit requirement that public health education include social justice subject matter in the curriculum of all schools of public health and all MPH programs sponsored by schools of medicine would stimulate new course development and enhancement of existing course content. Specific goals would be as follows:

- Develop and share curricular materials and instructional modules in acute and chronic disease epidemiology, environmental health, health policy, maternal and child health, nutrition, mental health, and international health that demonstrate the connection between social injustice and poor health.
- Design methods courses for research and analysis to increase understanding of the importance of social justice to improvements in health status. "Bringing disparities to public attention so they can be addressed is key to promoting social justice" (p. 187).[25]
- Mobilize ASPH to sponsor and support activities in the pedagogy of social justice through its Council on Education, Council on Minority Health, and other structures within the organization.
- Sponsor workshops for training in advocacy skills for communicating the growing body of knowledge about the social gradient in health to policymakers at local, state, and federal levels. The long-term goals would be to increase social and political will for support of policies that would address structural barriers to achieving social justice.
- Partner with other private groups and government units engaged in the analysis of the determinants of health inequalities to provide internships, practicum experiences, or other opportunities for education and training. Examples include participation in the project on health disparities at the Agency for Healthcare Research and Quality, evaluation of progress toward the goals of *Healthy People 2010* that address disparities, and the continued monitoring by Physicians for Human Rights of the goals outlined in *The Right to Equal Treatment*.[26]

Conclusion

Rudolf Virchow, the great German pathologist who fought on the side of the democrats in the March revolution of 1848, combined passion for social justice with scientific rigor. After the revolution of 1848, he established and edited the journal *Medicinische Reform* (*The Reform of Medicine*). In one of the early issues, he introduced the terms "public health" and "public health care" to the scientific literature, arguing that it is the responsibility of the state to create healthy conditions for the public and to provide public health services. He wrote,[27]

> Should medicine ever fulfill its great ends, it must enter into the larger political and social life of our time; it must indicate the barriers that obstruct the normal completion of the life-cycle and remove them. Should this ever come to pass, Medicine, what ever it may then be, will become the common good of all. It will cease to be medicine and will be absorbed into that general body of knowledge which is identified with power. (p. 561)

As the gap between rich and poor continues to grow, the barriers obstructing "the normal completion of the life-cycle" loom large indeed to those of us in public health. And, like Albert Schweitzer, we may think and feel that our "knowledge is pessimistic, but my willing and hoping are optimistic" (p. 242).[28] His pessimism came from feeling the "full weight of what we conceive to be the absence of purpose in the course of world events" (p. 242). His optimism derived from his confidence that "the spirit generated by truth is stronger than the force of circumstances" (p. 243).

Our duty to the next generation of public health professionals is to provide them as students and younger colleagues with ample opportunities to learn the truth about social justice and the social determinants of health to help surmount the barriers to equity in health. The challenge to educators in public health is to provide curricula and practicum experiences in supportive educational environments that enable our students to grow into their ideals.

References

1. Rawls J. A theory of justice. Cambridge, Mass: Belknap Press, Harvard University Press, 1971.
2. The International Bill of Human Rights. Available at: http://www1.umn.edu/humanrts/instree/auob.htm. Accessed January 26, 2005.
3. International Declaration of Health Rights. Baltimore, Md.: Johns Hopkins University, Bloomberg School of Public Health. Available at: http://www.jhsph.edu/Alumni/Declaration. Accessed January 26, 2005.
4. Rollins School of Public Health, Emory University. Available at: http://www.sph.emory.edu/COMMENCEMENT/2001/2001declaration.html. Accessed January 26, 2005.
5. Branch WT Jr. Supporting the moral development of medical students. J Gen Intern Med 2000;15:503–8.
6. Adler NE, Boyce T, Chesney M, et al. Socioeconomic status and health: the challenge of the gradient. Am Psychol 1994;49:15–24.
7. Marmot M. Inequalities in health. N Engl J Med 2001;345:134–6.
8. Marmot M. Economic and social determinants of disease. Bull WHO 2001;79:988–9.

9. Adler, NE. Looking beyond the borders of the health sector: the socioeconomic determinants of health. In: Rubin ER, Schappert SL, eds. Meeting health needs in the 21st century. Washington, D.C.: Association of Academic Health Centers, 2003.

10. van den Hazel P. Speech at conference of Policy Interpretation Network on Children's Health and Environment, Amsterdam, 2003. Available at: htth://www.pinche.hvdgm.nl/resource/pdf/amsterdam_opening_speech.pdf. Accessed January 26, 2005.

11. University of Minnesota Human Rights Library. Available at: http://www1.umn.edu/humanrts/edumat/IHRIP/circle/modules/module14.htm. Accessed January 26, 2005.

12. WHO definition of health. Available at: http://www.who.int/about/definition/en/. Accessed February 20, 2005.

13. Charter of the United Nations. Available at: http://www1.umn.edu/humanrts/instree/auncharter.html. Accessed January 26, 2005.

14. Universal Declaration of Human Rights. Available at: http://www1.umn.edu/humanrts/instree/b1udhr.htm. Accessed January 26, 2005.

15. International Covenant on Economic, Social and Cultural Rights. Available at: http://www1.umn.edu/humanrts/instree/b2esc.htm. Accessed January 26, 2005.

16. Declaration of Alma-Ata, 1978. Available at: http://www.euro.who.int/AboutWHO/Policy/20010827_1. Accessed January 26, 2005.

17. Lalonde M. A new perspective on the health of Canadians: a working document. Ottawa, Canada: Health Canada, 1974.

18. Black report 1980. Available at: http://bmj.bmjjournals.com/cgi/content/full/325/7364/DC2. Accessed January 26, 2005.

19. Committee for the Study of the Future of Public Health, Institute of Medicine. The future of public health. Washington, D.C.: National Academies Press, 1988.

20. Institute of Medicine. The future of the public's health in the 21st century. Washington, D.C.: National Academies Press, 2002.

21. Council on Education for Public Health. Accredited schools and programs. Available at: http://www.ceph.org. Accessed January 26, 2005.

22. Sow MK. 2002 Annual data report. Washington, D.C.: Association of Schools of Public Health, April 2003.

23. Bowen WG, Bok D. The shape of the river: long-term consequences of considering race in college and university admissions. Princeton, N.J.: Princeton University Press, 1998.

24. Gostin LO, Mann J. Towards the development of a human rights impact assessment for the formulation and evaluation of public health policies. J Health Hum Rights 1994;1:59–80.

25. Healton C, Nelson K. Reversal of misfortune: viewing tobacco as a social justice issue. Am J Public Health 2004;94:186–91.

26. The right to equal treatment. A report by the Panel on Racial and Ethnic Disparities in Medical Care. Boston, Mass.: Physicians for Human Rights, 2003.

27. Virchow R. De Einheitsbestrebunger in der Wissenschaftlichen, quoted in Strauss MB. Familiar medical quotations. Boston, Mass.: Little, Brown and Company, 1968.

28. Schweitzer A. Out of my life and thought. Baltimore, Md.: Johns Hopkins University Press, 1998.

26

RESEARCHING CRITICAL QUESTIONS ON SOCIAL JUSTICE AND PUBLIC HEALTH: AN ECOSOCIAL PERSPECTIVE

Nancy Krieger

> When I give food to the poor, they call me a saint.
> When I ask why the poor have no food, they call me a communist.
> —Dom Helder Camara (1909–1999), Archbishop of Recife, Brazil[1]

Introduction

Questioning the existence of injustice is central to work for social justice. Asking about its causes and consequences is at once both a practical necessity and a vital act of imagination and hope, premised on the insight that what is need not always be. Once the question is raised, critical and creative work can and must be done to expose why the injustice exists, including who gains and who loses and how it wreaks its woe, thereby generating knowledge useful for both rectifying harm and creating just and sustainable solutions.

Translated into issues of social justice and public health, critical research questions necessarily focus on

1. What is the evidence that social injustice harms health?
2. What can be done to prevent this harm?

Straightforward as these questions may seem, the answers are far from simple. As shown in figure 26–1, important debates swirl around the existence and magnitude of and solutions to social inequalities in health. While many of these disputes are polarized between "right" and "left" political analyses, as exemplified by arguments about individualistic versus structural explanations for social inequalities in health,[2,3] or risk associated with various commercial products, such as tobacco[3,4] or organochlorines,[5] not all are. Critical debates also occur among proponents of social justice deeply concerned about social inequalities in health, as evident in controversies over how to study the contribution of socioeconomic deprivation to racial/ethnic disparities in health[6,7] and whether, and if so, why, income inequality harms health.[8,9] The complexities of problems encompassed in social injustices in health and of conducting valid research on their causes means that both legitimate and manufactured disagreements can give rise to conflicting claims.

Complexity, however, is not an excuse for inaction—especially because inaction inevitably translates into shoring up the status quo. The challenge instead is to devise a useful research agenda for social justice in public health. Four key reasons to develop such an agenda are as follows:

1. *Ignorance forestalls action.* Two adages suffice: "If you don't ask, you don't know," and "If you don't know, you can't act"; the converse is: "No data, no problem."[10]

2. *The "facts" never "speak for themselves."* Instead, research findings must be critically evaluated in relation to (a) the theoretical frameworks researchers use; (b) the rigor with which we conceptualize, operationalize, analyze, and interpret the relevant constructs and data; and (c) the intellectual honesty we muster to address thoughtfully the likely limitations of any given study and implications for the conclusions reached.[10–13]

3. *Specificity matters.* The overarching hypothesis that social injustice harms health in no way implies that each and every type of injustice is causally related to each and every type of health outcome, or that such relationships are static. Consider, after all, the marked class shift in smoking over the twentieth century in industrialized nations, which went from being concentrated chiefly among more affluent sectors of the populations to becoming most prevalent among more impoverished groups.[4,14] Explaining the actual current and changing population distributions of disease, including social inequalities in health, thus constitutes a core test of both etiologic hypotheses and the efficacy of policies and interventions intended to improve the public's health.[11,12]

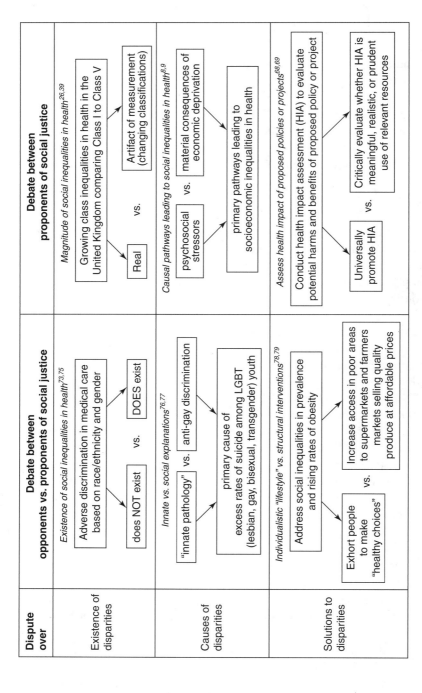

Figure 26-1 Why rigorous research on social justice and population health is necessary: case examples of disputes regarding existence, causes, and solutions to social inequalities in health.

4. *Research can exacerbate and even generate, rather than help rectify, social inequalities in health.* This sorry statement is readily illustrated by the blatant examples of scientific racism and eugenics.[11,15,16] Also of concern are more subtle and insidious examples whereby studies focus on characteristics of the dispossessed but not their context—as has occurred, for example, in research on homelessness and health that identifies causes of homelessness in characteristics of the homeless without considering the characteristics of the housing market.[17,18]

Testing claims about the causes and consequences of and solutions to social inequalities in health is thus necessitated by both the problematic legacy and critical potential of public health research.

In this chapter, I discuss a proposal for a public health research agenda that advances issues of social justice and includes four components: theory, monitoring, etiology, and prevention. Drawing on ecosocial theory[11,12] and the proposition that social justice is the foundation of public health,[19] I define these components as follows:

1. *Theory:* Research to clarify and develop the theoretical frameworks used to explain and guide research on and actions to address social inequalities in health
2. *Monitoring:* Research to assess the magnitude of and to improve methods for routinely documenting social inequalities in health, including whether these injustices in health are increasing or decreasing over time
3. *Etiology:* Research to test hypotheses about the causes of social inequalities in the population distribution of (a) health status (disease, disability, death, and well-being), and (b) access to and provision of appropriate health care
4. *Prevention:* Research to develop, evaluate, and improve methods to assess (a) efforts explicitly intended to address social inequalities in health, and (b) the beneficial and adverse health consequences of "non-health" policies and programs with social justice implications, including economic, trade, labor, housing, educational, transportation, agriculture, and military policies.

For each component, I delineate broad principles and provide specific examples, recognizing that the work of developing specific hypotheses and analytic designs requires substantive and detailed knowledge conjoined with overarching ideas.

Theory: Research to Sharpen Ideas, Analysis, and Explanations

Why theory? Consider the model of determinants of population health—including social inequalities in health—shown in figure 26-2. This model, centered on the distribution and level of population health, appeared in the U.S. federal report "Shaping a Health Statistics Vision for the 21st Century,"[20] with the express purpose of identifying the kinds of data that should be routinely obtained to permit monitoring and investigation of the public's health. Note its concern with context, time, and place and its attention to political, economic, social, cultural, physical, ecological, public health, and medical factors shaping population health. Its inclusion of these myriad determinants and its concern with injustice is not accidental but rather is structured by its explicit reliance on theories of population health.[12,20,21] This is what theory can do: It can provide insight into and encourage us to test our ideas about the workings of our world (and universe) by envisioning causal relationships between specified domains of phenomena, including links between social injustice and health, and suggesting ways to test whether the hypothesized relationships in fact exist.[12,13]

The ecosocial theory of disease distribution that I have been developing,[11,12,21] for example, calls attention to four constructs posited to be useful for determining "who and what drives population patterns of health, disease, and well-being, including social inequalities in health" (p. 672).[12] Aiding conceptualization of social injustices in health as biological expressions of social inequality, these constructs are as follows:

1. *Embodiment*, referring to how we literally incorporate, biologically, the material and social world in which we live
2. *Pathways of embodiment*, referring to how processes of embodiment are shaped simultaneously by histories of societal arrangements of power and property and by constraints and possibilities of our evolved biology, including gene expression, and not just gene frequency
3. *Cumulative interplay of exposure, susceptibility, and resistance across the life course*, referring to the importance of timing and accumulation of, as well as responses to, embodied exposures
4. *Accountability and agency*, referring not only to the institutions and persons responsible for generating or perpetuating social inequalities in health but also to the public health researchers for the theories used to explain or ignore these injustices.

By using such a theory, one can begin systematically to select, for example, among determinants presented in figure 26-2 to diagram diverse

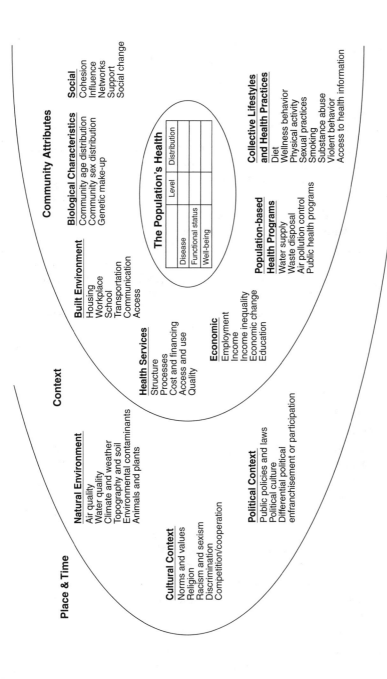

Figure 26-2 Determinants of population health. (Presented in the 2002 U.S. federal report: Shaping a health statistics vision for the 21st century.[20])

pathways of embodiment conceivably leading to social disparities in health and to discern whether additional determinants should be included. This is because theory enables perception of gaps, rather than drawing on only what has already been documented.

Ecosocial theory, however, is only one of several theories of disease distribution that explicitly link issues of social justice and public health with others. Although it is beyond the scope of this chapter to explicate these theories (see Krieger[12] for a review of the principal theories used in social epidemiology), others include social production of disease, political economy of health, and health and human rights—all of which importantly emphasize societal determinants but tend to leave biology relatively opaque.[2,3,12,21,22] Additional more biologically or psychologically oriented theories not inherently focused on social injustice but nevertheless often drawn on in research concerned with social inequalities in health include life course perspective, human and social ecology, social psychology, and various psychosocial theories focused on health behaviors.[23–25]

Also germane are frameworks explicitly focused on social justice and social change but not inherently concerned with health, including critical social theory, feminism, antiracist theories, postcolonialism, poststructuralism, Marxist theories, and theories of justice.[2,3,25–28] Critical issues raised by these latter theories include defining (and debating) definitions of "social justice," "social injustice," "equity," and "inequity,"[26–28] all constructs highly relevant to the claims that social injustice in health exists and that social justice is the foundation of public health.[2,3,19,21,22,25–27] Although these diverse ideas are beyond the scope of this chapter to elaborate, at issue are fundamental notions of (a) distributive and procedural justice; (b) the constellation of indivisible social, economic, political, civil, and cultural rights core to a human rights framework; and (c) the actions of states plus private and public institutions to oppose or condone exploitation and to protect, promote, or violate human rights.[22,26–28]

Yet, to date, little systematic research has been conducted on similarities, differences, and deficiencies of these diverse contemporary theories that explicitly—and all too often implicitly—inform research on social injustice and health. Indeed, given the dominance of the biomedical paradigm and its positivist emphasis on individual "lifestyles" and faulty genes,[3,12,29,30] many public health researchers are often untrained in theories of disease distribution, let alone theories of justice. They are thus unaware of their potential usefulness for sharpening not only research questions but also the design, analysis, and interpretation of public health investigations, interventions, and evaluations. Contemporary scholarship in science studies, however, highlights that advances in scientific understanding are achieved more often through refinement—and replacement—of concepts and ways of thinking, rather than by novel discoveries per se.[11,30] Research on characterizing and improving theories for social justice and public health is thus well warranted—and sorely needed, precisely because it is rarely explicitly funded!

Monitoring: Research to Document the Extent of, and Trends in, Social Inequalities in Health

Research to improve monitoring of social inequalities in health is likewise urgently required. Without routine monitoring, it is not possible to assess the extent of these injustices in public health, whether they are becoming worse or diminishing over time, or their relationship to changes in their presumed societal determinants.

A prerequisite for tracking health outcomes and their determinants, however, is having a functioning public health monitoring infrastructure.[10,20,31,32] This entails systems that (a) can accurately and comprehensively document incident and/or prevalent cases (plus ensure confidentiality of this information), and (b) have access to relevant denominator data (such as from the census) to compute the desired rates. Also important is the capacity to link to data on relevant societal determinants of health, as suggested in figure 26–2. Accomplishing any of these tasks is difficult, and even more so when public health agencies lack funds to provide essential services. Thus, in addition to generating social disparities in health, social injustice further compounds the problem by reducing the resources required to monitor its adverse effects on population health.[10]

Three types of research involving monitoring and social injustices in health are needed, as follows:

1. *Research on the categories used to classify and the methods used to enumerate societal groups* whose differential rates and risks constitute evidence of social injustice in health. At issue is how these categories are conceptualized and operationalized (such as regarding class, race/ethnicity, gender, sexuality, nationality, immigrant status, and disability),[33] plus problems with misclassification and biased ascertainment. Underscoring the need for research on these issues is, for example, one recent methodologic study demonstrating how misclassification and the undercount together led to serious understatement of U.S. mortality rates in the 1980s among American Indians and Asian and Pacific Islanders compared with white Americans[34]; how these problems affect contemporary data, especially given changes in U.S. census classification of race/ethnicity, remains unknown.

2. *Research on contextual data to augment public health monitoring data gathered on individuals* to permit linkage to relevant data that cannot be reduced to individual-level characteristics. The need for such inquiry is suggested by results of the U.S. Public Health Disparities Geocoding Project, which found that choice and level of area-based socioeconomic measures matter, with the census tract poverty measure most sensitive to expected socioeconomic gradients in health, while ZIP code–level measures often missed—and in some cases reversed—these gradients.[35,36]

3. *Research on the measures used to compare health status across societal groups*, regarding both the choice of outcomes (such as debates over whether to use such summary measures as disability-adjusted life years [DALYs][37,38]) and the type of contrast (such as relative versus absolute risk, or comparing only the extremes versus the full distribution).[39] Indicating the need for such research are studies demonstrating, for example, that while women may on average have longer life expectancy than men, they often have the same or fewer years of healthy life expectancy,[40] and that the magnitude of socioeconomic inequalities in health among women is less than that among men if absolute rates are compared but that the magnitudes are similar if relative risks are compared.[41]

Together, these diverse examples suggest that the use of different methods can lead to very different understandings of who disproportionately endures burdens of ill health. If the impact of injustice on health is to be accurately assessed, context-specific research on diverse approaches to monitoring social disparities in health is essential.

Etiology: Investigating the Determinants of, and Deterrents to, Social Inequalities in Health Status and Health Care

Although theory can provide critical insight into connections between injustice and health and monitoring can provide evidence of social disparities in health, etiologic research is required to determine if hypothesized determinants in fact explain the actual population distribution of health and social inequalities in health—over time and both within and across societies.

Critical Questions for Research on Social Justice and Public Health

Questions linking social injustice to population patterns of health, disease, and well-being are distinguished by their emphasis on societal accountability—for both the injustice at issue and its rectification. To show that poverty and ill health are causally connected due to constraints imposed by structural inequality rather than individual failure—that is, a social justice versus victim-blaming explanation[2,3,26,27,42]—requires evidence, not just ideological debate.

Three theoretically driven overarching questions useful for explicitly articulating issues of accountability and agency can thus be useful for guiding etiologic research on social injustice and health. Some of these questions and their derivatives have been examined in public health research, but many have not, suggesting that much remains to be done.[2,3,12,21,43,44] These questions are as follows:

1. *How does prioritizing capital accumulation over human need and ecosystem sustainability affect health status and health care?* At issue are neoliberal economic policies, injurious workplace organization and exposure to occupational hazards, inadequate pay scales, environmental pollution, unaffordable housing, privatization of health care, costly pharmaceuticals, and rampant commodification of virtually every human activity, need, and desire.

2. *What is the public health impact of state policies enforcing these priorities?* Included are policies that govern (a) regulation or deregulation of corporations, the real estate industry, the insurance industry, and interest rates; (b) enactment or repeal (or enforcement or neglect) of tax codes, trade agreements, labor laws, and environmental laws; (c) absolute and relative levels of spending on social and health programs compared with prison systems and the military; and (d) diplomatic relations with, economic domination of, and even invasion of countries abroad.

3. *What is the impact of impoverishment, and of violation of economic, social, political, civil, and cultural rights, singularly and combined, on population distributions of health and health care?* For example, what are the health consequences of: experiencing economic and noneconomic forms of racial discrimination; being sexually or physically abused by a family member or intimate partner or on account of belonging to a sexual minority (such as lesbian, gay, bisexual, transgender, or transsexual); or experiencing unjust repression and violence at the hands of agents of the state or paramilitary groups?

Although these questions importantly focus on societal determinants of health, they nevertheless offer little guidance on how to move from these determinants to their manifestation in population inequities in health. To the extent that evidence is needed on magnitude of harm caused, let alone mechanisms by which harm is caused (including to refute explanations embracing only individualized "risk factors"), more specificity is required.

Refining the Research Question: An Ecosocial Approach

One way to develop a systematic approach to refining research questions addressing links between injustice and population health is perhaps to consider key socially structured and biologically contingent pathways by which inequality can become embodied, across the life course, as delineated using an ecosocial perspective.[11,12,16,21] These pathways—potentially multilevel and multitemporal—involve adverse exposure to:

1. Economic and social deprivation
2. Toxic substances, pathogens, and hazardous conditions
3. Discrimination and other socially inflicted trauma (mental, physical, and sexual, directly experienced or witnessed, from verbal threats to violent acts)
4. Targeted marketing of commodities that can harm health, such as "junk" food and psychoactive substances (alcohol, tobacco, and other licit and illicit drugs)
5. Inadequate or degrading medical care.

Also relevant are health consequences of people's responses to being subjected to these structural, ecological, institutional, and interpersonal manifestations of inequality. These responses—each with their own set of potential health impacts—can range from internalized oppression and harmful use of psychoactive substances to reflective coping, active resistance, and community organizing to rectify inequity and promote human rights, social justice, and ecologically sustainable economies.

Translating these general concerns into specific research questions requires rigorously elaborating relevant hypotheses, generating valid study designs, and choosing or, if necessary, developing apt measures and analytic methods. In each and every case, scrupulous attention must be paid to issues of:

1. Etiologic period (time from exposure to when the outcome is manifested)
2. Type, level, and timing of measurement: of the exposure(s), outcome(s), and other covariates
3. Specificity (or not) of the exposure–outcome relationship
4. Historical trends in the occurrence of the exposures and outcomes under study.

Moreover, if current and changing patterns of population health and social inequalities in health are to be explained, then attention to the specifics of changing exposures—and not just "inequality" per se—is clearly warranted.[12,44]

Exemplifying why conceptual and operational clarity is critical is research that demonstrates what happens if the relevant social groups or exposures are misspecified. For example, measure social class only at the individual, rather than household level, and key trends in social inequalities in women's health will be missed.[45,46] Measure economic resources only in adulthood, not in childhood, and the cumulative impact of economic deprivation will remain invisible.[23,44,45,47] Measure household resources, but ignore neighborhood or regional economic conditions, and important contextual determinants will be missed.[35,36,48–50] Measure racial/ethnic identity, but ignore direct and indirect measures of racial discrimination, and the toll of racism on health will remain unknown.[6,16,51] Measure sex, gender, and sexuality, but omit data on current and past histories of sexual and/or gendered violence, and explanations of somatic and mental health will be incomplete.[21,52,53]

Case Example: Excess Hypertension Among African-Americans

How might this way of thinking be used to generate specific research questions? Consider, as one example, the case of excess rates of hypertension among the U.S. black population compared with not only the U.S. white population but also other populations of West African descent, whether in West Africa, the Caribbean, or elsewhere, reflecting histories of the intercontinental slave trade and contemporary migration.[16,51,54] Research illuminating the impact of injustice on population distributions of hypertension—conceptualized as a biological expression of racial inequality[16,51,55]—could fruitfully be historical, international, contemporary, and local.[16,51,54–58]

To offer one approach to concretizing such a broad research agenda, figure 26-3 illustrates a selection of possible hypotheses relevant to investigating injustice in relation to black–white disparities in blood pressure among working-age adults, generated using the list of pathways prompted by an ecosocial perspective.[11,12,21] These pathways, conjoining social and biological phenomena, explicitly involve structural, ecological, institutional, and interpersonal expressions of inequality, experienced and embodied across the life course. Thus, as diagrammed, conditions such as economic deprivation and racial discrimination can increase the risk of hypertension via pathways involving lead exposure, damaged kidneys, excessive body mass index, unmanaged hypertension due to lack of access to adequate health care, and increased allostatic load[16,51,54–61]—with the last of these defined as *"the wear and tear of the body and brain resulting from chronic overactivity or inactivity of physiological systems that are normally involved in adaptation to environmental challenge"* (italics in original) (p. 37).[61] To investigate any of these hypotheses would require adequate measures of both exposures and outcomes, plus numerous covariates. Highlighting the need for both

**Hypotheses involving structural, ecological,
institutional, and interpersonal expressions of inequality**

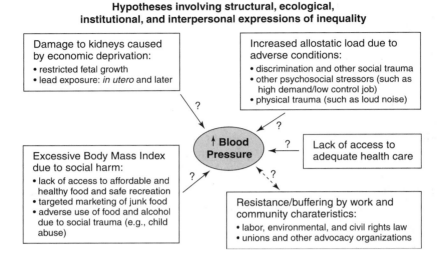

Figure 26-3 Case example: social inequalities in the population distribution of hypertension—selected hypotheses that could be systematically explored, involving multilevel pathways of embodiment across the life course.[16,51,54–61]

methodologic and etiologic research, moreover, the necessity for rigorous methodological research for developing, say, valid self-report measures of racial discrimination,[16,51,57] or of the body burden of lead,[60] cannot be minimized.

Clearly, no one study could ever realistically address even the restricted set of pathways proposed in figure 26-3. The point is not that a focus on injustice means any given investigation should measure "everything"—that would be unrealistic and absurd. Instead, the aim should be to use relevant theories concerned with social inequalities in health to consider systematically the choice of hypotheses, study design, measured variables, and unmeasured covariates likely to be important, as well as potential confounders and possibilities of selection bias. Equally key is identifying whose input would be helpful in sorting out these questions. Depending on the study hypothesis and sources of data, valuable input can likely be gained from academic researchers, public health practitioners, policymakers, and global, national, and community-based advocacy organizations, including members of groups whose experiences of inequality led them to bear the burden of the particular health problem under study.[2,3,21,22,25,26,43] By situating the knowledge and conduct of any given investigation within its broader societal context,[12,13,30] odds are that researchers will be better positioned to understand and convey the meanings and limitations of their study results.

Prevention: Research to Develop, Evaluate, and Improve Methods to Assess the Health Impact of Programs and Policies Involving Issues of Social Justice

The content of the questions for prevention research differ from those of etiologic research, but when it comes to addressing links between injustice and health, some common principles apply. These principles include not only conceptualizing relevant pathways at multiple levels, in relation to relevant timeframes, but also asking who gains from as well as who is harmed by injustice.[2,3,21,25–27,42–44] If social injustice were simply a matter of ignorance, increasing knowledge would be sufficient to render the world more equitable—yet many of those firmly holding on to power and privilege are highly educated persons. A corollary is that if it were easy to challenge privilege and rectify injustice, the world would already be a very different place.

Research on prevention and social inequalities in health tends to focus on two distinct topics: (a) prevention, health promotion, and advocacy efforts explicitly focused on health, and (b) the health impact of policies and programs originating outside of public health effort. Typically, research on designing, implementing, and evaluating explicitly health-oriented interventions is organized around social units whose physical and social conditions reflect (and generate) broader social inequities, such as workplaces, schools, and communities.[24–26,50] Examples include research on promoting workers' health by simultaneously addressing occupational hazards and health behaviors, increasing access to clean water, reducing exposure to airborne pollutants and cigarette smoke, increasing safer sex and condom use, reducing harm associated with use of licit and illicit drugs, and increasing access to health services.[25,26,43,62]

Also relevant is research to develop vaccines for, plus pharmacological agents to treat, the myriad infectious and parasitic diseases that disproportionately affect impoverished populations worldwide.[63,64] Research likewise is needed to develop more options for safe, effective, affordable, and user-friendly contraceptives, including barrier methods to curtail the spread of sexually transmitted infections.[53,65] Recommending this type of research in no way contradicts understandable concerns regarding commonplace and often-hyped suggestions that technological "magic bullets," improved health care, and public health programs can by themselves improve health without addressing the social injustices that create social disparities in health.[2,3] As the historical record and contemporary efforts make clear, however, the development of potentially life-saving technologies, therapies, and health interventions are nevertheless one component of a critical research agenda for social justice and public health; neglecting these concerns can lead to what has been termed "public health nihilism"[66] and forgo closing gaps created by elite research programs that have long ignored "unprofitable" diseases affecting those bearing the brunt of social injustices in health.

Importantly, although diverse kinds of public health interventions can ethically be randomized among or between members of a designated community (such as type of prevention message that is used), others cannot (such as the provision of clean water). One implication is that the randomized clinical trial (RCT) paradigm cannot be the sole standard for evidence on what makes a difference for addressing social disparities in health. This is because the RCT design cannot be used for critical determinants that can be changed but cannot be not randomized.[67] For this reason, research to evaluate the successes—and failures—of advocacy initiatives designed not for "research" but to improve people's lives[21,25,43] is also critically needed.

Also necessary is prevention-oriented research on the impact of policies and programs that affect health but that were not explicitly conceived or implemented in relation to public health concerns. Examples include policies on taxation, trade, labor, immigration, transportation, urban development, education, housing, and antipoverty programs, among others. Although concerns about the impact of such "non-health" policies on population health are not new, new attention to the promise of research on this topic for prevention of social inequalities in health is coalescing under the rubric of "health impact assessment" (HIA).[68,69] The conduct of HIAs could potentially (a) enhance recognition of societal determinants of health and of intersectoral responsibility for health, and (b) call attention to how "non-health" policies and programs have the potential to reduce—or exacerbate—social inequalities in health.[68] Even as HIA offers promise as a new avenue of prevention research promoting links between social justice and health, important questions remain about both the process and possible pitfalls, including feasibility and costs of generating valid estimates of likely health impacts.[68]

Conclusion

Clearly, many questions can be asked about the links between social injustice and health. Determining whether such research should be conducted, and which types of questions should be prioritized, necessitates critical attention to principles of social justice and human rights. Concern for these principles is essential from the first glimmers of a research idea all the way through to creating the study team, designing the study, getting it funded, collecting the data, testing hypotheses, and interpreting and disseminating results. It likewise necessitates collective strategizing to ensure that both public and private sponsors forthrightly fund research on social injustice and health. Suggesting this is possible are the myriad efforts that have led to the requirements that every institute at the U.S. National Institutes of Health develop a strategic plan to address health disparities.[70]

The conceptual and methodological rigor required—and developed—for research linking social justice and public health refutes the oft-asserted conservative canard that advocacy and rigorous science are incompatible.[71-73] Instead, given the lives at stake, research tackling social inequities in health has the responsibility to use the best knowledge and methods available.[2,3,18,21,43,44,47,74] It is this hard-won knowledge, secured by dedicated and inspired effort to investigate determinants of and remedies for social inequalities in health, that public health researchers can uniquely bring to the proverbial table—one contribution among many to create a more just, caring, and sustainable world.

References

1. Lecumberri B. Brazil's Helder Camara, champion of poor, dies at 90. Agence France Presse, August 28, 1999. Available at: http://www.hartford-hwp.com/archives/42/084. html. Accessed January 27, 2005.
2. Navarro V, ed. The political economy of social inequalities: consequences for health and quality of life. Amityville, N.Y.: Baywood Publishing Company, 2002.
3. Tesh SN. Hidden arguments: political ideology and disease prevention policy. New Brunswick, N.J.: Rutgers University Press, 1988.
4. Kluger R. Ashes to ashes: America's hundred-year cigarette war, the public health, and the unabashed triumph of Philip Morris. New York, N.Y.: Alfred A. Knopf, 1996.
5. Thornton J. Pandora's poison: chlorine, health, and a new environmental strategy. Cambridge, Mass.: MIT Press, 2000.
6. Krieger N. Does racism harm health? did child abuse exist before 1962?—on explicit questions, critical science, and current controversies: an ecosocial perspective. Am J Public Health 2003;93:194–9.
7. Kaufman JS, Cooper RS. Seeking causal explanations in social epidemiology. Am J Epidemiol 1999;150:113–20.
8. Lynch JW, Davey Smith G, Kaplan GA, et al. Income inequality and mortality: importance to health of individual incomes, psychological environment, or material conditions. BMJ 2000;320:1200–4.
9. Marmot M, Wilkinson RG. Psychosocial and material pathways in the relation between income and health: a response to Lynch et al. BMJ 2001;322:1233–6.
10. Krieger N. The making of public health data: paradigms, politics, and policy. J Public Health Policy 1992;13:412–27.
11. Krieger N. Epidemiology and the web of causation: has anyone seen the spider? Soc Sci Med 1994;39:887–903.
12. Krieger N. Theories for social epidemiology in the 21st century: an ecosocial perspective. Int J Epidemiol 2001;30:668–77.
13. Haraway DJ. Situated knowledge: the science question in feminism and the privilege of partial perspective. In: Haraway DJ. Simians, Cyborgs and women: the reinvention of nature. New York, N.Y.: Routledge Press, 1991:183–201.

14. Stellman SD, Resnicow K. Tobacco smoking, cancer and social class. In: Kogevinas M, Pearce N, Susser M, Boffetta P, eds. Social inequalities and cancer. Lyon, France: International Agency for Research on Cancer, 1997:229–50 (IARC scientific publication no. 138).

15. Kevles DJ. In the name of eugenics: genetics and the uses of human heredity. Cambridge, Mass.: Harvard University Press, 1995.

16. Krieger N. Discrimination and health. In: Berkman L, Kawachi I, eds. Social epidemiology. New York, N.Y.: Oxford University Press, 2000:36–75.

17. Sclar ED. Homelessness and housing policy: a game of musical chairs. Am J Public Health 1990;80:1039–40.

18. Schwartz S, Carpenter KM. The right answer to the wrong question: consequences of type III error for public health research. Am J Public Health 1999;89:1175–80.

19. Krieger N, Birn AE. A vision of social justice as the foundation of public health: commemorating 150 years of the spirit of 1848. Am J Public Health 1998;88:1603–6.

20. U.S. Department of Health and Human Services Data Council, Centers for Disease Control and Prevention, National Center for Health Statistics, National Committee on Vital and Health Statistics. Shaping a health statistics vision for the 21st century: final report. Washington, D.C.: National Center for Health Statistics, 2003.

21. Krieger N, ed. Embodying inequality: epidemiologic perspectives. Amityville, N.Y.: Baywood Publishing, 2004.

22. Gruskin S, Tarantola D. Health and human rights. In: Detels R, McEwen J, Beaglehole R, et al, eds. The Oxford textbook of public health. 4th ed. New York, N.Y.: Oxford University Press, 2001:311–35.

23. Ben-Shlomo Y, Kuh DH. A lifecourse approach to chronic disease epidemiology: conceptual models, empirical challenges, and interdisciplinary perspectives. Int J Epidemiol 2002;31:285–93.

24. Schneiderman N, Speers MA, Silva JM, et al, eds. Integrating behavioral and social sciences with public health. Washington, D.C.: American Psychological Association, 2001.

25. Wallerstein N, Duran B. The conceptual, historical, and practice roots of community based participatory research. In: Minkler M, Wallerstein N, eds. Community based participatory research for health. San Francisco, Calif.: Jossey-Bass, 2003:27–52.

26. Evans T, Whitehead M, Diderichsen F, et al, eds. Challenging inequities in health: from ethics to action. Oxford, U.K.: Oxford University Press, 2001.

27. Doyal L, Gough I. A theory of human need. New York, N.Y.: Guilford Press, 1991.

28. Miller D. Principles of social justice. Cambridge, Mass.: Harvard University Press, 1999.

29. Lock M, Gordon D, eds. Biomedicine examined. Dordrecht, the Netherlands: Kluwer Academic Publishers, 1988.

30. Rosenberg CE, Golden J, eds. Framing disease: studies in cultural history. New Brunswick, N.J.: Rutgers University Press, 1992.

31. Krieger N, Chen JT, Ebel G. Can we monitor socioeconomic inequalities in health? A survey of U.S. health departments' data collection and reporting practices. Public Health Rep 1997;112:481–91.

32. Braveman P, Starfield B, Geiger HJ. World health report 2000: how it removes equity from the agenda for public health monitoring and policy. BMJ 2001;323:678–81.

33. Krieger N. A glossary for social epidemiology. J Epidemiol Commun Health 2001;55:693–700.

34. Rosenberg HM, Maurer JD, Sorlie PD, et al. Quality of death rates by race and Hispanic origin: a summary of current research, 1999. National Center for Health Statistics, Vital Health Stat 2(128), 1999.

35. Krieger N, Chen JT, Waterman PD, Rehkopf DH, Subramanian SV. Painting a truer picture of US socioeconomic and racial/ethnic health inequalities: The Public Health Disparities Geocoding Project. Am J Public Health 2005;95:312–23.

36. Krieger N, Waterman PD, Chen JT, Rehkopf DH, Subramanian SV. The Public Health Disparities Geocoding Project Monograph. Available at: http://www.hsph. harvard.edu/thegeocodingproject. Accessed January 27, 2005.

37. Ezzati M, Lopez AD, Rodgers A, et al. Selected major risk factors and global and regional burden of disease. Lancet 2002;360:1347–60.

38. Reidpath DD, Allotey PA, Kouame A, et al. Measuring health in a vacuum: examining the disability weight of the DALY. Health Policy Plan 2003;18:351–6.

39. Wagstaff A, Paci P, van Doorslaer E. On the measurement of inequalities in health. Soc Sci Med 1991;33:545–57.

40. Mathers CD, Murray CJL, Lopez AD, et al. Global patterns of health life expectancy for older women. J Women's Aging 2002;14:99–117.

41. Mustard CA, Etches J. Gender differences in socioeconomic inequality in mortality. J Epidemiol Commun Health 2003;57:974–80.

42. Crawford R. You are dangerous to your health: the ideology and politics of victim blaming. Int J Health Services 1977;7:663–80.

43. Hofrichter R, ed. Health and social justice: politics, ideology and inequity in the distribution of disease—a public health reader. San Francisco, Calif.: Jossey-Bass, 2003.

44. Davey Smith G, ed. Health inequalities: lifecourse approaches. Bristol, U.K.: University of Bristol Policy Press, 2003.

45. Krieger N, Williams D, Moss N. Measuring social class in US public health research: concepts, methodologies and guidelines. Annu Rev Public Health 1997;18:341–78.

46. Cooper H. Investigating socio-economic explanations for gender and ethnic inequalities in health. Soc Sci Med 2002;54:693–706.

47. Graham H. Building an inter-disciplinary science of health inequalities: the example of lifecourse research. Soc Sci Med 2002;55:2005–16.

48. O'Campo P. Invited commentary: advancing theory and methods for multilevel models of residential neighborhoods and health. Am J Epidemiol 2003;157:9–13.

49. Macintyre S, Ellaway A, Cummins S. Place effects on health: how can we conceptualise, operationalise and measure them? Soc Sci Med 2002;55:125–39.

50. Kawachi I, Berkman LF, eds. Neighborhoods and health. New York, N.Y.: Oxford University Press, 2003.

51. Williams DR. Race, socioeconomic status, and health. The added effects of racism and discrimination. Ann N Y Acad Sci 1999;896:173–88.

52. Krug E, Dahlberg L, Mercy J, et al, eds. World report on violence and health. Geneva, Switzerland: World Health Organization, 2002.

53. Doyal L. What makes women sick? Gender and the political economy of health. New Brunswick, N.J.: Rutgers University Press, 1995.

54. Cruikshank JK, Mbanya JC, Wilks R, et al. Sick genes, sick individuals or sick populations with chronic disease? The emergence of diabetes and high blood pressure in African-Origin populations. Int J Epidemiol 2001;30:111–7.

55. Krieger N. Refiguring "race": epidemiology, racialized biology, and biological expressions of race relations. Int J Health Serv 2000;30:211–6.

56. Krieger N, Sidney S. Racial discrimination and blood pressure: the CARDIA study of young black and white adults. Am J Public Health 1996;86:1370–8.

57. Clark R, Anderson NB, Clark VR, et al. Racism as a stressor for African Americans: a biopsychosocial model. Am Psychol 1999;54:805–16.

58. Elliott P. High blood pressure in the community. In: Bulpitt CJ, ed. Handbook of hypertension, vol 20: epidemiology of hypertension. Amsterdam, the Netherlands: Elsevier, 2000:1–18.

59. Lopes AA, Port FK. The low birth weight hypothesis as a plausible explanation for the black/white differences in hypertension, non-insulin-dependent diabetes, and end-stage renal disease. Am J Kidney Dis 1995;25:350–6.

60. Vupputuri S, He J, Munter P, et al. Blood lead level is associated with elevated blood pressure in blacks. Hypertension 2003;41:463–8.

61. McEwen BS. Stress, adaptation, and disease: allostasis and allostatic load. Ann N Y Acad Sci 1998;840:33–44.

62. Sorensen G, Emmons K, Stoddard A, et al. Do social influences contribute to occupational differences in smoking behavior? Am J Health Promotion 2002;16:135–41.

63. Trouiller P, Olliaro P, Torreele E, et al. Drug development for neglected diseases: a deficient market and a public-health policy failure. Lancet 2002;359:2188–94.

64. Farmer P. Infections and inequalities: the modern plagues. Berkeley, Calif.: University of California Press, 1999.

65. Reaves ND. Unresolved issues in contraceptive health policy. Health Care Women Int 2002;23:854–60.

66. Fairchild A, Oppenheimer G. Public health nihilism vs pragmatism: history, politics, and the control of tuberculosis. Am J Public Health 1998;88:1105–17.

67. Davey Smith G, Ebrahim S, Frankel S. How policy informs the evidence: "evidence based" thinking can lead to debased policy making. BMJ 2001;322:184–5.

68. Krieger N, Northridge M, Gruskin S, et al. Assessing health impact assessment: multidisciplinary and international perspectives. J Epidemiol Commun Health 2003; 57:659–62.

69. Scott-Samuel A. Health impact assessment: an idea whose time has come. BMJ 1996;313:183–4.

70. National Center on Minority Health and Health Disparities. NIH strategic plan and budget to reduce and ultimately eliminate health disparities. FY 2002. Washington, D.C.: National Institutes of Health, U.S. Department of Health and Human Services, 2003.

71. Savitz DA, Poole C, Miller WC. Reassessing the role of epidemiology in public health. Am J Public Health 1999;89:1158–61.

72. Rothman KJ, Adami H-O, Trichopolous D. Should the mission of epidemiology include the eradication of poverty? Lancet 1998;352:810–3.

73. Satel SL. PC, M.D.: How political correctness is corrupting medicine. New York, N.Y.: Basic Books, 2000.

74. Krieger N. Questioning epidemiology: objectivity, advocacy, and socially responsible science. Am J Public Health 1999;1151–3.

75. Smedley BD, Stith AY, Nelson AR, eds. Unequal treatment: confronting racial and ethnic disparities in health care. Committee on Understanding and Eliminating Racial and Ethnic Disparities in Health Care, Board on Health Sciences Policy, Institute of Medicine. Washington, D.C.: National Academies Press, 2003.

76. Erwin K. Interpreting the evidence: competing paradigms and the emergence of lesbian and gay suicide as a "social fact." Int J Health Serv 1993;23:437–53.

77. Herrell R, Goldberg J, True WR, et al. Sexual orientation and suicidality: a co-twin control study in adult men. Arch Gen Psychiatry 1999;56:867–74.
78. U.S. Department of Health and Human Services. Steps to a healthier US initiative. Available at: http://www.healthierus.gov/. Accessed January 27, 2005.
79. Nestle M. Food politics: how the food industry influences nutrition and health. Berkeley, Calif.: University of California Press, 2002.

27

PROTECTING HUMAN RIGHTS THROUGH INTERNATIONAL AND NATIONAL LAW

Peter Weiss and Henry A. Freedman

Introduction

International and national law can play a critical role in protecting human rights, and thereby reducing social injustice, because law is perhaps the primary system through which the state and international community seek to enforce social norms. Human rights is not a creation of the twentieth century. Antigone, in Sophocles' play of that name from the fifth century B.C.E., defies a royal decree forbidding the burial of her brother Polyneices by relying on "the unwritten and unfailing laws of heaven" whose "life is not of today or yesterday, but from all time."[1]

The notion of a supreme law that confers on individuals rights transcending those found in the codes of laws of their nations is a constant theme running through the writings of all major cultures for the past 2,500 years. Heaven as the source of rights came gradually to be complemented by nature (human as well as societal and environmental)—hence the reference to "the laws of nature and of nature's God," which precedes the definition of the inalienable rights ("life, liberty, and the pursuit of happiness") in the United States Declaration of Independence in 1776.

The fundamental law of the United States, the 1789 Constitution, and the 1791 Bill of Rights (the first 10 amendments to the Constitution) imposed few positive obligations on the government, and none related to economic or social rights. Interestingly enough, the codification of international human rights began about the same time, with the branch of human rights law dealing with the obligations of combatants, known as humanitarian law or by its Latin name, *jus in bello.* These obligations of omission and commission created, if only indirectly, concomitant rights in the persons and institutions to be protected. In 1782, the United States and Prussia signed a treaty of amity and commerce that provided that, should war break out between them, all women and children, scholars of every faculty, cultivators of the earth, artisans, manufacturers and fishermen, unarmed and inhabiting unfortified towns, villages or places, and, in general, all others whose occupations were for the common subsistence and benefit of mankind should be allowed to continue their respective employment and should not be molested in their persons.[2] This represents the increasingly ignored principle that civilians are not legitimate targets in war,[3] which forms the bedrock of subsequent international treaties, including the Hague Conventions of 1899 and 1907 and the Geneva Conventions of 1949.[4]

Meanwhile, in the United States, constitutional amendments following the Civil War (1861–1865) prohibited slavery and provided that no state shall "deprive any person of life, liberty, or property, without due process of law; nor deny . . . the equal protection of the laws."[5] These provisions have proved crucial in securing certain social and economic rights but do not affirmatively provide for those rights.

Because of the federal structure of the United States, each of the 50 states is also an important source of rights. However, only the constitution of New York State imposes a sufficiently explicit affirmative state obligation to provide for the poor that meaningful court enforcement has been obtained. Other states have either no provision for economic and social rights or a limited provision easily satisfied by whatever a state does.

The United Nations Charter, which came into force in 1945, constitutes a treaty binding on all of its original and future members. Many people remember that, in its first paragraph, "We the Peoples of the United Nations" commit ourselves to "save succeeding generations from the scourge of war" (Preamble). But few recall that in its second paragraph, this commitment is extended to reaffirming "faith in fundamental human rights, in the dignity and worth of the human person, in the equal rights of men and women" (Preamble) and that one of the purposes of the United Nations, as defined in its charter, is "promoting and encouraging respect for human rights" (Article 1[3]).[6]

How International and National Law Can Reduce Social Injustice

International Law

The United Nations Charter is like a *matrioshka,* a Russian nesting doll, producing document after document of greater particularity, but of smaller scope, than its predecessor. Thus, in 1948, under the leadership of Eleanor Roosevelt and with the approval of the United States, the United Nations adopted the first comprehensive, nonmilitary, code of human rights, the Universal Declaration of Human Rights (UDHR), which contains articles dealing with economic, social, and cultural rights, including social security, education, and a standard of living adequate for health and well-being, including food, clothing, housing, medical care, and necessary social services.[7] Mothers and children, whether born in or out of wedlock, are entitled to special care and assistance.

Eight years later, two covenants—the International Covenant on Economic, Social and Cultural Rights (ICESCR)[8] and the International Covenant on Civil and Political Rights (ICCPR)[9]—provided greater detail on the rights described in the UDHR and made signatory nations responsible for recognizing and implementing these rights. Thus, nations are required to recognize the right to safe and healthy working conditions, punish employers who employ children and young persons in harmful work, and recognize "the right of everyone to the enjoyment of the highest attainable standard of physical and mental health" (ICESCR, Article 12[1]). Signatory nations agree to achieve the full realization of the last of these rights by reducing infant mortality; improving environmental and industrial hygiene; preventing, treating, and controlling epidemic, endemic, occupational, and other diseases; and ensuring access of sick people to medical services. This last clause, which could sound like a mandate for universal health care, may explain why the United States has never ratified ICESCR, although it did finally ratify ICCPR in 1982. However, the United States is a member of the World Health Organization and has therefore accepted—albeit not in the form of a treaty—the principle that "the enjoyment of the highest attainable standard of health is one of the fundamental rights of every human being."[10]

Another important source of state obligations in the economic and social sphere is the Charter of the Organization of American States,[11] ratified by the United States in 1951. By its terms, the member states pledge themselves "to accelerate their economic and social development" (Article 31) and to achieve "equitable distribution of national income . . . modernization of rural life, protection of man's potential through the extension and application of modern medical science, proper nutrition . . . adequate housing for all sectors of the population, and urban conditions that offer the opportunity for a healthful, productive, and full life"(Article 31).

The framers of the UDHR and of the two covenants made no distinction between two sets of human rights. In identical preambles to the two conventions, they declared that there were two sets of rights that were completely interdependent and could only be achieved together: (a) civil and political rights; and (b) economic, social, and cultural rights. Unfortunately, many judges, policymakers, and academics have insisted on making a distinction between these two sets of rights. During the Cold War, the capitalist West generally regarded the ICCPR rights as real and enforceable and the ICESCR as "aspirational" and unenforceable, whereas the socialist East took the opposite view. The Western view now prevails worldwide, except for Cuba, North Korea, and, to some extent, China. Even the reality of ICCPR leaves much to be desired in many countries, including, particularly since the terrorist attacks of September 2001, the United States and some of its NATO allies.

The time may be here to transform the right to health and other social and economic rights from abstract concepts into legally enforceable instruments. Many courts, and particularly those in the United States, still refuse to treat ICESCR as "real." They adhere to the notion that such rights can only be progressively implemented as resources become available, ignoring that government resources are allocated by politicians according to their own sense of values and priorities. But this is by no means true for the rest of the world. The "case law" page of ESCR-NET lists about 90 recent cases from 12 countries and some international and regional human rights bodies that deal with such economic, social, and cultural rights as social security, health, housing, and education. They involve decisions based on ICESCR and national constitutions.

The most famous of these cases is the Grootboom case, which was decided by the Constitutional Court of South Africa in 2000.[12] It involved an appeal by a community of squatters for assistance from the provincial and municipal authorities under two sections of the South African Constitution dealing with the right to housing and with children's right to basic shelter. The order of the Supreme Court included the construction and operation of 20 permanent toilets, the installation and operation of 20 water taps, and the provision of building material up to a value of 760 rands (US$130), to all households.

On the precedent of this case, the Constitutional Court in 2001 decided the case of *Treatment Action Campaign v. Minister of Health*.[13] This decision affirmed an order by a lower court to provide the retroviral drug nevirapine to all HIV-positive pregnant women in South Africa, probably saving tens of thousands of lives.

Among other cases involving public health and social justice are the following:

- In *Maria Isabel Chamorro Santamaria et al. v. the Ministry of the Economy and the National Treasury*,[14] the Supreme Court of Costa Rica decided that the national treasury had sufficient funds to provide the plaintiffs with the social services that had previously been denied to them.
- In *Paschim Banga Khet Samit v. State of West Bengal*, a case brought by a plaintiff who fell off a train and was denied emergency medical

treatment in six government hospitals, the Supreme Court of India awarded compensation to the plaintiff and issued a detailed set of orders to the state government designed to improve the availability of medical services in West Bengal.

- In *Jorge Odir v. Miranda Cortez,* the Inter-American Commission for Human Rights affirmed the right to health in the American Convention on Human Rights. It also requested the government of El Salvador to immediately supply retroviral medication to the petitioners with HIV/AIDS, a request that was later given the force of law by the Supreme Court of El Salvador.
- In *Shela Zia v. Wapda PLD,* the Supreme Court of Pakistan, following the precedent set by the Supreme Court of India of accepting direct petitions from citizens who considered their human rights violated, held that it lacked the expertise to decide whether a proposed power station would constitute a serious health hazard but ordered the government to establish a commission of internationally known and recognized scientists to evaluate the petitioners' claim.

In addition to national tribunals and regional ones, such as the Inter-American Commission and Court for Human Rights or the European Court of Human Rights, questions of humanitarian law that implicate social injustice are subject to litigation in international tribunals. The International Court of Justice (ICJ) did so in the case brought by Nicaragua against the United States in 1984 concerning the activities of the U.S.-sponsored contras. More recently, in the nuclear weapons case, the ICJ held that "a threat or use of nuclear weapons should be compatible with the requirements of the international law applicable in armed conflict, particularly those of the principles and rules of international humanitarian law."[15] However, cases involving violation of human rights or humanitarian law rarely come before the ICJ.

By contrast, the International Criminal Court, still in its infancy, is likely to eventually have a docket dealing precisely with the principles of international humanitarian law to which the ICJ referred in the Nuclear Weapons Case. Its jurisdiction is limited, for the time being, to "the crime of genocide, war crimes, and crimes against humanity."[16]

National Law in the United States

Because social and economic rights are not mentioned in the U.S. Constitution, progressive forces have succeeded in addressing social justice and human rights issues through federal and state legislation. A key step was the 1935 Social Security Act, which created federal retirement and survivor's benefits (and later disability benefits) and the unemployment insurance program—with all of these benefits based on earnings history, not current economic need. The Act also provided matching funds for state welfare programs for the elderly and Aid to Families with Dependent Children (AFDC)—largely for families missing one parent. Eligibility for these programs was based, in contrast, on current financial need and satisfaction of other factors. In 1935, the U.S. Congress was dominated by senators from the South. To ensure that the federal government would not use these programs to promote a civil rights agenda, Congress afforded the states enormous discretion in setting eligibility and benefits. As time passed, administration of these programs was often permeated by arbitrariness and racial discrimination.

In recent years, legislatures have stripped legal rights from many social welfare programs, program rules and administration have narrowed eligibility and made application for programs and compliance with program requirements more difficult, tax revenues needed to fund programs have been eliminated, judges have been increasingly hostile to claims, and much of the public—including many of those who have been harmed—have believed that poverty and other social ills are the sole responsibility of the individual, not the consequence of economic forces or government policy. Although significant progress is being made in many other areas of human rights, poverty, with its severe impact on health, remains endemic, especially among racial and ethnic minorities and single mothers and children.[7]

In 1965, the U.S. Congress created the Medicare program to provide health care for seniors and people with disabilities eligible for Social Security benefits and a state-federal program to fund health care for certain needy families, seniors, and persons with disabilities. The federal government assumed responsibility for the needs-based cash assistance programs for the elderly and disabled in 1974, now called the Supplemental Security Income (SSI) program. AFDC served as the nation's major welfare program until 1996.

Creative lawyering in the late 1960s effected profound changes in welfare programs through two U.S. Supreme Court cases that established a legal "entitlement" to assistance:

- In *King v. Smith*, Alabama had denied AFDC to a mother who had recently had sexual relations with a man who was not the father of her child. Alabama's policy was one of several used, especially by the Southern states, to exclude many people of color and others considered "unworthy." In 1968, a unanimous U.S. Supreme Court ruled that Alabama could not exclude people for whom matching funds were available under federal law. This decision led to rapid growth of welfare rolls and a substantial increase in the percentage of minority individuals on them.
- Two years later, in *Goldberg v. Kelly,* the Supreme Court applied the Constitutional Due Process clause in ruling that welfare benefits could not be terminated unless advance notice was given and an opportunity for an in-person hearing provided. The court adopted the argument raised by

progressive lawyers and scholars that government benefits created with explicit eligibility conditions were a form of "property"—a "statutory entitlement" that could not be taken away without due process of law. This transformed state welfare administration, reducing arbitrariness and increasing accountability. Still, bureaucracies were too large and complex, social and political hostility to those in poverty were too great, and the ability of many welfare recipients to assert and defend their rights too hampered for complete rationality and fairness to be achieved.

During the 1980s and 1990s, social programs came under increasing attack, with charges that they nourished antisocial behavior and long-term impoverishment. One major trend was replacing federally created individual "entitlements" with "block grants" to the states, devolving to state and local authorities the power to set standards and rules. The 1996 legislation that replaced AFDC with the block grant Temporary Assistance to Needy Families Program explicitly stated that there was no provision for an "entitlement" to benefits. This legislation gave the states far greater discretion but imposed rigorous work requirements. Welfare rolls decreased because of a growing economy, much-harsher eligibility requirements, and services to assist people to get jobs.

Just as there is no explicit constitutional right to subsistence (except in New York), there is no right to shelter or to health care. Still, lawyers have aggressively and creatively enforced statutory rights in health care and housing programs. Many states have constitutional provisions ensuring rights to public education, and lawyers have had some success in forcing states to address severe underfunding of education in many local school districts. Nonetheless, the combination of tax cutting and state constitutional provisions forbidding budget deficits is making it difficult for public officials to provide for education, much less other social needs not mentioned in state constitutions.

Greater success has been achieved in promoting civil rights. The U.S. Supreme Court declared racial segregation in education to be unconstitutional in 1954. Congress passed legislation prohibiting racial segregation in employment, transportation, and many other areas, and profound changes have occurred in U.S. society as a result. Unfortunately, segregation in housing and education has persisted in much of the United States, and persons of color are still far more likely to be poor. On the other hand, despite major efforts by conservative forces, the U.S. Supreme Court ruled in 2003 that public colleges could take race into account in seeking to achieve a more diversified student body.

Constitutional decisions and legislation have also barred many forms of discrimination against women, and women have truly taken a far more significant role in business, politics, and sports than they had before. Reproductive rights have faced a much more rocky road, with only a narrow U.S. Supreme Court majority continuing to uphold a woman's right to abortion, while social forces and restrictive legislation have made availability of abortion much more limited.

Much progress has been made in eliminating various forms of discrimination on the basis of sexual orientation, with gay marriage ruled valid by one state's highest court, and a recent Supreme Court decision allowing criminal prosecution of sodomy overturned by the current Supreme Court. In addition, the rights of persons with disabilities have been recognized by Congress, with the result that public facilities and programs are far more accessible to persons with disabilities and employers are required to make reasonable accommodations for disabilities.

Rights, however, are meaningful only if there are courts to enforce them and lawyers to assert them, and there are reasons to be concerned about both at the present time. During the past decade, a bare majority of the U.S. Supreme Court has issued a series of decisions imposing barriers to asserting claims of rights, particularly against the states.

At the same time, there are hardly enough lawyers to enforce rights. While the Supreme Court has found a constitutional due process right to counsel in criminal cases, no equivalent right has been found for most civil cases. There is, however, a rich history of rights lawyering that has made a profound difference in U.S. society. Privately supported groups, such as the Center for Constitutional Rights, the American Civil Liberties Union, the NAACP Legal Defense Fund, and other groups with an ethnic, women's, or sexual orientation focus, have largely focused on civil liberties and civil rights. Lawyers have joined together to defend rights in relatively radical groups, such as the National Lawyers Guild. Mainstream bar associations, including the American Bar Association, have become increasingly involved in many fights for civil liberties and civil rights. The passage of federal and state antidiscrimination laws has brought government lawyers into court to enforce rights. Because these organizations are reliant almost entirely on private contributions, they can maintain their impact and independence only if foundations and individuals are willing to continue their financial support.

Publicly funded legal aid efforts have focused on defending individuals in the marketplace and in their dealings with government agencies. The privately supported legal aid societies in the earlier parts of the twentieth century provided limited assistance in individual cases. An entirely new approach—law reform to end poverty—was articulated in the late 1960s when the federal legal services program was created as a part of President Lyndon Johnson's War on Poverty.

Federal funds were used both to establish local offices and open a variety of national and state support centers to provide leadership to the local offices. The

15 national support centers, scattered about the country, each focused on a specific area of the law, such as the Welfare Law Center and the National Health Law Program. Many of them developed the legal theories and brought the cases that have made such a mark on the legal landscape; for example, the Welfare Law Center was the source of the welfare cases described earlier. Because much of this work challenged powerful economic interests, especially large growers, or government bureaucracies, the legal services program was controversial from the outset. In 1995, power in Congress shifted sharply to the political right. Funding was slashed, with national and state support eliminated entirely. In addition, local programs were subjected to a variety of new restrictions. These included a flat prohibition on class actions, which eliminated much "high impact" work; any representation of most people who were not U.S. citizens; and any use of privately raised money for work that they could not perform with federal funds.

An Agenda for Action

As with every other social goal, the path to its achievement must include at least three elements: education, advocacy, and litigation.

International

Education on the right to health can begin with at least two WHO publications: *25 Questions & Answers on Health & Human Rights* answers such questions as, What are human rights? What is meant by the right to health? What is meant by a rights-based approach to health? And how can poor countries with resource limitations be held to the same standards as rich countries? The other publication, *The Right to Health*, is a lovely comic book aimed at the primary school level.

As for advocacy, WHO's Section on Ethics and Health (ETH/SDE) published in October 2003 "Health and Human Rights," a paper setting out an ambitious program designed to advance WHO's health agenda to fulfill rights rather than needs. The three objectives of the program are to support governments in integrating a human rights–based approach to health development, to strengthen WHO's capacity to integrate a human rights–based approach in its work, and to advance the right to health in international law and international development processes.[17] There is much that health workers worldwide can do to promote this program, either by working with WHO or by undertaking their own projects.

WHO is not the only United Nations specialized agency to embark on a project to transform needs into rights. The Food and Agriculture Organization

(FAO) has established an Intergovernmental Working Group "to elaborate a set of voluntary guidelines to support the progressive realization of the right to adequate food."[18]

In addition, interest in promoting international economic and social rights is burgeoning in civil society organizations in the United States and abroad, as illustrated by the following examples:

- Africa Action (www.africaaction.org), a merger of three leading Africa advocacy groups based in the United States, is leading a campaign with the slogan "Africa's Right to Health."
- The Center for Economic and Social Rights (www.cesr.org), established in New York in 1993, implements projects in the United States and abroad that challenge economic injustice as a violation of international human rights law.
- ESCR-NET, a project financed by The Ford Foundation, keeps hundreds of human rights activists from many countries in communication via the Internet, exchanging information and ideas about developments concerning economic, social, and cultural rights. In 2003, it held its first international conference in Thailand, with the theme "Creating New Paths Toward Social Justice."
- The Philadelphia-based Kensington Welfare Rights Union (www.kwru.org) organized a "Poor People's March for Economic Human Rights" from Mississippi to Washington in 2003, on the fortieth anniversary of Dr. Martin Luther King's March on Washington. KWRU has links with economic human rights groups in other countries.
- The Center for Constitutional Rights (www.ccr-ny.org) has pioneered the use of international human rights in domestic courts since it helped to bring about the 1980 landmark decision in *Filartiga v. Pena* under the Alien Tort Claims Act. The center has been a long-time advocate for economic and social rights and has made consistent use of international law in litigation.

In the United States

As in the international arena, improvement in social and economic rights will require education, advocacy, and litigation by an unprecedented number of people. The forces seeking to turn back the clock, and restrict wealth and well-being to the few, have been growing more powerful and have been setting the agenda, but united efforts by caring people can turn that situation around.

Fortunately, for those seeking to educate themselves on issues of health care rights and the broad range of economic and social justice issues, the challenge is choosing among the many resources available. Despite the rapidly evolving political and economic climate, updated information is available on many websites. Some sites are more neutral, focusing on academic and government reports and data; an excellent starting point for social welfare information is the Finance Project (www.financeprojectinfo.org). Other sites designed to support those advocating for progressive improvements in policy at either the federal or state level are the Coalition on Human Needs, (www.chn.org), the Center for Community Change (www.communitychange.org), and the Sargent Shriver National Center on Poverty Law (www.povertylaw.org). Sites with a particular focus on health advocacy information include Families USA (www.familiesusa.org) and the National Health Law Program (www.healthlaw.org). Other groups have focused on issues of race, such as the Poverty and Race Research Action Council (www.prrac.org) and the Applied Research Center (www.arc.org). Very useful information on budget and tax policy may be found at the Center on Budget Policies and Priorities (www.cbpp.org).

Concerned persons can therefore educate themselves quickly, but the challenge for them is how to make change happen. There is much they can do.

First, advocacy organizations and coalitions are already hard at work in most states and in Washington, D.C., trying to move officials, legislatures, and the United States Congress to preserve and improve health care and other vital rights. They need volunteers and they need funds; many of the websites noted earlier can provide information on such efforts. The religious community has been a steadfast advocate for social and economic justice; useful entry points for a wealth of leads on various issues and campaigns are the National Council of the Churches of Christ in the USA (www.ncccusa.org), Catholic Charities USA (www.catholiccharitiesusa.org), and the Religious Action Center of Reform Judaism (www.rac.org). For more information on grassroots organizing concerning social justice, one can consult the Center for Community Change page, noted earlier, and the Low Income Networking and Communication Project, (www.lincproject.org), a program of the Welfare Law Center (www.welfarelaw.org).

Organizers in low-income communities are increasingly focusing on voter mobilization in recognition of the critical role played by politicians; anyone seriously interested in effecting change in American policies has to become involved in the political process and demand that candidates and elected officials account for their positions on issues of social and economic justice. Anyone can write letters to elected officials and the editors of newspapers and magazines about policies currently being discussed or debated.

Another critical area for advocacy efforts is to stop the U.S. Supreme Court and lower federal courts from emasculating federal laws that protect rights. Many civil rights lawyers and academics have launched ambitious campaigns to alert the public to the dangers of judicial law making that erases rights-creating legislation and to take effective action that can begin to restore the federal courts as a bastion of individual rights.

Finally, there is litigation that must be pursued. Many critical laws and constitutional requirements are not being enforced. Energetic and creative enforcement of current entitlements is needed in benefit programs, such as Medicaid and the Food Stamp Program; in federal and state laws protecting wages, working conditions, and the right to organize; in laws prohibiting discrimination on the basis of race, ethnicity, sex, citizenship, sexual orientation, and disability; and in the constitution's due process clause. Such advocacy will help many individuals, promote rationality and fairness in decision making, and educate the public and the judiciary about the needs to enforce those rights and challenge prejudice and stereotypes.

As noted earlier, there are far too few lawyers available to enforce these rights. While the federal government provides limited financial support for civil legal aid services for the indigent through the Legal Services Corporation (www.lsc.gov), the restrictions on that program have limited its ability to enforce these rights on a broad scale. Concerned individuals can search out organizations pursuing matters of the most interest to them and volunteer time, especially if the person is legally trained, and individuals can contribute financially. In addition, they can become engaged politically, at the local, state, and federal levels, to oppose the right's relentless attack on public funding for civil legal services.

Conclusion

For a variety of reasons, including the decline in civil liberties following 9/11 and the triumph of free-market capitalism over socialism and social democracy, the pursuit of human rights has fallen on bad times. However, the idea of enforceable economic, social, and cultural rights is beginning to take root here and in some other countries. In the United States, it is beginning to permeate civil society. Eventually, it will enter into the political and judicial life of this country. It is the only sure bulwark against social injustice. Lawyers must go to court, victims of social injustice must take to the streets, and activists must lobby their elected representatives. These are the paths for fighting social injustice and achieving human rights.

References

1. Encyclopedia Britannica. Great Books of the Western World, Vol. 5, p. 135.
2. Friedman L, ed. The law of war, a documentary history. New York, N.Y.: Random House, 1972:150.
3. Gnaedinger A, Director-General of the International Committee of the Red Cross. The protection of civilians in armed conflict. Statement to the United Nations Security

Council, December 10, 2002. Available at: http://www/icrc.org/web/eng/siteeng0.nsf/iwpList99/153DFC452D5CBA7FC1256C8C0054F214. Accessed January 28, 2005.

4. Available at: http://www.yale.edu.lawweb/Avalon/lawofwar/lawwar.htm. Accessed January 28, 2005.

5. U.S. Constitution, Amendments XIII and XIV.

6. United Nations Charter. Available at: http://www.un.org/aboutun/charter. Accessed April 14, 2005.

7. Universal Declaration of Human Rights. Available at: http://www.unhchr.ch/udhr/lang/eng.htm. Accessed January 28, 2005.

8. International Covenant on Economic, Social and Cultural Rights. Available at: http://www.unhchr.ch/html/menu3/b/a_cescr.htm. Accessed January 28, 2005.

9. International Covenant on Civil and Political Rights. Available at: http://www.unhchr.ch/html/menu3/b/a_ccpr.htm. Accessed January 28, 2005.

10. World Health Organization Constitution. Available at: http://www.who.int/about/en. Accessed April 14, 2005.

11. Available at: http://www.oad/juridico/english/charter/html. Accessed January 28, 2005.

12. *Grootboom v. Government of the Republic of South Africa and others*, Constitutional Court—CCT 38/00. Available at: http://www.concourt.gov.za/judgment.php?case_id=11987. Accessed May 21, 2005.

13. Constitutional Court of South Africa—CCT 08/02. Discussed at: http://www.nigerianet.org. Accessed May 21, 2005.

14. For this and the three cases that follow, as well as other economic and social rights cases, see: http://www.escrnet.org/EngGeneral/. Accessed May 21, 2005.

15. Legality of the threat or use of nuclear weapons, general list no. 95, Advisory Opinion of 8 July 1996, par. 105(D). Available at: http://www.icj-cij.org/icjwww/icases/iunan/iunanframe.htm. Accessed April 14, 2005.

16. Rome Statute of the International Criminal Court. Available at: http://www.un.org/law/icc/. Accessed May 26, 2005.

17. Health and Human Rights Strategy Unit, World Health Organization. Health and human rights publication series no. 1. Geneva, Switzerland: World health Organization, July 2002.

18. Available at: http://www.fav.org/righttofood/en/highlight_5159Gen.html. Accessed January 28, 2005.

28

PROMOTING EQUITABLE AND SUSTAINABLE HUMAN DEVELOPMENT

Richard Jolly

Introduction

Progress toward social justice as it affects public health requires actions, within each country and internationally, to reduce the extremes of social injustice outside of health and health services.

Income inequalities in the world today have never been higher, especially the gaps of income between the poorest and the richest countries. Within many countries, both rich and poor, the levels of inequality of income are also at record levels. Both dimensions of inequality present major problems for achieving equity in public health, which the World Health Organization (WHO) declared to be the priority for primary health care until 2020.

Notwithstanding these trends, it is a bad mistake to imagine that because income inequalities are wide and often growing, the possibilities of reducing social injustice in public health must remain a utopian dream. On a global scale, there have been major improvements in public health over the past 50 years, including unprecedented reductions in child mortality in almost all parts of the world and also, except for the impact of HIV/AIDS, increases in life expectancy. There have also been advances in many areas closely related to health: the adoption of human rights, the commitment to goals to reduce poverty and develop effective affordable strategies for improving living standards, and the demonstration, by many countries, of the practical politics of achieving these improvements in practice.

The possibilities of human progress are also demonstrated in the expansion of school enrollments and adult literacy and in advances in the status and empowerment of women and girls in most developing countries. The rates of these improvements over the past 50 years have generally exceeded anything achieved within developed countries during the early stages of their development or over the longer period of their economic and social advance. For example, all but 25 developing countries in 2002 had infant mortality rates below 100 per 1,000 live births—a rate achieved by only one industrial country, Norway, in 1900.[1] Seventy developing countries had achieved, by 2000, young child (under age 5) mortality rates below 70, the level achieved by the United States and the United Kingdom only by about 1940.[2]

Nevertheless, none of these advances gives any room for complacency. They stand as examples of what can be done, not as monuments to goals that have been universally achieved. Given the unprecedented levels of wealth and income, the wide gaps between the potential and actual achievements in public health in the world today are a scandal, as are the gaps in other major areas of human existence. The situation is all the more outrageous given the unprecedented public awareness and media outreach, which makes these disparities in human conditions increasingly evident. Global injustice represents not only violations of human rights but also missed opportunities on a prodigious scale. These missed opportunities signify failures of the obligations of governments to enable their citizens—and especially their children—to achieve the highest possible standard of health. These failures also involve less-emphasized violations of the obligations of developed countries to assist developing countries in advancing health and education.

This chapter explores the broader economic and political issues involved in such social injustice—and in ending it. It analyzes the economic and social challenges of moving toward greater social justice in public health—in the context of today's world of social injustice, with particular emphasis on actions that developing countries can take to accelerate advance. The chapter then considers the priority actions required of the developed countries to assist this process. The chapter concludes with a discussion of priorities to meet the broader and longer-term challenge of reducing social injustice on a global scale and enabling all countries to move towards patterns of more sustainable human development.

Requirements for Greater Social Justice in Public Health

Most people in the health sector—physicians, public health workers, policymakers, patients, and others—recognize the need for broader economic and social action if health is to flourish. Even so, many myths abound. There are narrow and specific views that this broader action is mostly of changes within the medical sector—ensuring public or private finance for hospitals, providing access to pharmaceuticals at lower prices, or supporting longer-run medical research and technological discoveries, such as new treatments for HIV/AIDS or a vaccine for malaria. Even those who accept that many of the most important supportive actions for health lie outside basic medicine may also be thinking too narrowly. Basic education, clean water, and adequate sanitation are certainly important, but they are not the only priorities for improving health on a broader scale.

Such misperceptions and oversimplifications help to direct attention to a range of much broader issues. These issues can be found in the experience of countries that have demonstrated the possibility of making rapid progress in the health of their populations, even in situations of severe economic constraints. Examples are as diverse as Malaysia and Tunisia, Sri Lanka and Mauritius, China and Cuba, Costa Rica and Barbados. All of these countries have made advances in health, mostly linked to general economic advance, but also combined with other changes that have reduced poverty and brought greater social justice. Economic growth has played a part in developing countries, precisely because the countries and their populations have been lacking in the household, community, and government resources required for progress in public health. But economic growth alone has never been enough. Changes have also been needed in economic and social structures, laws and institutions, and norms and practices to help lay the foundations for advance to improved public health and greater social justice.[3-6]

Economic growth with structural change, thus, involves three priorities, which have been much discussed in recent years:

1. Economic growth that benefits the poor
2. Social policies incorporating strong commitments to social justice, beginning with commitments to the goals of education and health for all, including gender equality on the road to universality
3. Long-term measures for economic and environmental sustainability.

Although implementing such strategies is challenging, a number of countries have demonstrated substantial progress along these lines over the past 20 years. In Africa, Botswana, Mauritius, and Tunisia stand out as impressive examples of human and social success[3]—with South Africa more recently demonstrating commitment and creativity in the pursuit of social justice in public health as well as in related areas, such as by proclaiming access to safe drinking water and sanitation as human rights. Tragically, the surge in HIV/AIDS has set back much—but not all—of this progress.

In Asia, China, Malaysia, Sri Lanka, Vietnam, and some states of India, such as Kerala and Tamil Nadu, have demonstrated the possibilities of combining accelerated economic growth with policies and institutional changes to reduce rapidly poverty, malnutrition, and major causes of ill health. Although inequalities of income have often risen, there is no doubt that the numbers and the proportions of people in poverty have fallen sharply in the past two decades. Over a longer period, Korea and Taiwan have demonstrated the possibility and desirability of combining economic growth with redistributive measures, as well as showing strong commitments to public health and education for all. From an economic point of view, the examples of Korea and Taiwan are of special interest because they illustrate how long-term sustained economic growth can be achieved using policy instruments that differ sharply from the neoliberal orthodoxy, which has been so strongly promoted by the Bretton Woods Institutions since 1980.

In Latin America, Costa Rica stands out as a country that has for 50 years combined strong democratic commitments with policies of public health and universal education. A special feature of Costa Rica's development has been its constitution, adopted in 1948, which prevents the country from having an army. This measure has saved billions of dollars on military expenditures, enabling Costa Rica to spend markedly more on health and education than most other countries of Central and South America and the Caribbean. Not surprisingly, Costa Rica has some of the best economic and social indicators in Latin America. But there are others. Barbados and, in a different way, Cuba also represent countries that have achieved high levels of social development and equality, relative to their income levels.

Three More Myths

The experiences of these countries help to lay to rest other myths—for example, that social justice always comes with high costs in economic efficiency and must therefore be abandoned or postponed in developing countries. The early experiences of Korea, Mauritius, Taiwan, and Tunisia show this to be a false dichotomy. Skillfully pursued, equity and greater social justice can contribute substantively to economic growth, productivity, and efficiency.

A second myth is that there is a clear tradeoff between development and human rights. Here, the experience of various countries is less clear. There is no evidence that a tradeoff is inevitable, but neither is there strong evidence that support for human rights always enhances economic growth and development. Rather, there is increasing realization that human rights and expanded freedoms are integral parts of development.[4,7] Development should thus be pursued in ways that are consistent with human rights and in ways that progressively further their attainment.

A third, and final, myth is that human goals and human development are luxuries that must await the time when countries become rich enough to afford them. This myth is contradicted by the already-mentioned experiences of several countries. Human goals and human development—and the pursuit of public health and education for all—are less a matter of resources than of priorities. Of course, the amount of resources available to support them depends in some measure on the level of a country's development, and this, in turn, affects somewhat the quality of schools and teachers and of health services and health professionals. But the commitment to achieve health and education for all need not be delayed until the highest possible standards can be guaranteed. The experience of some of the most successful countries—for example, Sri Lanka, which eradicated malaria in the late 1940s—demonstrates that early progress to these human goals helps lay the foundation for many other forms of economic and social progress.

A related requirement for social justice is the need for people to be at the center of development. People need to be empowered to take charge of their own lives—and their own health. This implies the need for strengthening human capabilities as a matter of development strategy. There needs to be a focus on strengthening human capabilities by education and on strengthening other capabilities by ensuring opportunities for people to earn and produce adequate income. Access to both health services and such related services as safe water and basic sanitation are also important for strengthening capabilities.

This need to start with people and to put people at the center is much more than a semantic point. Many well-intentioned projects have failed in health, water supply, agricultural production, and education because people have not been put at the center of planning or execution. So one can see water pumps, ploughs, and tractors lying rusting on the sidelines or, in other cases, captured by a local interest group that has seized most of the benefits.

Putting People at the Center

In recent years, much has been learned about practical ways of achieving a human-centered approach and a methodology for achieving this has been developed and applied in many countries. This is human development. Some 120 countries have prepared national human development reports, analyzing the situation and needs of their populations within a human development perspective and reaching conclusions for policy action.

Human development focuses on development as the strengthening of human capabilities and the expansion of human choices, to enable people to live the lives they have reason to value.* The essential capabilities are defined by reference to human rights and by concerns for equity within countries between women and men, between girls and boys, and among ethnic, religious, and geographic groups. These broad concerns for equity also bring in concerns for sustainability by emphasizing equity between the present population of countries and future generations.

The impact of the human development approach has been reinforced, nationally and internationally, by the use of four human development indices. Each has been consciously designed to shift attention from the narrowness and inadequacies of gross national product (GNP) as a measure of national advance and human well-being. In place of GNP, human development focuses on the Human Development Index (HDI), a combined measure of three fundamentals of human life in any particular country or region: (a) longevity, (b) knowledge, and (c) access to a reasonable standard of living. Longevity is measured by life expectancy. Knowledge is measured by a combination of the proportion of the population who are literate and the proportion of children who are enrolled in school. Access to a reasonable standard of living is measured by a modified statistic of income, which gives greatest weight to income up to about the world average and relatively less weight to levels of income above this level.

There are three related measures:

1. The Gender Development Index (GDI), which applies the HDI measure only to the females in a country
2. The Gender Empowerment Measure (GEM), which measures the proportion of women in the leadership of each country—in parliament, in senior management and administrative positions, and among its scientists and technologists
3. The Human Poverty Index (HPI), which focuses on deprivation reflected by the following human-development indicators: the proportion of a country's population with life expectancy below 40, the proportion illiterate, the proportion without access to health care, the proportion without adequate access to safe water, and the proportion of children underweight for age.

The Millennium Development Goals for Poverty Reduction

In 2000, a major step toward generating commitments and action toward the reduction of poverty on a global scale was taken at the Millennium Summit, convened at the United Nations. The Summit involved the participation of

---

*Full definitions of human development and the indices will be found on pp. 27–29 and 340–349 of reference 5.

147 heads of state or government and senior representatives of another 30 countries. They agreed to a Millennium Declaration, with eight Millennium Development Goals (MDGs), focused on a halving of the proportion of people in poverty in all countries by 2015.[8] (Seven of these goals are listed below. The eighth MDG is described later in this chapter.) (See table 21-7 on p. 394.)

1. Eradicating extreme poverty and hunger by 2015, halving between 1990 and 2015 the proportion of people with incomes below $1 per day and the proportion of people who suffer from hunger
2. Achieving universal primary education, by ensuring that, by 2015, girls and boys alike in all countries can complete basic primary education
3. Promoting gender equality and empowerment of women, by eliminating gender disparities in primary and secondary education, preferably by 2005, and in all levels of education by 2010
4. Reducing child mortality by two-thirds of its 1990 level by 2015
5. Improving maternal and reproductive health, including the reduction of the 1990 maternal mortality ratio by three-fourths by 2015
6. In order to combat HIV/AIDS, malaria, and other diseases, halting, by 2015, in each country the rise of (a) HIV/AIDS—and beginning to reduce its transmission; and (b) malaria and other major diseases—and beginning to reduce their occurrence
7. Ensuring environmental sustainability by integrating principles of sustainable development into country policies and programs and (a) to reverse the loss of environmental resources, (b) to halve, by 2015, the proportion of people without access to safe drinking water and adequate sanitation, and (c) to achieve, by 2020, a significant improvement in the lives of at least 100 million slum-dwellers (p. 2).[5]

What is the likelihood that measures to achieve these well-intentioned international goals will be seriously implemented at the national and international levels? Judged by the record of previous global goals set by the United Nations, the probability is better than is commonly recognized. Since the 1960s, when President John Kennedy first proposed a decade for development and the goal of accelerating economic growth in developing countries, the United Nations has set 50 goals relating to economic and social development. Some goals, such as the eradication of smallpox in the 1960s and 1970s and the expansion of immunization coverage in the 1980s (to achieve 80 percent coverage in developing countries by 1990), have had a major impact on global health, with almost all countries taking action and many achieving the goal on time or soon after.

Other goals, such as reducing child mortality, increasing life expectancy, the iodizing of salt, and expanding education, have had a considerable impact—often achieved by one-third or more of the population of many developing countries. In contrast, a few goals, such as accelerating economic growth in the 50 or so poorest and least developed countries and reducing maternal mortality in the 1990s, have had hardly any impact. Revealingly, the goals set in 1970 to raise development assistance from developed to developing countries to a level of 0.7 percent of GDP as soon as possible has had little impact. Most developed countries have failed miserably in meeting this goal, with overseas development assistance falling from 0.33 percent in 1990 to 0.22 percent in 2001—from less than one-half the goal in 1990 to less than one-third in 2001. However, four developed countries—Denmark, the Netherlands, Norway, and Sweden—rapidly achieved this goal and have consistently maintained it for more than 30 years. (See figure 21-1 on p. 384.)

The possibility of the MDGs being achieved was analyzed by the United Nations Development Program in its "Human Development Report, 2003" (HDR 2003). The prospects for this vary enormously among different countries and regions, among different goals, and by different assumptions made about the extent to which recent action toward the goals is accelerated.

HDR 2003 analyzes the prospects of countries in different regions of the world. Apart from countries in East Asia and the Pacific—including China, where extreme income poverty has already been halved in the last decade or so and significant progress has been made on other goals—the need for accelerated action is urgent. In Arab countries and in Latin America and the Caribbean, achieving the goals will generally be challenging but possible. However, as HDR 2003 states[5]:

> For other developing regions achieving the MDGs will be a huge challenge. Unless things improve, it will take sub-Saharan Africa until 2129 to achieve universal primary education, until 2147 to halve extreme poverty and until 2165 to cut child mortality by two thirds. For hunger, no date can be set because the region's situation continues to worsen. Though South Asia has made faster progress, substantial improvements will be required in most areas if the Goals are to be met. (p. 33)

This analysis led the HDR 2003 to identify two groups of countries that require urgent changes in their course: (a) 60 countries that combine low human development and poor performance toward the goals (top-priority and high-priority countries); and (b) countries that are progressing well toward the goals, on average, but with large segments of poor people being left behind. Each country needs to prepare its own analysis and strategy, which many countries have already done or are doing. However, one can identify four broad priorities for action that almost all developing countries need to take if they are to be successful in accelerating action toward the goals and in reaching them by the target date or soon after:

1. *Developing and implementing decentralized approaches* for many goals to ensure participation of all communities and to ensure that women and men—and older children—can guide the process and outcomes in relation to their own perceptions of needs
2. *Setting budget priorities and providing adequate resources* in support of action toward the goals
3. *Developing and implementing new approaches to deal with conflict and corruption* to ensure that resources allocated in support of the goals are not captured or diverted by existing power groups
4. *Monitoring progress*—not only to ensure technical and administrative support, but also to motivate and gain the support of the population as a whole and to act as a watchdog for diversion or lagging of support.

Priority Actions Required of the Developed Countries

The role of the developed countries in assisting or facilitating developing countries in achieving the MDGs is another topic shrouded in myths, which have been maintained—often vociferously—by various political parties or factions within leading developed countries. Three of the myths are as follows:

1. *Myth 1: Developed countries can, and need to, do little.* Globalization provides markets and opportunities for each developing country that wishes to make use of its benefits, as China, Korea, and some other countries have demonstrated. Other developing countries need only follow the same path.
2. *Myth 2: While governments can do little, the private sector can do much.* If developing countries open their doors to foreign investment, their economies will take off, providing the resources and the economic dynamism for improvements in living standards, accompanied by reductions in poverty and progress toward the MDGs.
3. *Myth 3 (almost the opposite of Myth 1): The main role of developed countries is to provide aid.* With aid, developing countries will have the resources to accelerate action toward the MDGs. Without aid, the task will be impossible for a high proportion of developing countries, especially the poorest.

All three myths represent extremes. Each may have a grain of truth, but each is overwhelmingly wrong. Actually, developed countries are of enormous importance for the economic and social prospects of developing countries, especially for accelerating progress toward the MDGs. Most important is their role in the creation of an enabling global environment—or in obstructing its creation. An enabling global environment makes possible trade, investment flows on fair conditions, debt relief for the heavily indebted developing countries, and their access to technology and development assistance on fair and reasonable terms, especially for the poorest and least-developed countries.

The eighth MDG deals precisely with these issues, calling for the strengthening of "a global partnership for development," comprising seven components (pp. 2–3)[5]:

1. Developing further an open, rule-based, predictable, non-discriminatory trading and financial system, both nationally and internationally
2. Addressing the special needs of the least-developed countries, with tariff- and quota-free access for exports, enhanced programs of debt relief and cancellation of official bilateral debt, and more generous aid for countries committed to poverty reduction
3. Addressing the special needs of land-locked and small-island developing countries
4. Dealing comprehensively with the debt problems of developing countries through national and international measures to order to make debt sustainable in the long term
5. Developing and implementing strategies for decent and productive work for youth
6. Providing access to affordable essential drugs in developing countries, in cooperation with pharmaceutical companies
7. Making available the benefits of new technologies, especially information and communication technologies, in cooperation with the private sector.

Implementation of these priority measures by developed countries would do much to enable most developing countries to accelerate their economic and social advance and, as part of this, progress toward the MDGs. It would, however, represent fundamental changes from policies pursued by the major industrial countries over the past few decades.

The eighth MDG is the only goal that is not quantified and has no time-bound targets. Past experience does not give much cause for optimism. Goals for aid, agreed to in a succession of global conferences over the past four decades, have been among those goals that have been least implemented. And commitments to open developed country markets to exports from developing countries have often not been kept. Recent experience of the United States raising tariffs and of Europe and the United States failing to phase out farming subsidies, as required by the World Trade Organization, augur badly for the fulfillment of the eighth MDG.

This said, the Millennium Summit launched some important initiatives, which offer real hope that international action for poverty reduction is gaining momentum:

- Many developing countries have publicly committed themselves to the MDGs, at least in rhetoric, and have prepared poverty reduction strategy papers (PRSPs) for negotiation with donors for aid.
- The World Bank and UN agencies have established new mechanisms for working together in support of poverty reduction. At the country level, the PRSPs are increasingly used as the framework for development assistance and debt relief, linked directly to increased support for poverty reduction.
- Most significantly, there is a new spirit of commitment among many donor governments, especially those of Europe. Official development assistance is rising, both absolutely and as a percentage of national income— although at 0.25 percent, it is still far below the UN target level of 0.7 percent, and less than three-fourths of the level it averaged during the 1980–1992 period.
- Many analyses have been performed nationally and internationally to map out what it will take to achieve the goals—in resources, broader strategy, and sector-by-sector action. The largest and most publicized of these analyses has been done by the Millennium Project Task Force, which produced a major report to the Secretary General of the United Nations in 2005.[9]

By 2005, one-third of the period had elapsed from the year when the MDGs were established (2000) to the target year for their achievement (2015). An assessment of progress was provided in the Millennium Project Task Force report, which concluded that the goal of halving poverty by 2015 was doable, but only with the implementation of the following critical measures:

- Each country needs to prepare a "PRSP for MDG plan," specifying the actions required to achieve the MDGs. The important new element in this approach to the PRSPs is that the analysis would start by asking what it would take to achieve the goals, nationally and in international support—not what was the most that could be done with the resources likely to be available.
- National programs need to emphasize "scaling up" sufficiently to achieve the MDGs, reaching out to the whole population—not being content with limited operations.

- Donor partnerships need to focus on mobilizing and maintaining the support needed for these PRSPs for MDGs. But the Task Force report recognized that not every country is ready for action. Some are caught in conflict, others are failing in other ways. The report accordingly suggested immediate concentration in 2005 on at least a dozen "fast track" countries, for rapid scale-up, on the basis of their good governance and absorptive capacity.
- Additional support needs to be provided for some "quick-win" options:

  1. The free mass distribution of bed nets for protection against malaria together with effective antimalarial medicines in regions of malaria transmission;
  2. Ending user fees for primary schools and essential health services;
  3. Successful completion of the "3-by-5 campaign" to bring 3 million AIDS patients in developing countries onto antiretroviral treatment by 2005; and
  4. Expansion of school meals programs to cover all children in hunger "hot spots," using locally produced foods and massive support for small-holder farmers.

Realism always conflicts with vision in assessing the likelihood of such proposals being accepted and implemented. The Task Force report called for a Decade of Bold Ambitions, and estimated that the full implementation of its proposals would require a doubling of development assistance by 2006 and further increases to reach 0.54 percent of national income in the high-income countries by 2015. The report calls for (a) concentration of this aid on low-income countries, (b) improvements in the quality of aid, and (c) other increases to cover the need for global scientific research and technological development to address the special needs of the poor in areas of health, agriculture, natural resource and environmental management, energy, and climate.

Reducing Social Injustice Globally and Facilitating Sustainable Human Development

Inequalities of power, income, and living standards have long been part of the world's structures. But many people do not realize the extent to which inequalities of income and power among countries have grown over the past 200 years. In 1820, in the early years of the Industrial Revolution, average income in the United States was estimated to be about three times that of India and China; income in Great Britain then was estimated to be a little higher than that in the United States. Since then, the gaps in average income between the richest and the poorest countries have grown substantially. By 1870, the gap between the richest and the poorest country was about 7:1; by 1913, 11:1; and by 1950, 35:1. Over the past 50 years, the gap between the richest and poorest country has widened further to more than 70:1.[10] The World Bank, in 2002, stated that the gaps between the richest and the poorest 20 countries had doubled from 1970 to 2000, from 19:1 to 37:1.[11]

Even these extremes among countries understate income disparities between the richest and the poorest people in the world. The richest 1 percent of people worldwide receive as much as the bottom 57 percent. Thus, less than 50 million of the world's richest people receive the same income as 2.7 billion of the world's poor. Worldwide, the ratio between the average income of the top 5 percent and the bottom 5 percent increased from 78:1 in 1988 to 1:114 in 1993.

These inequalities reflect and reinforce a frame of social and economic injustice on a global scale that acts as a major obstacle to the achievement of public health for all and achievement of the MDGs for poverty reduction. Some advance is possible. And progress toward the MDGs will certainly lay the foundation for further economic and social development in developing countries, as a first step in strengthening human capabilities among their populations. Nevertheless, this will not go far to decrease the present levels of global inequality and social injustice. Further decrease will need to await reductions of power, income disparities, and control on an international scale, which, in turn, will require broader and more fundamental actions.

In the present political climate, such actions seem so unlikely that it is difficult to imagine that they can be realistic options. Yet perceptions can and do change. Many argue that the roots of terrorism and global instability are found in—or at least build on—deep reactions in many developing countries to what is seen as social injustice and economic and other inequalities on a global scale. If such views were to become more widely accepted in the developed countries, a range of actions to alter the global economic imbalances would be possible,

At the end of the 1990s, the historian David Landes expressed the challenge as follows:

> The old division of the world into two power blocs, East and West, has subsided. Now the big challenge and threat is the gap in wealth and health that separates rich and poor. These are often styled North and South, because the division is geographic; but a more accurate signifier would be the West and the Rest, because the division is also historical. Here is the greatest single problem and danger facing the world in the Third Millennium. The only worry that comes close to it is environmental deterioration, and the two are intimately connected, indeed are one.[12]

Conclusion

Ending health and social injustice on a global scale requires a range of fundamental actions, many far beyond what is at present politically acceptable in the developed countries. This is not an argument for inaction or acceptance of poor public health and social injustice. Much can be done and has been done in recent decades, achieving important measures of progress, in both health and human development. The actions required for ending social injustice as it affects health go far beyond those of the health sector. Priority actions extend to many aspects of economic and social policy, nationally and internationally. Many of these priority actions involve specialist knowledge in other fields beyond medicine and public health—although as with public health, the broader issues are too important and fundamental to be left entirely to the experts. Thus, those involved in the health sector need to be aware of the broader challenges and to press and mobilize for action so that social justice can be achieved and public health attained—to ensure the conditions in which people can be healthy.

References

1. Mitchell BR. European historical statistics, 1750–1970. London, England: Macmillan, 1978.
2. UNICEF. State of the world's children 1989. Oxford, U.K.: Oxford University Press, 1989:84.
3. United Nations Development Program. Human development report 1997: human development to eradicate poverty. New York, N.Y.: Oxford University Press, 1997.
4. United Nations Development Program. Human development report 2000: human rights and human development. New York, N.Y.: Oxford University Press, 2000.
5. United Nations Development Program. Human development report 2003, millennium development goals: a compact among nations to end human poverty. New York, N.Y.: Oxford University Press, 2003.
6. Mehrotra S, Jolly R. Development with a human face: experiences in social achievement and economic growth. Oxford, U.K.: Clarendon Press, 1997.
7. Sen A. Development as freedom. New York, N.Y.: Random House, 1999.
8. Available at: www.un.org/millennium/summit. Accessed January 28, 2005.
9. United Nations Development Program. Investing in development: a practical plan to achieve the millennium development goals, overview. UN Millennium Project, Report to the Secretary General. New York, N.Y.: United Nations Development Program, 2005.
10. UNDP. Human development report 1999. New York, N.Y.: Oxford University Press, 1999.
11. World Bank. World development report, 2003: sustainable development in a dynamic world: transforming institutions, growth and quality of life. New York, N.Y.: Oxford University Press, 2002:183.
12. Landes D. The wealth and poverty of nations: why some are so rich and some so poor. New York, N.Y.: W.W. Norton, 1999: xx.

Further Reading

Annan K. We the peoples: the role of the United Nations in the 21st century. New York, N.Y.: United Nations, 2000.

Commission on global governance, our global neighbourhood. New York, N.Y.: Oxford University Press, 1995.

Mehrotra S, Jolly R, eds. Development with a human face: experiences in social achievement and economic growth. Oxford, U.K.: Clarendon Press, 1999.

United Nations Development Program. Human development report 2003, millennium development goals: a compact among nations to end human poverty. New York, N.Y.: Oxford University Press, 2003.

UNICEF. Progress since the world summit for children: a statistical review. New York, N.Y.: UNICEF, 2001.

UNICEF. The state of the world's children 2003. New York, N.Y.: UNICEF, 2003.

United Nations. Millennium declaration. New York, N.Y.: United Nations, 2000.

United Nations. The world's women: trends and statistics. New York, N.Y.: United Nations, 2000.

World Bank. World development report 2000/2001: attacking poverty. New York, N.Y.: Oxford University Press, 2000.

World Health Organization. The world health report 1998: life in the 21st century: a vision for all. Geneva, Switzerland: World Health Organization, 1998.

World Health Organization. The world health report 2002, reducing risk and promoting healthy life. Geneva, Switzerland: World Health Organization, 2002.

APPENDIX: SOME ORGANIZATIONS ADDRESSING SOCIAL INJUSTICE

ACORN (Association of Community Organizations for Reform Now)
88 Third Avenue
Brooklyn, NY 11217
Tel: 718-246-7900
Website: www.acorn.org

The nation's largest community organization of low- and moderate-income families, with over 150,000 member families organized into 750 neighborhood chapters in more than 60 cities across the country.

American Civil Liberties Union
125 Broad Street, 18th Floor
New York, NY 10004
Tel: 888-567-2258
Website: www.aclu.org

Works daily in courts, legislatures, and communities to defend and preserve the individual rights and liberties guaranteed to every person under the U.S. Constitution and laws.

American Public Health Association
800 I Street NW
Washington, DC 20001-3701
Tel: 202-777-2742
Website: www.apha.org

The oldest and largest organization of public health professionals in the world, representing more than 50,000 members from over 50 occupations of public health. Brings together researchers, health service providers, administrators, teachers, and other health workers in a unique, multidisciplinary environment of professional exchange, study, and action. Actively serves the public, its members, and the public health profession through its scientific and practice programs, publications, annual meeting, awards program, educational services, and advocacy efforts.

Amnesty International
1 Easton Street
London WC1X 0DW
United Kingdom
Tel: 44 20-7413-5500
Website: www.amnesty.org

Amnesty International USA
5 Penn Plaza, 14th Floor
New York, NY 10001
Tel: 212-807-8400
Website: www.amnestyusa.org

Worldwide movement of people who campaign for internationally recognized human rights. Undertakes research and action focused on preventing and ending grave abuses of the rights to physical and mental integrity, freedom of conscience and expression, and freedom from discrimination, within the context of its work to promote all human rights.

Center for Constitutional Rights
666 Broadway, 7th Floor
New York, NY 10012
Tel: 212-614-6464
Website: www.ccr-ny.org

Dedicated to protecting and advancing the rights protected by the U.S. Constitution and the Universal Declaration of Human Rights.

Center for Defense Information
1779 Massachusetts Avenue NW
Washington, DC 20036-2019
Tel: 202-332-0600
Website: www.cdi.org

Strengthens security through international cooperation; reduced reliance on unilateral military power to resolve conflict; reduced reliance on nuclear weapons; a transformed and reformed military establishment; and prudent oversight of, and spending on, defense programs. Contributes alternative views on security to promote wide-ranging discourse and debate; educates the public and in-forms policymakers about issues of security policy, strategy, operators, weapon systems, and defense budgeting; and pursues creative solutions to the problems of today and tomorrow.

Center for Economic and Social Rights (CESR)
162 Montague Street, 2nd Floor
Brooklyn, NY 11201
Tel: 718-237-9145
Website: www.cesr.org

Promotes the universal right of every human being to housing, education, health, a healthy environment, food, work, and an adequate standard of living.

Center for Policy Analysis on Trade and Health (CPATH)
98 Seal Rock Drive
San Francisco, CA 94121-1437
Tel: 415-933-6204
Website: www.cpath.org

Protects and expands access to health care, water, and other vital human services. Links health, health care, and global trade communities to create economically and socially just, democratically accountable, and environmentally sustainable solutions to the negative effects of economic globalization.

Center for Reproductive Rights
120 Wall Street
New York, NY 10005
Tel: 917-637-3600
Website: www.reproductiverights.org

A nonprofit advocacy organization dedicated to promoting and defending women's reproductive rights worldwide.

Children's Defense Fund
25 E Street NW
Washington, DC 20001
Tel: 202-628-8787
Website: www.childrensdefense.org

Provides a strong, effective voice for all the children of America who cannot vote, lobby, or speak for themselves. Pays particular attention to the needs of poor and minority children and those with disabilities. Educates the nation about the needs of children and encourages preventive investment before they become ill or get into trouble, drop out of school, or suffer family breakdown.

Council for a Livable World
322 4th Street NE
Washington, DC 20002
Tel: 202-543-4100
Website: www.clw.org

An arms control organization that focuses on halting the spread of weapons of mass destruction, opposing a national missile defense system, cutting Pentagon waste, and reducing excessive arms exports. Also a political lobby that endorses political candidates.

Disabled Peoples International
748 Broadway
Winnipeg, Manitoba
Canada RG3 OX3
Tel: 204-287-8010
Website: www.dpi.org

A network of national organizations and assemblies of disabled people, established to promote human rights of disabled people through full participation, equalization of opportunity, and development. Operated by and on behalf of disabled people.

Disability Group, World Bank
Office of the Advisor on Disability
The World Bank
1818 H Street NW
Washington, DC 20433
Tel: 202-473-2922
Website: www.worldbank.org/disability

A key player in global disability issues as they relate to economic development and human rights. Issues papers and reports that form the base for an emerging field of disability in health and development.

Doctors for Global Health (DGH)
P.O. Box 1761
Decatur, GA 30031
Tel: 404-377-3566
Website: www.dghonline.org

A private, not-for-profit organization that promotes health, education, art, and other human rights throughout the world. Its mission is to improve health and foster other human rights with those most in need by accompanying communities, while educating and inspiring others to action.

Families USA
1334 G Street, NW
Washington, DC 20005
Tel: 202-628-3030
Website: www.familiesusa.org

A national nonprofit, nonpartisan organization dedicated to the achievement of high-quality, affordable health care for all Americans.

Federation of American Scientists
1717 K Street, NW
Washington, DC 20036
Tel: 202-546-3300
Website: www.fas.org

The oldest organization dedicated to ending the worldwide arms race and avoiding the use of nuclear weapons for any purpose.

Francis X. Bagnaud Center for Health and Human Rights
Harvard School of Public Health
651 Huntington Avenue, 7th Floor
Boston, MA 02115
Tel: 617-432-0656
Website: www.hsph.harvard.edu/fxbcenter

The first academic center to focus exclusively on health and human rights, it undertakes research, teaching, service, and policy development. Its three programs and directors are:

Program on International Health and Human Rights
Sofia Gruskin, Director
Program on Humanitarian Crises and Human Rights
Jennifer Leaning, Director
Program on Human Rights in Development
Steven Marks, Director

Gay Men's Health Crisis
119 West 24th Street
New York, NY 10011
Tel: 212-367-1000
Website: www.gmhc.org

Volunteer-supported and community-based organization committed to national leadership in the fight against AIDS. Works to reduces the spread of HIV infection, helps people with HIV maintain and improve their health and independence, and keeps the prevention, treatment, and cure of HIV an urgent national and local priority. Fights homophobia and affirms the individual dignity of all gay men and lesbians.

Global Lawyers and Physicians
Department of Health Law, Bioethics and Human Rights
Boston University of Public Health
715 Albany Street
Boston, MA 02118
Tel: 617-638-4626
Website: www.glphr.org

Works at the local, national, and international levels through collaboration and partnerships with individuals, nongovernment organizations, intergovernment organizations, and governments on issues such as the global implementation of the health-related provisions of the Universal Declaration of Human Rights and the Covenants on Civil and Political Rights and on Economic, Social, and Cultural Rights, with a focus on health and human rights, patient rights, and human experimentation.

Health Development Agency
Holborn Gate
330 High Holburn
London WC1V 7BA
United Kingdom
Tel: 44 20-7430-0850
Website: www.hda-online.org.uk

Reviews evidence on what works to reduce inequalities in health and gathers evidence and advises policymakers, practitioners, and others to transfer scientific knowledge.

Hesperian Foundation
1919 Addison Street, Suite 304
Berkeley, CA 94704
Tel: 510-845-1447
Website: www.hesperian.org

Promotes health and self-determination in poor communities worldwide by making health information accessible. Hesperian publications are written simply and include many illustrations so people with little formal education can understand, apply, and share medical information.

Institute of Medicine
500 Fifth Street, NW
Washington, DC 20001
Tel: 202-334-2352
Website: www.iom.edu

Chartered in 1970 as a component of the National Academy of Sciences, its mission is to serve as adviser to the nation to improve health. It provides unbiased, evidence-based, and authoritative information and advice concerning health and science policy to policy makers, professionals, leaders in every sector of society, and the public at large.

International Centre for Health and Society
Department of Epidemiology and Public Health, UCL
1-19 Torrington Place
London WC1E 6BT
United Kingdom
Tel: 44 20-7679-1708
Website: www.ucl.ac.uk/ichs

Performs research on the social, economic, and psychological determinants of health, with a focus on social inequalities, and proposes policies based on research findings.

International Health Cities Foundation
555 12th Street, 10th Floor
Oadland, CA 94607
Tel: 510-642-1715
Website: www.healthycities.org

The term *Healthy Cities* means that health is the result of much more than medical care. People are healthy when they live in nurturing environments and are involved in the life of their communities. The movement began with the World Health Organization. The IHCF facilitates linkages among people, issues, and resources in order to support the development of Healthy Cities initiatives.

International Physicians for the Prevention of Nuclear War
727 Massachusetts Avenue
Cambridge, MA 02139-3323
Tel: 617-868-5050
Website: www.ippnw.org

A nonpartisan, global federation of national medical organizations in 58 countries dedicated to research, education, and advocacy relevant to the prevention of nuclear war. Seeks to prevent all wars, promote nonviolent conflict resolution, and minimize the effects of war and preparations for war on health, development, and the environment.

International Society for Equity in Health
Department of Family and Community Health
University of Toronto
263 McCaul Street, Fifth Floor
Toronto, Ontario
Canada M5T 1W7
Tel: 416-978-3763
Website: www.iseqh.org/en/index.html

Promotes equity in health and health services internationally through education, research, publication, communication, and charitable support.

Lambda Legal
120 Wall Street, Suite 1500
New York, NY 10005-3904
Tel: 212-809-8585
Website: www.lambdalegal.org

A national organization committed to achieving full recognition of the civil rights of lesbians, gay men, bisexuals, transgender people, and people with HIV/AIDS through impact litigation, education, and public policy work.

Legal Aid Society
199 Water Street
New York, NY 10038
Tel: 212-577-3300
Website: www.legal-aid.org

A law firm for poor people located in New York. The first of many—founded more than 125 years ago. Provides a wide variety of legal services for people who cannot afford a lawyer.

Medact (IPPNW/United Kingdom)
The Grayston Center
28 Charles Square
London N1 6HT
United Kingdom
Tel: 44 20 7324 4733
Website: www.medact.org

An organization of health professionals challenging social and environmental barriers to health worldwide. It highlights the health effects of violent conflict, poverty, and environmental degradation, and, with others, acts to eradicate them.

Mental Disability Rights International
1156 15th Street NW, Suite 1001
Washington, DC 20005
Tel: 202-296-0800
Website: www.mdri.org

Promotes the human rights and full participation in society of people with mental disabilities worldwide. Documents human rights abuses, works for programmatic and policy reform, and trains social justice activists in many countries.

National Center for Lesbian Rights
870 Market Street, Suite 370
San Francisco, CA 94102
Tel: 415-392-6257
Website: www.nclrights.org

A national legal resource center that advances the rights and safety of lesbians and their families through litigation, public policy advocacy, free legal advice and counseling, and public education. Provides representation and resources to gay men and to bisexual and transgender individuals on key issues that also advance lesbian rights.

National Centre for Social Research
35 Northampton Square
London EC1V 0AX
United Kingdom
Tel: 44 20-7250-1866
Website: www.natcen.ac.uk

Designs, performs, and analyses research studies in social and public policy, including extensive research among the general public.

National Coalition for the Homeless
2201 P Street, NW
Washington, DC 20037

Tel: 202-462-4822
Website: www.nationalhomeless.org

With a mission to end homelessness, focuses work in areas of housing justice, economic justice, health care justice, and civil and voting rights. Approaches are grassroots organizing, public education, policy advocacy, technical assistance, and partnerships.

National Coalition for LGBT Health
1407 S Street NW
Washington, DC 20009
Tel: 202-797-3516
Website: www.lgbthealth.net

Improves the health and well-being of lesbian, gay, bisexual, and transgender individuals through advocacy at the national level that is focused on research, policy, education, and training.

National Gay and Lesbian Task Force
1325 Massachusetts Avenue NW,
Suite 600
Washington, DC 20005
Tel: 202-393-5177
Website: www.ngltf.org

Works for the civil rights of gay, lesbian, bisexual, and transgender people.

National Senior Citizens Law Center
1101 14th Street NW, Suite 400
Washington, DC 20005
Tel: 202-289-6976
Website: www.nsclc.org

Advocates nationwide to promote the independence and well-being of low-income elderly individuals and persons with disabilities, through litigation, legislative and agency representation, and assistance to attorneys and paralegals in field programs.

National Transgender Advocacy Coalition
PO Box 76027
Washington, DC 20013
Website: www.ntac.org

Works to reform societal attitudes and the law to achieve equal rights for transgender and other gender-diverse individuals.

Oxfam America
26 West Street
Boston, MA 02111
Tel: 617-482-1211
Website: www.oxfam.org

Oxfam Great Britain
274 Banbury Road
Oxford, OX2 7DZ
United Kingdom
Tel: 44 18-6531 1311
Website: www.oxfam.org.uk

Both promote rights to basic social services, sustainable livelihoods, life, and security as well as the right to equity and the right to be heard as integral components of poverty reduction.

Pan American Health Organization (PAHO)
(WHO Regional Office for the Americas)
525 Twenty-Third Street NW
Washington, DC 20037
Tel: 202-974-3000
Website: www.paho.org

An international public health agency with 100 years of experience in working to improve health and living standards of the countries of the Americas. Serves as the specialized organization for health of the Inter-American System. Also serves as the Regional Office for the Americas of the World Health Organization and enjoys international recognition as part of the United Nations System. PAHO operates the Equity, Health and Human Development Listserv (www.paho.org/english/dd/ikm/eq-list.htm), which shares public health information of international significance that enables policymakers, researchers, and practitioners to improve health, especially among disadvantaged populations.

Partners in Health
641 Huntington Avenue
Boston, MA 02115
Tel: 617-432-5256
Website: www.pih.org

An international charity organization that provides direct health care services and performs research and advocacy activities for sick and poor people.

Physicians for Global Survival (IPPNW/Canada)
208-145 Spruce Street
Ottawa, Ontario K1R 6P1
Canada
Tel: 613-233-1982
Website: www.pgs.ca

Educates and advocates for the abolition of nuclear weapons, the prevention of war, and the promotion of nonviolent means of conflict resolution and social justice.

Physicians for Human Rights
Two Arrow Street, Suite 301
Cambridge, MA 02138
Tel: 617-301-4200
Website: www.phrusa.org

Promotes health by protecting human rights. Using medical and scientific methods, investigates and exposes violations of human rights worldwide, and works to stop them. Supports institutions that hold perpetrators of human rights abuses, including health professionals, accountable for their actions. Educates health professionals and medical, public health, and nursing students and organizes them to become active in supporting a movement for human rights and creating a culture of human rights in the medical and scientific professions.

Physicians for a National Health Program
29 East Madison, Suite 602
Chicago, IL 60602
Tel: 312-782-6006
Website: www.pnhp.org

Advocates for a universal, comprehensive single-payer national health program. It has more than 10,000 members and chapters across the United States.

Physicians for Social Responsibility (IPPNW/USA)
1875 Connecticut Avenue NW, #1012
Washington, DC 20009
Tel: 202-667-4260
Website: www.psr.org

A leading public policy organization representing the medical and public health professions and concerned citizens, working together for nuclear disarmament, a healthful environment, and an end to the epidemic of gun violence.

Rehabilitation International
25 East 21st Street
New York, NY 10010
Tel: 212-420-1500
Website: www.rehab-international.org

The oldest and one of the largest international organizations covering all disabled populations. Organizes major regional and international conferences. Clearinghouse for information on disability advocacy and service groups worldwide.

Spirit of 1848 Listserv
Postings on social justice and public health
Web page: www.progressivehn.org
To subscribe: spiritof1848-subscribe@yahoogroups.com

Hosted by the Spirit of 1848: A Network linking Politics, Passion, and Public Health, a caucus of the American Public Health Association. A volunteer network whose mission is to "develop our thoughts, strategize, and enhance efforts to eliminate social inequalities in health."

United Nations Children's Fund (UNICEF)
3 United Nations Plaza
New York, NY 10017

Tel: 212-326-7025
Website: www.unicef.org

Supports health and survival of children and women, with priority for girls and the poorest, through its offices and programs in many countries.

Union of Concerned Scientists
2 Brattle Square
Cambridge, MA 02238-9105
Tel: 617-547-5552
Website: www.ucsusa.org

An independent nonprofit alliance of concerned citizens and scientists that augments rigorous scientific analysis with innovative thinking and committed citizen advocacy to build a cleaner, healthier environment and a safer world. Experts work together with citizens across the country to disseminate findings and alter policies in local communities and at the national level.

United Nations
New York, NY 10017
Tel: 212-963-1234
Website: www.un.org

According to the Charter, the United Nations has four purposes: to maintain international peace and security; to develop friendly relations among nations; to cooperate in solving international problems and in promoting respect for human rights; and to be a center for harmonizing the actions of nations. The United Nations is not a world government and it does not make laws. It does, however, provide the means to help resolve international conflicts and formulate policies on matters affecting all of us.

United Nations Educational, Scientific and Cultural Organization (UNESCO)
7, place de Fontenoy
75352 Paris 07 SP
France
Tel: 33 1-45 68-10 00
Website: www.unesco.org

Promotes international cooperation among its Member States and Associate Members in the fields of education, science, culture, and communication. Functions as a laboratory of ideas and a standard-setter to forge universal agreements on emerging ethical issues. Serves as a clearinghouse—for the dissemination and sharing of information and knowledge—while helping Member States to build their human and institutional capacities in diverse fields.

United Nations High Commissioner for Human Rights
1775 K Street NW, #300
Washington, DC 20006
Website: www.ohchr.org

Its vision is of a world in which the human rights of all are fully respected and enjoyed in conditions of global peace. The High Commissioner works to keep that vision to the forefront through constant encouragement of the international community and its Member States to uphold universally agreed-on human rights standards.

WITNESS
80 Hanson Place, 5th Floor
Brooklyn, NY 11217
Tel: 718-783-2000
Website: www.witness.org

A human rights program that strengthens local activists by providing them with video cameras and training in production and advocacy. Partner groups address injustice worldwide on many issues.

World Health Organization (WHO)
Avenue Appia 20
1211 Geneva 27
Switzerland
Tel: 41 22-791 21 11
Website: www.who.int

The United Nations' specialized agency for health. WHO's objective is the attainment by all peoples of the highest possible level of health—defined as a state of complete physical, mental, and social well-being and not merely the absence of disease or infirmity. In addition to PAHO (above), WHO has several other regional offices.

WHO Secretariat to the Commission on Social Inequalities in Health
Evidence for Information Cluster
World Health Organization
20 Avenue Appia
CH 1211 Geneva 27
Switzerland
Tel: 41 22-791 2111
Website: www.who.int

From 2005 to 2008, its focus will be on the political dimensions of addressing inequalities.

INDEX